DALLAS
RHINOPLASTY

Nasal Surgery by the Masters

DALLAS RHINOPLASTY

Nasal Surgery by the Masters

EDITED BY

Jack P. Gunter, M.D.

Clinical Professor, Departments of Plastic Surgery and Otolaryngology,
The University of Texas Southwestern Medical Center, Dallas, Texas

Rod J. Rohrich, M.D.

Professor and Chairman, Department of Plastic Surgery,
Holder of Crystal Charity Ball Distinguished Chair in Plastic Surgery
and the Betty and Warren Woodward Chair in Plastic and Reconstructive Surgery,
The University of Texas Southwestern Medical Center, Dallas, Texas

William P. Adams, Jr., M.D.

Assistant Professor, Department of Plastic Surgery,
The University of Texas Southwestern Medical Center, Dallas, Texas

Holly Smith, B.F.A.

Photographic Editor

Quality Medical Publishing, Inc.

ST. LOUIS, MISSOURI ▪ 2002

This book presents current scientific information and opinion pertinent to
medical professionals. It does not provide advice concerning specific diagnosis
and treatment of individual cases and is not intended for use by the layperson.
The authors and publisher will not be responsible or liable for actions taken
as a result of the opinions expressed in this book.

PUBLISHER   Karen Berger

ASSOCIATE EDITOR   Michelle Leaman

PROJECT MANAGER   Carolita Deter

PRODUCTION   Mary Stueck, Susan Trail, Carolyn Reich

INTERIOR DESIGN   Village Typographers, Inc.

COVER DESIGN   Diane M. Beasley, David Berger

LIBRARY OF CONGRESS CATALOGING-IN-PUBLICATION DATA

Dallas rhinoplasty : nasal surgery by the masters / edited by Jack P. Gunter,
Rod J. Rohrich, William P. Adams, Jr.
    p. ; cm.
  Includes bibliographical references and index.
  ISBN 1-57626-129-8
    1. Rhinoplasty—Congresses.   2. Nose—Surgery—Congresses.
  I. Gunter, Jack P., 1937-   . II. Rohrich, Rod J.   III. Adams, William P., Jr.
  IV. Dallas Rhinoplasty Symposium.
    [DNLM: 1. Rhinoplasty—methods.   WV 312 D145 2001]
  RD119.5.N67 D35 2001
  617.5′230592—dc21
                                                          2001019387

VT/VT/WW

5   4   3   2   1

Contributors

William P. Adams, Jr., M.D.
Assistant Professor, Department of Plastic Surgery, The University of Texas Southwestern Medical Center, Dallas, Texas

Scott Andochick, M.D., D.D.S.
Private practice, Frederick, Maryland

Tapan K. Bhattacharyya, M.Sc., Ph.D., D.Sc.
Research Specialist, Department of Otolaryngology—Head and Neck Surgery, University of Illinois, Chicago, Illinois

James D. Burt, M.B.B.S., F.R.A.C.S.
Plastic and Reconstructive Surgery Unit, St. Vincent's Hospital, Fitzroy, Victoria, Australia

H. Steve Byrd, M.D.
Clinical Professor and Vice Chairman, Department of Plastic Surgery, The University of Texas Southwestern Medical Center; Chief, Department of Plastic Surgery, Baylor University Medical Center, Dallas, Texas

Maria S. Chand, M.D.
Assistant Professor, Division of Otolaryngology—Head and Neck Surgery, Indiana University School of Medicine, Indianapolis, Indiana

Clifford P. Clark III, M.D.
Private practice, Winter Park, Florida

Mark B. Constantian, M.D.
Adjunct Assistant Professor of Surgery, Department of Plastic Surgery, Dartmouth Medical School, Hanover, New Hampshire

Steve Copit, M.D.
Private practice, Philadelphia, Pennsylvania

Mark A. Deuber, M.D.
Chief Resident, Department of Plastic Surgery, The University of Texas Southwestern Medical Center, Dallas, Texas

Ronald M. Friedman, M.D.
Private practice, Plano, Texas

Thomas Grosch, M.D.
Private practice, La Canada–Flintridge, California

Sanjay Grover, M.D.
Private practice, Beverly Hills, California

Ronald P. Gruber, M.D.
Clinical Assistant Professor, Department of Plastic Surgery, Stanford University, Stanford, California

Joseph M. Gryskiewicz, M.D.
Clinical Professor, University of Minnesota Academic Health Center, Minneapolis, Minnesota

Bahman Guyuron, M.D.
Clinical Professor, Department of Plastic and Reconstructive Surgery, Case Western Reserve University, Cleveland, Ohio

Jack P. Gunter, M.D.
Clinical Professor, Departments of Plastic Surgery and Otolaryngology, The University of Texas Southwestern Medical Center, Dallas, Texas

Richard Ha, M.D.
Chief Resident, Department of Plastic Surgery, The University of Texas Southwestern Medical Center, Dallas, Texas

Fred L. Hackney, M.D., D.D.S.
Clinical Instructor, Department of Plastic Surgery, The University of Texas Southwestern Medical Center, Dallas, Texas

Raymond J. Harshbarger, M.D.

Staff, Plastic Surgery, Brooke Army Medical Center, Fort Sam Houston, Texas

P. Craig Hobar, M.D.

Clinical Associate Professor, Department of Plastic Surgery, The University of Texas Southwestern Medical Center, Dallas, Texas

Larry H. Hollier, Jr., M.D.

Assistant Professor, Division of Plastic Surgery, Baylor College of Medicine, Houston, Texas

Thomas J. Hubbard, M.D.

Private practice, Suffolk, Virginia

Bang Huynh, M.D.

General Surgery Intern, Department of Surgery, The University of Texas Southwestern Medical Center, Dallas, Texas

Raymond V. Janevicius, M.D.

Clinical Assistant Professor, Department of Surgery, University of Illinois, Chicago, Illinois

Jeffrey M. Kenkel, M.D.

Associate Professor and Vice Chairman, Department of Plastic Surgery, The University of Texas Southwestern Medical Center, Dallas, Texas

Michael Klebuc, M.D.

Assistant Professor, Division of Plastic Surgery, Baylor College of Medicine, Houston, Texas

Jeffery K. Krueger, M.D.

Chief Resident, Department of Plastic Surgery, The University of Texas Southwestern Medical Center, Dallas, Texas

Wayne F. Larrabee, Jr., M.D.

Clinical Professor, Department of Otolaryngology— Head and Neck Surgery, University of Washington, Seattle, Washington

Bradley F. Marple, M.D.

Associate Professor, Department of Otolaryngology, Head and Neck Surgery, The University of Texas Southwestern Medical Center, Dallas, Texas

Royce A. Mueller, M.D.

Assistant Professor, Department of Otolaryngology and Maxillo-Facial Surgery, University of Nebraska Medical Center, Omaha, Nebraska

Arshad R. Muzaffar, M.D.

Fellow in Craniofacial Surgery, Children's Hospital and Regional Medical Center, University of Washington, Seattle, Washington

Robert M. Oneal, M.D.

Clinical Professor, Department of Surgery (Plastic Surgery), University of Michigan Medical Center, Ann Arbor, Michigan

Fernando Ortiz-Monasterio, M.D.

Professor Emeritus, Faculty of Medicine, Universidad Nacional Autónoma de México, Mexico City, Mexico

James F. Paul, D.D.S., M.D.

Private practice, Bettendorf, Iowa

George C. Peck, M.D.

Private practice, Livingston, New Jersey

George C. Peck, Jr., M.D.

Private practice, Livingston, New Jersey

Joseph Raniere, Jr., M.D.

Private practice, Jonesboro, Georgia

Brian J. Reagan, M.D.

Private practice, La Jolla, California

Rod J. Rohrich, M.D.

Professor and Chairman, Department of Plastic Surgery, Holder of the Crystal Charity Ball Distinguished Chair in Plastic Surgery and the Betty and Warren Woodward Chair in Plastic and Reconstructive Surgery, The University of Texas Southwestern Medical Center, Dallas, Texas

Ronald C. Russo, M.D.

Private practice, Colorado Springs, Colorado

Jack H. Sheen, M.D.

Clinical Professor of Plastic Surgery, Department of Surgery, University of Southern California; Associate Clinical Professor of Plastic Surgery, Department of Surgery, University of California, Los Angeles, California

Hashem Shemshadi, M.D.
Assistant Professor, Department of Plastic Surgery, Iran University, Tehran, Iran

Samuel Stal, M.D.
Associate Professor, Department of Surgery, Division of Plastic Surgery, Baylor College of Medicine, Houston, Texas

Patrick K. Sullivan, M.D.
Associate Professor of Plastic Surgery, Department of Surgery, Brown University School of Medicine, Providence, Rhode Island

M. Eugene Tardy, Jr., M.D.
Professor of Clinical Otolaryngology and Director, Division of Facial Plastic Surgery, University of Illinois; Instructor, Department of Otolaryngology, Northwestern University, Chicago, Illinois; Professor of Clinical Otolaryngology, Department of Otolaryngology/Head and Neck Surgery, Indiana University School of Medicine, Indianapolis, Indiana

John B. Tebbetts, M.D.
Private practice, Dallas, Texas

John F. Teichgraeber, M.D.
Professor, Department of Surgery, Division of Pediatric Surgery, University of Texas, Houston, Texas

Dean M. Toriumi, M.D.
Associate Professor and Director of Resident Research, Department of Otolaryngology—Head and Neck Surgery, University of Illinois, Chicago, Illinois

K. Glen Walton, M.D.
Private practice, Gainesville, Georgia

Deborah Watson, M.D.
Assistant Professor, Division of Otolaryngology—Head and Neck Surgery, University of California School of Medicine, San Diego, California

JACK P. GUNTER
A Tribute

*J*ack Gunter has been a close personal friend, confidant, and colleague for more than two decades. He has also been one of my role models as well as a father figure as I have struggled to learn the craft of plastic surgery. Jack is the consummate teacher who has encouraged, cajoled, and chided me and so many others to excel in what we do. It did not matter whether I was a resident or chairman of my own department; his only goal was to teach me to be more critical of my results so that I could become a better rhinoplasty surgeon. His instruction and guidance have been invaluable in shaping my career and practice.

Jack Gunter has been a major force in educating plastic surgeons about rhinoplasty. He has been an outspoken advocate of the open approach to nasal surgery and of precise preoperative nasal analysis and operative planning, so typified by his reliance on the Gunter graphics. This has been the hallmark of a Jack Gunter rhinoplasty.

This book is a tribute to Jack Gunter, a master surgeon whose passion for rhinoplasty has inspired us all to excellence. It is Jack's voice I hear every time I perform a rhinoplasty as he urges me and all of his students and colleagues to make each case "the best it can be."

R.J.R.

The following signatures have been contributed by the faculty of the Dallas Rhinoplasty Symposium over the past 17 years as a testimony to and in appreciation of Jack Gunter's many contributions in advancing the art and science of rhinoplasty.

William P. Adams Jr.

Fred J Hackney

George C Peck Jr.

George C. Peck Sr.

Patrick H Pownell

Rod J Rohrich

Thomas J Hubbard

Raymond Janusiruus

Robert W Sheffield

H. Steve Byrd

Bob Simons

Samuel Stol

Patrick K Sullivan

E Gaylon McCollough Jr.

Robert M Mc_Neal

Norman Pastorek

Dean M Toriumi

Preface

*T*he impetus for the Dallas Rhinoplasty Symposium and ultimately this book originated from my formative experiences as an otolaryngology resident at Tulane University. I was fortunate to work with Dr. Jack R. Anderson, one of the leading rhinoplasty surgeons in the country at that time. Dr. Anderson was an enthusiastic teacher who first ignited my interest in rhinoplasty and ultimately in plastic surgery.

Under Dr. Anderson's influence, my fascination with rhinoplasty grew rapidly and continues to this day. Otolaryngology allowed me to hone my skill in rhinoplasty but required that I treat patients with a wide range of head and neck problems, which was not always a satisfying experience for me. Given the same medications, some patients improved and others did not. I often wondered whether the treatment effected the change or whether it was attributable to psychological or environmental variables. I wanted more feedback and more control over the outcome. That is why I found plastic surgery so compelling. Plastic surgery, especially rhinoplasty, leaves no doubt; you can look at a patient and immediately see whether the results are good or bad. Also, plastic surgery appealed to my appreciation for things beautiful; it offered a unique opportunity to alter shape and form to achieve a superior aesthetic result.

After finishing my residency at Tulane, I served a 1-year National Institute of Health Facial Plastic Surgery fellowship under the direction of Dr. John T. Dickinson at Mercy Hospital in Pittsburgh. There I learned the basics of reconstructive surgery using flaps and grafts. On completion of my fellowship I joined the faculty of the Division of Otolaryngology at The University of Texas Southwestern Medical Center in Dallas where I staffed and operated on as many facial plastic surgery cases as possible. Of all the cases in which I was involved, rhinoplasty remained the most intriguing and challenging. After 7 years at the university, serving 3 of those years as chairman of the Division of Otolaryngology, I resigned to go into private practice and to devote all of my time to facial plastic surgery. At that time the conflict between otolaryngologists and plastic surgeons had developed into a turf war, and I felt that to pursue my interest in plastic surgery I needed to become board certified in plastic surgery. That decision led me to the University of Michigan where I completed a plastic surgery residency under the tutelage of Drs. Reed O. Dingman and William C. Grabb before returning once again to private practice in Dallas.

While at the University of Michigan, I met Dr. Robert Oneal who shared my special interest in rhinoplasty and my concern that residents were not receiving sufficient training in this area. We discussed the merits of starting a rhinoplasty symposium for residents and decided it would be a worthwhile endeavor. On returning to Dallas I approached Dr. Fritz E. Barton, then chairman of the Division of Plastic Surgery at The University of Texas Southwestern Medical Center in Dallas, about starting a rhinoplasty symposium for plastic surgery and otolaryngology residents at that institution. He offered enthusiastic support and financial backing to turn this dream into a reality. The first symposium was held in 1984.

The Dallas Rhinoplasty Symposium, now in its eighteenth year, offers a unique experience because of its emphasis on cadaver dissections, its colorful faculty, and its mix of plastic surgery and otolaryngology attendees. It has served to provide surgeons with a better understanding of nasal anatomy and to foster acceptance of different approaches for treating difficult problems. It is noted for the camaraderie of the faculty and the lively and animated panel discussions. The fact that rhinoplasty continues to challenge the skill of both new and experienced surgeons partially accounts for the success of the symposium. But its success is also due in large part to its role as a catalyst in introducing new ideas and innovative techniques to the specialty.

Open rhinoplasty is one such technique that was introduced early on at our symposium. Today open rhinoplasty is widely accepted and preferred by many, but that was not always the case. Only a few of the faculty used the open approach when the symposium first began. In fact, I had just started performing open rhinoplasty and at the beginning many of the faculty would come a day early to watch me operate. Afterwards we would proceed to a conference room where the faculty members shared new techniques they had been developing and any problems they were encountering.

The free exchange of ideas has characterized this symposium from its outset. Faculty and participants have been encouraged to question ideas and openly disagree. They responded enthusiastically with lively debate. We felt that the audience should be aware that even the experts disagree on how to best handle complex situations.

Panel discussions have always been one of the highlights of the meeting. One reason for this is that it has always been a requirement that all panelists who present a case must include an operative diagram in the presentation to pictorially show their surgical technique. This has clearly contributed to the understanding of the operation by the audience and faculty and is the reason that the diagrams are used in this book to illustrate the operation on all case reports. In the beginning the panels reflected a great diversity of opinion, but over the years we noted an increasing commonality. Thereafter we made a concerted effort to invite guests who represented different approaches. Many fondly remember the pitched verbal battles between Dr. Jack Sheen, one of the first and most enjoyable guests, and Dr. John Tebbetts. In one energetic discussion Dr. Tebbetts asked Dr. Sheen if he had ever tried an open rhinoplasty. Dr. Sheen replied no. Dr. Tebbetts then asked, "How do you know you wouldn't like it?" Dr. Sheen quickly retorted, "John, I have never jumped off a 15-story building but I know I would not like it." Today, however, despite our quest to profile opposing views, it is difficult to find faculty who primarily use the endonasal approach to rhinoplasty.

The first faculty members were all young Turks at the beginning of their careers. Dr. Oneal and I represented the most seasoned contributors. Over the years many notable rhinoplasty surgeons have developed from this core group, among them Drs. Rod Rohrich, Steve Byrd, Sam Stal, and John Tebbetts; today they number among the best teachers of rhinoplasty along with the many outside experts who have come to share their wisdom.

Numerous advances have taken place since I first watched Dr. Anderson perform rhinoplasty and these have been well represented in our symposium. Dr. Sheen was a catalyst for many of the seminal developments that have taken place in rhinoplasty, providing better analysis combined with innovative solutions to common problems. His concepts of augmentation and his use of spreader grafts and tip grafts have immeasurably improved our art. We have also benefited from the teaching of the open approach. It has advanced our understanding of nasal anatomy and nasal surgery because we can readily visualize the problems confronting us. We have learned from our rhinoplasty colleagues in plastic surgery and otolaryngology who have come together for an honest dialogue, freely presenting their ideas and exploring the potential for new techniques and improved results in rhinoplasty.

This book, *Dallas Rhinoplasty: Nasal Surgery by the Masters,* co-edited by Rod J. Rohrich, my long-time colleague and friend, and William P. Adams, Jr., a new educator with the zeal and energy to become an expert rhinoplastic surgeon and teacher, is the culmination of the efforts of those who have participated in the Dallas Rhinoplasty Symposium and reflects the growth in knowledge and expertise over the past two decades. In keeping with the tradition of the symposium, we hope that it will stimulate more accurate analyses of problems and encourage innovation and individualization of treatment approaches with the ultimate goal of improving the care we provide our patients and enhancing the quality of our results.

Jack P. Gunter

*T*he Dallas Rhinoplasty Symposium has come to be recognized as a teaching model. For plastic surgeons and otolaryngologists it represents the premier source of innovative changes and technical advances in rhinoplasty. It is considered one of the most successful "hands on" educational symposia in the United States because it delivers what it promises: cutting-edge information about basic and complex issues in nasal surgery taught by master surgeons in the field. Furthermore, it offers a dynamic, entertaining, and challenging learning experience.

This symposium was the brainchild of Jack Gunter. It grew out of his observation that plastic surgery residents were lacking in experience and exposure to the basic anatomy and surgical concepts key to successful rhinoplasty. Rhinoplasty remains one of the most challenging procedures to master; it is also difficult to teach, particularly when performed via an endonasal approach. Trained in otolaryngology and plastic surgery, Jack recognized the problems inherent in teaching rhinoplasty to plastic surgery residents. This prompted him to champion the open approach for nasal surgery and to teach plastic surgery residents the art of rhinoplasty.

Initially the symposium was designed primarily as a gross anatomy course. It became clear from working in the anatomy laboratory that there was a lot of confusion about basic rhinoplasty, even among talented, experienced surgeons. Therefore we used the laboratory experience to develop consistent nasal anatomy terminology and to establish basic principles and guidelines for functional nasal evaluation, preoperative planning, and surgical technique. These guidelines and the lessons learned in those original anatomy courses have become guiding principles for this teaching experience today. The clear focus is on accurate preoperative diagnosis and planning.

It became obvious to those of us who attended the first course either as faculty or residents that this symposium provided a unique venue for sharing information about this complex topic. During the first years the meeting was intentionally kept small to foster a camaraderie and develop a standard of educational excellence. The intimacy of this experience allowed better focus and creativity. What began as a small group of Texas plastic surgery residents gradually expanded to include both otolaryngology residents and young and experienced practicing plastic surgery and otolaryngology physicians. The faculty also grew to include leading national and international experts. The ability to extend the reach of this teaching opportunity was due in large part to the support of The University of Texas Southwestern Medical School Department of Plastic Surgery that pledged the use of its conference facilities, anatomy laboratory, and cadaver materials as well as its organizational skills to attract participants from a broad audience.

The initial presentations evolved from simple slide presentations with photocopied handouts to computerized PowerPoint shows with multiple standardized views of patients and more formalized training materials and educational tools. Foremost among these tools have been the Gunter graphics, which have evolved over time and now represent the standard for graphically demonstrating how a rhinoplasty is done. The anatomy laboratory training was initially supplemented by a small laboratory manual and then with video and digital tapes and interactive laser disks; for the past 6 years course participants have also benefited from watching live surgery by the leaders in rhinoplasty. Some of the outstanding aspects of this meeting include:

- Panel discussions by a dedicated faculty enthusiastically debating and evaluating divergent options, opinions, and philosophies
- Focus on primary rhinoplasty and basic principles that are applicable to more difficult problems
- Consensus on rhinoplasty terminology and standardization of patient presentations and photography, which have become standard for every meeting on rhinoplasty
- Emphasis on the cadaver laboratory, the fine points of nasal anatomy, and proportional analysis of the nose and face

Now all of these educational materials and the comprehensive learning and clinical wisdom from this symposium have been embodied in *Dallas Rhinoplasty: Nasal Surgery by the Masters* and a complementary set of CD-ROMs. This book is an outgrowth of the symposium whose name it bears. Similar to the teaching course that inspired it, it provides a comprehensive approach to basic and advanced rhinoplasty. It captures the strengths of our course, the point/counterpoint of ideas, and the anatomic knowledge and basic principles that are the foundation of this teaching experience. The accompanying CD-ROMs provide a dynamic supplement to the written material with its anatomic dissections and demonstrations of surgical technique. Topics covered in the book range from basic terminology, anatomic discussions, and incision approaches to tip grafting, alar resection, and septoplasty. Divided into nine parts, the book provides comprehensive information on anatomy, analysis and planning, the nasal tip, the nasal dorsum, and the septum as well as special problems such as secondary rhinoplasty, traumatic deformities, and the deviated nose. The final two sections focus on special considerations and advances and on the personal approaches of some of the master surgeons who have contributed significantly to the craft of rhinoplasty. Key points and clinical caveats are highlighted in each chapter. The Gunter graphics are a unifying element throughout the book, providing a unique roadmap to the planning behind the surgery.

In retrospect, Jack Gunter's vision has proved not only innovative but intuitive. Although his initial intention was to provide a forum for educating plastic surgery residents about rhinoplasty, the symposium has reached a larger audience and has had a far greater educational impact than originally anticipated. It is now a source of ongoing education and information for residents and experienced plastic surgeons and otolaryngologists nationally and internationally.

The incredible success of the Dallas Rhinoplasty Symposium is due in large part to Jack Gunter's innate understanding that people need to share information, experiences, and problems to grow and to learn. The entire rhinoplasty faculty is available throughout the meeting for informal discussions with participants and other faculty members. This has fostered camaraderie among the faculty and life-long friendships. But most important, it has fostered excellence in rhinoplasty. Because of Jack's constructive and critical analysis, this symposium has helped the faculty as well as the participants to become better rhinoplasty surgeons, helping them to refine their skills, expand their understanding of nasal anatomy, and improve their understanding of how to analyze the nose proportionally and convert that evaluation into the best possible care for the patient.

This rhinoplasty course is a history of a successful idea that was nurtured in a receptive environment by individuals who cared deeply about education and rhinoplasty.

Rod J. Rohrich
Robert M. Oneal
Samuel Stal

Acknowledgments

We gratefully acknowledge and thank our publisher and the staff at Quality Medical Publishing, Inc., specifically Karen Berger, owner and publisher, Carolita Deter, project manager, and Michelle Leaman, associate editor, for their untiring efforts and quest for excellence in medical publishing. They were instrumental in transforming this text from a dream to reality.

We thank all our contributing authors and our entire staff, faculty, and residents at The University of Texas Southwestern Medical Center Department of Plastic Surgery for helping to make this educational text possible, especially Joann Hughes for her secretarial assistance and Barbara Porter for helping in the final manuscript preparation and obtaining copyright permission from the *Journal of Plastic and Reconstructive Surgery.* Lippincott–Williams & Wilkins generously allowed us to use several articles previously published in the journal. We greatly appreciate the operating room staff at Zale Lipshy University Hospital, Dallas Day Surgery Center, and Surgicenter Southwest for their patience as we defined and refined our rhinoplasty techniques.

We owe a great debt of gratitude to the following at The University of Texas Southwestern Medical Center who have contributed to the Dallas Rhinoplasty Symposium over the past 18 years as we evolved from a basic course in rhinoplasty to the refinements of live surgery and panel discussions that culminated in *Dallas Rhinoplasty: Nasal Surgery by the Masters*—the Continuing Medical Education Department, the Medical Television Department (especially the director, Andy Guynn), and the Anatomy Department for providing the anatomic specimens for the laboratory.

Finally, we express our appreciation to Diane Sinn, administrative manager at The University of Texas Southwestern Medical Center, and to Marilyn Jackson, assistant to Dr. Jack Gunter, for their time and effort in organizing the numerous meetings necessary to produce this text and to Holly Smith for her superb efforts in digitalization of the photographs and Gunter graphics that gave the entire book a uniform look of excellence.

Contents

■ VOLUME I ■

PART THREE
Nasal Tip

Section 1 ▪ THE BASICS

PART FIVE

Septum

◾ **VOLUME II** ◾

PART SIX

Secondary Rhinoplasty

PART SEVEN

Traumatic Deformities and the Deviated Septum

PART EIGHT
Special Considerations and Advances

PART NINE
Personal Approaches

DALLAS RHINOPLASTY

Nasal Surgery by the Masters

Secondary Rhinoplasty

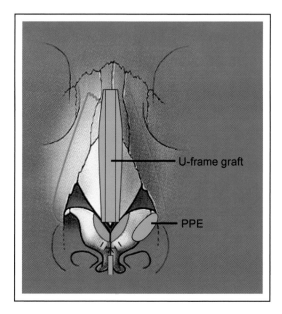

38

Structural Grafting in Secondary Rhinoplasty

Deborah Watson, M.D. ▪ Dean M. Toriumi, M.D.

Deformities occurring after rhinoplasty result from many factors, including faulty preoperative diagnosis, incorrect selection of surgical technique, flawed execution of surgical maneuvers, and unfavorable healing. Both structural and functional deformities can be caused by aggressive resection of the nasal skeleton with failure to maintain or reconstruct the supporting framework. If the supportive nasal structures are altered and no attempts are made to reconstitute them, contractile forces within the nasal tissue are likely to deform the desired postoperative results during the healing process.

---

*Aggressive resection of the nasal skeleton and failure to maintain
or reconstruct the supporting framework can result in structural and
functional deformities.*

Major supportive mechanisms of the nose can be distorted and interrupted by rhinoplasty procedures. Any incisions made through major supporting structures of the nose require reconstitution so that structural support is maintained. The integrity of the entire bony-cartilaginous nasal framework should also be respected during these procedures. This framework functions as the basic scaffold for the skin–soft tissue envelope (SSTE) and affects draping of the SSTE. The character of the SSTE also affects its own contour over the nasal framework. Thick, sebaceous skin may not satisfactorily conform to the postsurgical framework, whereas thin skin will adjust readily to the new scaffold. In this latter case a precise, symmetric, and stable framework is necessary to prevent visible irregularities.

Any incisions made through major supporting structures of the nose require reconstitution so that structural support is maintained.

To correct structural or functional deformities after previous rhinoplasty, a reconstructive approach should be followed during the revision procedure. Attention must be directed to achieving a more normal and aesthetically balanced nasal shape, reestablishing nasal support, and restoring adequate tip projection. Appropriate correction of nasal deformities relies on a variety of struts, grafts, and stabilizing sutures to reconstitute a supportive framework that can provide the desired nasal contour and withstand the contractile forces of healing.

Secondary rhinoplasty is frequently performed using precise pocket grafting via the endonasal approach. This is particularly useful for patients with isolated deformities. For example, a concavity along the lateral nasal wall can be corrected with an onlay cartilage graft placed through a small intranasal incision into a precise pocket. Alternatively, placement of structural grafts using precise suture fixation is afforded by the external rhinoplasty approach. Structural grafting is beneficial for severe functional deficits and nasal deformities resulting from a loss of integrity of the lower third tripod complex. The external rhinoplasty approach provides maximal surgical exposure and allows precise execution of any surgical maneuvers.[1-3]

Correction of nasal deformities involves a variety of struts, grafts, and stabilizing sutures to reconstitute a supportive framework.

In secondary rhinoplasty patients careful examination of the deformed cartilaginous and bony framework is critical for diagnosis and surgical planning. The upper, middle, and lower thirds of the nose should be assessed independently of one another for a thorough analysis. The internal nasal architecture and its relationship to the external scaffold must also be assessed for complete analysis of functional deficits.

The deformed cartilaginous and bony framework must be examined closely to ensure proper diagnosis and surgical planning.

It is important to realize that contour changes resulting from scar contracture may take many months or even years to occur. Another significant point that should be addressed in secondary rhinoplasty patients is the presence of a scar tissue layer beneath the SSTE without normal tissue planes. Dissection and elevation of the SSTE are more difficult and therefore must be performed in the supraperichondrial/periosteal plane with care and patience to preserve the vascular integrity of the flap.

Dissection and elevation of the SSTE must be performed in the supraperichondrial/periosteal plane.

When reduction of the nasal structural framework is aggressive and the resection is out of proportion to the size of the overlying SSTE, a dead space is created between the two components. This tissue void often becomes filled with scar tissue, producing amorphous contours of the lower nasal third and a potential parrot-beak deformity.

SECONDARY DEFORMITIES

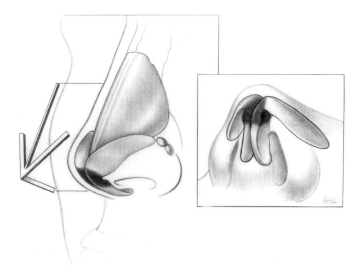

The lower third of the nose can be likened to a tripod-supporting structure comprising the conjoined medial crura and both lateral crura. The intermediate crura provide a transitional support between the medial and lateral crura.[4,5] The conjoined medial crura form one leg of the tripod and the lateral crura the other two legs. The caudal margin of the intermediate crura flares laterally to act as a transitional structure between the medial and lateral crura (see insert). The divergent and angulated intermediate crura (shaded area) contribute to the double break of the infratip lobule. This continuity of the tripod framework should be preserved during any rhinoplasty procedure. Application of grafts and reorientation of tissue may be necessary to achieve this. If the integrity of the tripod structure has been maintained, favorable long-term results are more likely than if the tripod structure has been compromised. The strengthened framework should resist the deforming forces of scar contracture and leave aesthetic and functional quality uncompromised.[6]

Reestablishment of tip projection is a common goal in secondary rhinoplasty. Tip support is easily altered by previous surgical manipulation, producing an asymmetric tip, buckled cartilages, columellar retraction, or alar retraction. Knowledge of the major tip support mechanisms and the expertise to create a stable structural framework of the lower third of the nose are critical. Components of major tip support include (1) length and strength of the lower lateral cartilages, (2) attachment of the cephalic margin of the lateral crura to the caudal margin of the upper lateral cartilages, and (3) ligamentous attachments between the conjoined medial crura and caudal septum.[2] The nasal septum itself should also be considered a major support structure of the nose.

Reestablishing tip projection is dependent on knowing the components of major tip support and how to preserve or reconstitute them.

When loss of tip support occurs, several physical changes are evident over time. There is a loss of tip projection, the alae flare laterally, the columella bows inferiorly, and the alar rims retract superiorly.[2] In addition, the domes may rotate superiorly if they are weakened by excessive trimming. The domal region is particularly vulnerable to unpredictable healing if resection of the anterior septal angle accompanies domal manipulation. Loss of tip projection can result from using a complete transfixion incision because this tends to sever the ligamentous attachments between the caudal septum and the medial crura footplates. If the cephalic portion of the lateral crura is overresected, the arch of the lower lateral cartilage is weakened and can result in bossae formation.

Loss of tip support can cause a loss in tip projection, flaring of the ala laterally, bowing of the columella inferiorly, and retraction of the alar rims superiorly.

FUNCTIONAL NASAL DEFICITS

Nasal obstruction due to nasal valve collapse is usually related to deficiencies in the structural support of the lateral nasal wall. Nasal airflow may create negative airway pressure that can collapse a weakened lateral nasal wall, resulting in airway obstruction.

Internal Nasal Valve Collapse

The internal nasal valve is the anatomic area bounded by the caudal margin of the upper lateral cartilage, nasal septum, floor of the nose, and occasionally the large inferior turbinates.[7] Internal nasal valve collapse is frequently seen after reductive rhinoplasty procedures. Collapse of the internal nasal valve is usually diagnosed when excessive medialization of the caudal margin of the upper lateral cartilage is noted with the negative pressure created during nasal inspiration. There is also evidence of medial collapse in the supra-alar region. By lateralizing this collapsed region with an instrument such as a nasal speculum or performing the Cottle maneuver (lateralizing the cheek and nasal wall with lateral digital pressure), improvement in nasal breathing is observed.[8]

Excessive medialization of the caudal margin of the upper lateral cartilage when negative pressure is created during nasal inspiration usually leads to the diagnosis of internal valve collapse.

Correcting internal nasal valve collapse is usually directed at repositioning the upper lateral cartilages or applying structural grafts to support the lateral nasal wall. Traditionally spreader grafts have been used to correct internal nasal valve collapse. When properly placed, these grafts will lateralize the upper lateral cartilages while increasing the width of the middle nasal vault.[9] Different structural grafts to reestablish support of the lateral nasal wall have been described in the literature.[10-13] Many of these grafts support the weakened upper lateral cartilages and lateralize the caudal upper lateral cartilage where the internal nasal valve is located.

Spreader grafts frequently are used to correct internal nasal valve collapse.

Internal nasal valve collapse can also result from contracted scars in the area of the nasal valve, excessive vestibular skin resection, or strictures that developed from poorly approximated endonasal incisions. Correction of these functional defects include removal of the scar tissue followed by Z-plasty, local mucosal flaps,[14] or replacement of the inner lining defect with a composite skin-cartilage graft obtained from the auricle.[3] The cartilaginous component of the graft provides support and decreases the likelihood of graft shrinkage.

Internal nasal valve collapse can also result from contracted scars in the area of the nasal valve.

External Nasal Valve Collapse

This form of lateral wall collapse involves collapse of the nostril margin, or alar lobule, during mild to moderate nasal inspiration.[15] The effect is typically seen in patients with narrow nostrils and overprojection of the nasal tip[5,9] and is actually more commonly found in nonoperated noses than noses having undergone previous surgery. When present, the external nasal valve collapse can be corrected with several techniques. The nasal tip can be de-projected to create oval-shaped nostrils instead of slitlike ones. In addition, structural grafts can be placed into the alar lobule for added support.

When external nasal valve collapse occurs during mild to moderate nasal inspiration, it signifies an unsupported nostril margin.

AUTOLOGOUS GRAFTING MATERIAL

Autologous cartilage grafts are preferred for reconstruction of secondary rhinoplasty patients.[2,3] Using nonautologous and synthetic material increases the risk for inflammation, infection, extrusion, and development of excess scar tissue under the SSTE.

The principal source of cartilage is the septum. It is easy to harvest, is sturdy, and can be easily sculpted. When the supply of septal cartilage is inadequate, conchal cartilage is harvested. Auricular cartilage, however, tends to be less rigid and more delicate compared with septal cartilage. Another source is costal cartilage. Harvesting costal cartilage entails significantly more surgical effort and is associated with greater operative risks. To add to its shortcomings, costal cartilage has the unfortunate tendency to warp over time if not carved correctly.[16]

The principal source of cartilage is the septum, but when the supply of septal cartilage is inadequate, conchal cartilage is harvested.

Calvaria and iliac crest are donor site possibilities for nasal bone grafting. Calvaria, a membranous type of bone, can be harvested with less patient morbidity and is less prone to resorption than is endochondral bone (i.e., iliac crest).[17] In selected patients segments of bone from the vomer or the perpendicular plate of the ethmoid can be used. Mazzola and Felisati[3] describe a batten bone graft harvested from the perpendicular plate of the ethmoid and used as a splint for a deviated septum. In general, bone grafts need to be placed in direct contact with nasal bones to ensure stability. To fix them into position intraoperatively, a small screw or sutures placed through carefully drilled holes are recommended.[3] An indication for using a bone graft is naso-frontal angle defects caused by overreduction of the nasal dorsum or post-traumatic deformities. These grafts can also suffice as alternatives to cartilage grafts when the nasal pyramid has been altered by excessive removal of the nasal bones.

Calvaria can be used for nasal bone grafting.

Softening the minor irregularities and edges of onlay grafts adds a finishing touch to the structural nasal framework before the SSTE is draped over. This technique can be accomplished with in situ trimming of the grafts or with camouflage grafting composed of either perichondrium, which is dissected off the posterior surface of the conchal cartilage, or superficial temporalis fascia. A small sheet of either perichondrium or fascia is gently draped over an underlying structural component and tacked down with 6-0 Monocryl sutures. Camouflage grafts are also advantageous for patients with thin nasal skin. The hard edges of the nasal scaffolding are muted by these grafts.

Camouflage grafts composed of perichondrium or fascia are used to soften the minor irregularities and edges of structural grafts.

STRUCTURAL GRAFTING IN MAJOR NASAL RECONSTRUCTION

Complex nasal reconstruction is frequently performed via the external rhinoplasty approach and often entails a columellar strut, lateral crural graft, tip graft, and dorsal augmentation to rebuild the nasal framework. External rhinoplasty affords full visualization of the lower third and middle vault structures to ensure proper diagnosis. To support a weakened columella, a cartilaginous strut graft is placed in a pocket dissected between the medial crura, and a mattress suture is used to fixate the strut into position.

To support a weakened columella, a cartilaginous strut graft is placed between the medial crura.

While the surgeon attends to the lower third of the nose, the contours of the lateral crura and domal region are analyzed for asymmetries. At times it is necessary to shave both cartilage and scar tissue to remove deforming protrusions. If any of the structural limbs of the tripod are weakened, lateral crural grafts are warranted. They should be carved into the proper configuration and then attached with mattress sutures to the remnant edge of the cartilage or vestibular skin.

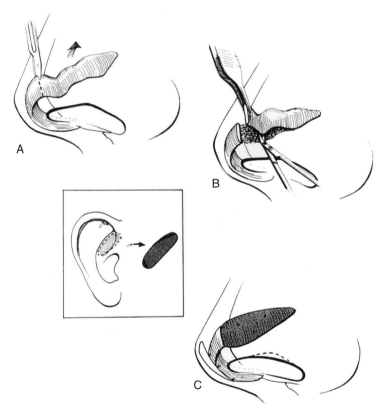

Reconstruction of the lateral crura

The deformed or weakened segment of the lateral crura *(A)* is incised while preserving the underlying vestibular skin. The buckled lateral crural segment *(B)* is carefully dissected from the vestibular skin. The graft *(C)* is sutured to the free edge of the remnant lateral crus with 6-0 PDS suture; the graft is then sutured to the vestibular skin with several 5-0 chromic mattress sutures.

Tip projection and a bidomal tip contour can be reestablished by positioning shield-shaped tip graft. A "unitip" deformity can be corrected by using a tip graft to set interdomal distance.

After the domes have been dissected apart, the tip graft can be sutured to both domes to hold them in a lateral position. This maneuver helps to correct the unitip deformity. "Pinched" domes form a unitip deformity *(A)*. Domes are dissected apart and sutured to the tip graft in a lateral position *(B)*.

Tip projection and a bidomal tip contour can be reestablished with a tip graft.

To reconstruct the middle vault, spreader grafts can be used to set middle vault width and reposition the upper lateral cartilages. Spreader grafts can be placed either through small intranasal incisions into submucosal tunnels or via the external rhinoplasty approach.

Augmentation of the dorsum can be achieved with an autologous cartilage graft. Small dorsal irregularities or excessively thin dorsal skin can be improved with an acellular dermal graft (AlloDerm, LifeCell Corp., Boston, Mass.).

An autologous cartilage graft can be used to augment the dorsum.

Columellar Strut Grafts

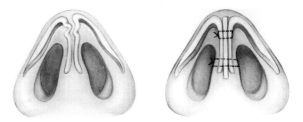

A sutured-in-place columella strut can be used to support weakened medial crura and to stabilize the base of the nose.[1] This also preserves tip projection, corrects buckling of the intermediate crura, and improves tip symmetry.[2] The columella strut is placed in a well-defined pocket that is dissected between the medial crura but does not extend to the nasal spine. If the strut is placed on the nasal spine, the strut may click on it and eventually create tip asymmetry.[2] The strut is sutured into position with a precisely placed 4-0 chromic mattress suture. The mattress suture is placed near the junction between the medial and intermediate crura to avoid distortion of the normal divergence of the caudal margins of the intermediate crura as they approach the domes.

The columellar strut preserves tip projection, corrects buckling of the intermediate crura, and improves tip symmetry.

Tip Graft

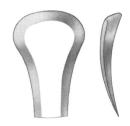

The shield-shaped tip graft can be carved from autologous septal or auricular cartilage. Several sculpting principles should be followed: the superior edge of the graft should be thicker and wider, all edges should be beveled, and the thinnest dimension should be at the base. The tip graft varies from 8 to 12 mm in superior width, 8 to 15 mm in length, and 1 to 3 mm in thickness.[6] The leading edge is the thickest portion of the graft. Note how the leading edge is rounded off to permit a smooth transition to the surrounding structures. The grafts are cut slightly longer to allow in situ carving of the graft once it is sutured into position. Final sculpting of the graft is usually done after it has been sutured into place.

> *The tip graft varies from 8 to 12 mm in superior width, 8 to 15 mm*
> *in length, and 1 to 3 mm in thickness.*

Correct positioning of this graft over a stable medial crural–columellar strut complex will improve tip projection and contour. The graft is secured to the caudal margins of the medial and intermediate crura with 6-0 Monocryl or PDS. These stabilizing sutures are placed bilaterally near the base and near the junction between the middle and upper third of the tip graft.[6] To create a flat surface and proper alignment for the tip graft, conservative trimming (<2 mm) of the caudal margin of the medial or intermediate crura may be necessary.[2]

> *Correct positioning of the tip graft over a stable medial crural–*
> *columellar strut complex will improve tip projection and contour.*

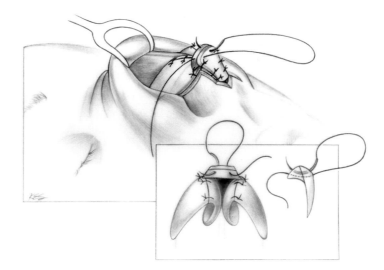

A buttress or cap graft placed behind the leading edge of the tip graft will provide support to weaker, more pliable grafts and will also serve to camouflage the leading edge of the tip graft. Note how the mattress suture fixes the cap graft to the leading edge of the tip graft with the knot tied behind the graft. Two additional sutures are used to fix the lateral aspect of the cap graft to the caudal margin of the lateral crura; this prevents excessive cephalic rotation of the tip graft under the tension of skin closure. Buttress grafts are sutured to the tip graft and to both domes so that the dead space between the leading edge of the tip graft and the existing domes is obliterated.

> *A buttress graft placed behind the leading edge of the tip graft will*
> *provide support for weaker, more pliable grafts.*

A longer tip graft can provide additional stability and can be used to increase tip projection by positioning the leading edge of the graft 1 to 2 mm above the existing domes.

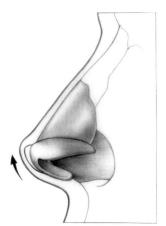

A shorter tip graft placed on the intermediate crura and domes will reestablish a double break; however, the shorter tip graft will not significantly increase tip projection. In addition, tip grafts are frequently used to camouflage asymmetries of the domal region. Asymmetries and nasal tip bifidity can be corrected by suturing the graft to the caudal margin of the intermediate or medial crura.[6]

Tip grafts are ideal for camouflaging asymmetries of the domal region.

Spreader Grafts

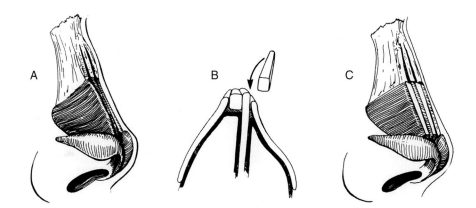

A narrow middle vault after rhinoplasty is often associated with inferomedial collapse of the upper lateral cartilages toward the septum *(A)*. A consequence of this deformity is nasal airway obstruction at the internal nasal valve. Supportive cartilaginous spreader grafts can be used to set proper middle vault width and reposition collapsed upper lateral cartilages. The grafts should measure approximately 3 × 20 mm each[3] and are placed in a narrow subperichondrial pocket that is made on either side of the septum at the level of the upper lateral cartilages *(B)*. They are secured into position with two horizontal 5-0 PDS sutures. Spreader grafts placed into submucosal tunnels will create a cantilever effect and lateralize the upper lateral cartilages. However, if the upper lateral cartilages are freed from the septum and spreader grafts are sutured into position, the lateralizing effect on the upper lateral cartilages is less pronounced *(C)*.

A narrow middle vault after rhinoplasty is often associated with inferomedial collapse of the upper lateral cartilages toward the septum.

Alar Batten Grafts

Alar batten grafts are convex cartilage grafts that are placed into a precise pocket at the location of maximal lateral wall collapse or supra-alar pinching.[5] As healing occurs, the contractile forces will attempt to medialize and compress the graft; therefore it is important to orient the grafts with the convex surface facing laterally to withstand the forces of scar contracture and the forces of inspiration.[18]

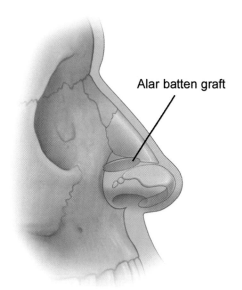

Alar batten graft

These grafts are appropriate for either internal or external nasal valve collapse. In cases of internal nasal valve collapse the alar batten grafts are positioned into a precise pocket at the point of maximal lateral wall collapse, which usually corresponds to the caudal margin of the upper lateral cartilages and the cephalic margin of the lateral crura. This region tends to undergo volume reduction during rhinoplasty procedures and may be weakened during the rhinoplasty operation.

Alar batten grafts are indicated for internal or external nasal valve collapse; they are positioned into a precise pocket at the point of maximal lateral wall collapse.

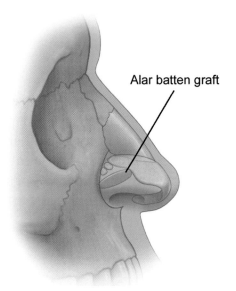

Alar batten graft

Alar batten grafts are also excellent for correcting external nasal valve collapse secondary to cephalically positioned lateral crura. Patients with malpositioned lateral crura also have weak alar lobules because of the lack of cartilaginous support. Placing the grafts in a caudal location to the lateral crura will provide the required support to prevent collapse of the external nasal valve.

Autologous cartilage best suited for these grafts is curved septal cartilage or auricular cartilage harvested from the cavum or cymba concha. A convexity of the graft is beneficial; it should also be strong enough to prevent lateral nasal wall collapse under negative inspiratory forces. The graft is carved into a rectangular shape to extend from the piriform aperture to the middle or lateral third of the lateral crura. A length of 10 to 15 mm and a width of 4 to 8 mm are standard.[18]

Alar batten grafts can be placed via an endonasal or external rhinoplasty approach. The common denominator is the creation of a precise surgical pocket in the subcutaneous plane at the site of maximal lateral wall collapse. Once inserted the graft should fit snugly without shifting in the dissected pocket. Too small a pocket, however, may force the graft to curl on itself and produce a deformity. Grafts placed endonasally usually do not require a stabilizing suture.

With the external rhinoplasty approach the lateral aspects of the lower lateral crura should be left undissected; this will allow creation of the precise pocket required for graft placement. If there is any evidence of graft mobility, then it should be sutured to the lateral third of the lateral crura.[18]

Lateral Crural Grafts

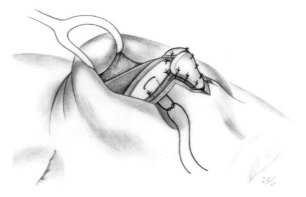

Weakened lateral crura from previous surgery can produce external valve collapse, create alar sidewall asymmetries, and cause inward bowing of the alar margin. Strengthening of the alar sidewall and lateral crura relies on the application of an anatomically positioned lateral crural graft placed over the weakened lateral crura to support them. Conchal cartilage is most ideal for these grafts. After they are carved into the appropriate shape, they are secured to the surface of the lateral crura with through-and-through 5-0 chromic mattress sutures.

Weakened lateral crura contribute to external valve collapse but can be strengthened with a lateral crural graft.

Composite Graft

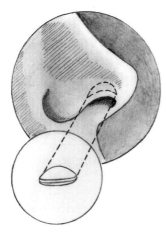

Alar retraction often results from aggressive resection of the lateral crus or vertical interruption of the alar cartilage. The resultant soft tissue void and weakened cartilage permit cephalic retraction of the alar margin by scar contracture.[19] Correction of alar notching can be accomplished by interposing a composite graft of full-thickness skin attached to auricular cartilage into a tissue pocket created on the internal alar side. This pocket is positioned slightly cephalad to the alar retraction and directly in line with the point of maximal notching.

Alar retraction usually results from aggressive resection of the lateral crus or vertical interruption of the alar cartilage.

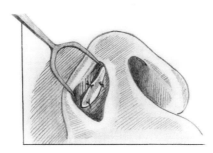

To initiate development of the surgical pocket, an incision is made several millimeters from the alar margin on the internal vestibular surface. The vestibular skin must be undermined and carefully unfurled to accommodate the graft. The preferred auricular donor site is just medial and inferior to the inferior crus on the anterolateral surface of the auricle.[19] The donor site is easily approximated without deformity using 5-0 nylon sutures. The composite graft can be fashioned into a fusiform shape of an appropriate size to reverse the notched alar defect. It is secured with four 5-0 chromic sutures to the peripheral edges of the predissected vestibular tissue pocket.

POSTOPERATIVE CARE AND FOLLOW-UP

If the external approach is used, the transcolumellar sutures should be removed 5 days after surgery and the incision supported with flesh-colored tape (Steri-Strip) for a couple of weeks to keep tension off the incision.

Postoperative edema may be more evident after the external approach than the endonasal approach. Edema in the supratip region can be treated with subdermal injections (0.1 to 0.2 ml) of triamcinolone acetonide, 10 mg/ml. These injections can be started 2 weeks after surgery and should not be performed more often than once a month. Frequent injections of higher concentrations of triamcinolone acetonide or superficial injections into the dermis may result in dermal atrophy.[6] With proper plane dissection rarely are steroid injections necessary.

It is essential to follow patients for many years to ascertain the healing/contractile effects and determine the success or failure of the reconstruction. The "shrink-wrap" effect of the SSTE will be more prominent years postoperatively. A stable framework will hopefully prevent functional deformities.

Long-term findings of greater than 5 years have been reported by the senior author.[6] Patients who had undergone external rhinoplasty were evaluated. Preservation of the desired nasal contours and framework was evident, and palpation of the nasal tip demonstrated excellent support of the tripod structure (consisting of the medial crural–columellar strut complex and tip graft). Occasionally a visible edge of cartilage was evident in a few cases involving dome division; however, domes are rarely ever divided anymore. Today separate dome binding sutures are used as well as an interdomal suture to establish tip width.

■ KEY POINTS

- ■ Preservation of the structural nasal framework during rhinoplasty procedures is critical for successful long-term results. Any intraoperative weakening of the nasal support mechanisms should be reconstituted at the time of surgery.

- ■ Use of the external rhinoplasty approach for secondary rhinoplasty permits direct visualization, accurate diagnosis, and precise execution of surgical maneuvers.

- ■ Functional nasal defects include internal and external nasal valve collapse and are corrected with spreader grafts and alar batten grafts, respectively.

■ Reconstructive efforts requiring grafting in secondary rhinoplasty are typically performed using autologous cartilage grafts.

■ A variety of autologous materials can be harvested for nasal reconstruction. Probably the most frequently used grafts originate from septal and conchal cartilage.

■ A sutured-in-place columellar strut can correct a retracted columella, reestablish nasal support mechanisms, and preserve tip projection.

■ A well-sculpted and positioned tip graft will add to the stability of the medial crural–columellar strut complex, increase tip projection, reestablish normal domal contours, and hide tip asymmetries.

■ Spreader grafts can correct nasal airway obstruction caused by inferomedial collapse of upper lateral cartilages as well as narrow middle vault and internal nasal valve deformity by widening the angle between the septum and upper lateral cartilage. Spreader grafts applied endonasally into precise submucosal pockets are more effective for functional correction of internal nasal valve collapse than spreader grafts applied after freeing the upper lateral cartilages from the dorsal margin of the septum.

■ Alar batten grafts are appropriate for correction of either internal or external nasal valve collapse and can be used in conjunction with spreader grafts. The precise placement of the grafts into a snug pocket dictates its success.

■ Lateral crural grafts can correct external nasal valve collapse but are used primarily for improving contour of the lower third of the nose. They are able to restore alar sidewall strength, symmetry, and shape because of their placement directly over the lateral crura.

■ Alar retraction can be corrected with an auricular skin/cartilage composite graft placed superior to the point of maximal notching on the internal vestibular side.

REFERENCES

1. Anderson JR. A reasoned approach to nasal base surgery. Arch Otolaryngol 110:349-358, 1984.
2. Johnson CMJ, Toriumi DM. Open Structure Rhinoplasty. Philadelphia: WB Saunders, 1990.
3. Mazzola RF, Felisati G. Secondary rhinoplasty: Analysis of the deformity and guidelines for management. Facial Plast Surg 13:163-177, 1997.
4. Sheen JH, Sheen AP. Aesthetic Rhinoplasty, 2nd ed. St Louis: Quality Medical Publishing, 1998 (reprint of 1987 ed.).
5. Tardy ME, Garner ET. Inspiratory nasal obstruction secondary to alar and nasal valve collapse: Technique for repair using autologous cartilage. Operative Tech Otolaryngol Head Neck Surg 1:215-218, 1990.

6. Toriumi DM, Johnson CMJ. Open structure rhinoplasty: Featured technical points and long-term follow-up. Facial Plast Surg Clin North Am 1:1-22, 1993.

7. Kasperbauer JL, Kern EB. Nasal valve physiology: Implications in nasal surgery. Otolaryngol Clin North Am 20:699-719, 1987.

8. Heinberg CE, Kern EB. The Cottle sign: An aid in the physical diagnosis of nasal airflow disturbance. Int Rhinol 11:89-94, 1973.

9. Sheen JH. Spreader graft: A method of reconstructing the roof of the middle nasal vault following rhinoplasty. Plast Reconstr Surg 73:230-237, 1984.

10. Beekhuis GJ. Nasal obstruction after rhinoplasty: Etiology and techniques for correction. Laryngoscope 86:540-548, 1976.

11. Constantian MB, Clardy RB. The relative importance of septal and nasal valvular surgery in correcting airway obstruction in primary and secondary rhinoplasty. Plast Reconstr Surg 98: 38-54, 1996.

12. Goode RL. Surgery of the incompetent nasal valve. Laryngoscope 95:546-555, 1985.

13. Stucker FJ, Hoasjoe DK. Nasal reconstruction with conchal cartilage: Correcting valve and lateral nasal collapse. Arch Otolaryngol Head Neck Surg 120:653-658, 1994.

14. Kern EB. Surgery of the nasal valve. In Rees TD, ed. Rhinoplasty: Discussion With the Experts. St Louis: Mosby–Yearbook, 1995, pp 209-222.

15. Constantian MB. The incompetent external nasal valve: Pathophysiology and treatment in primary and secondary rhinoplasty. Plast Reconstr Surg 93:919-931, 1994.

16. Von Mangoldt F. Reconstruction of saddlenose by cartilage overlay. Plast Reconstr Surg 46: 498-501, 1970.

17. Zins JE, Whitaker L. Membranous versus endochondral bone: Implications for craniofacial reconstruction. Plast Reconstr Surg 72:778-785, 1983.

18. Toriumi DM, Josen J, Weinberger M, Tardy ME. Use of alar batten grafts for correction of nasal valve collapse. Arch Otolaryngol Head Neck Surg 123:802-808, 1997.

19. Tardy ME, Toriumi DM. Alar retraction: Composite graft correction. Facial Plast Surg 6:101-106, 1989.

39

The Graft-Depleted Patient

Mark B. Constantian, M.D. • Arshad R. Muzaffar, M.D.

Not so long ago primary rhinoplasty was essentially a reduction operation (for which thin-skinned patients were ideal candidates and from which patients with thick or sebaceous skin were often excluded), and secondary rhinoplasty was limited to the occasional patient whose primary operation had not been properly completed. All this has changed over the past few decades, largely because of the influence of Sheen,[1,2] Peck,[3] Rees,[4] and many of the contributors to this book. Furthermore, a new paradigm of rhinoplasty is emerging that conceptualizes nasal surgery not as a reduction operation but rather a procedure in which reduction of some skeletal structures and augmentation of others (skeletally deficient) can rebalance the nose and maximize both function and aesthetics. Secondary rhinoplasty in the patient with an untouched septum or ear has thus become much more common, particularly when the surgeon understands that the volume of the skin sleeve changes very little and that reconstruction consists of supplying adequate skeletal support for the investing soft tissues and the airways.[5]

But what does one do with the 60-year-old patient who has had four prior open rhinoplasties during which material was harvested from the ears and septum and who yields only small fragments of ear cartilage and remnants of fibrous tissue? Obviously the rules of the game must change.

As more surgeons become familiar with various autologous donor sites, a group of secondary rhinoplasty patients is emerging with donor site depletion who have already had septoplasty or one or more auricular, calvarial, iliac, or rib grafts harvested. Some patients further limit the surgeon's options by prohibiting donor sites that are painful (e.g., iliac crest) or frightening (e.g., calvarium). Even the primary rhinoplasty patient may be donor-site depleted if the septum is bony and yields minimal usable cartilage (a circumstance that is more likely to occur in the non-Caucasian nose or the posttraumatic nose). Thus the surgeon faced with these patients must be familiar with techniques that permit acceptable functional and aesthetic results with suboptimal or minimal graft material.

> *Graft donor site depletion may significantly limit the surgical options for framework modification in secondary and some primary rhinoplasty patients.*

In the last 3 years the senior author (M.B.C.) has performed secondary rhinoplasties in 206 patients, of whom 141 (or 76%) were donor-site depleted. In addition, 17% of the primary rhinoplasty patients had nasal septa that were at least 75% bony and supplied insufficient cartilaginous graft material for the usual reconstructive techniques. I use Sheen's techniques,[1,2] essentially without modifications, or other methods previously described.[5-9] Nasal airflow was routinely measured in all patients undergoing functional nasal surgery by anterior, active mask rhinomanometry following the use of 1% phenylephrine spray to eliminate nasal cycling and mucosal factors,[6,7,10] essentially following the protocol established by Kern.[10] The data presented herein were derived from the first 123 patients. Nasal airflow (in milliliters) was calculated from the geometric mean of independent measurements of each nasal airway during a 14-second test period (geometric mean = $V_R \times V_L$).

OPERATIVE TECHNIQUES

In many cases satisfactory results can be obtained despite insufficient or suboptimal graft material if the surgeon observes the following guidelines:

1. Internal valvular reconstruction can be accomplished using either spreader grafts[11] or dorsal grafts[12] with equivalent functional effects. Geometric mean nasal airflow doubles with either graft type (n = 48, mean airflow 296 ± 123 ml/ 14 sec [preoperatively] to 776 ± 401 ml/14 sec [postoperatively], $p < 0.0001$).[6,7,13,14]

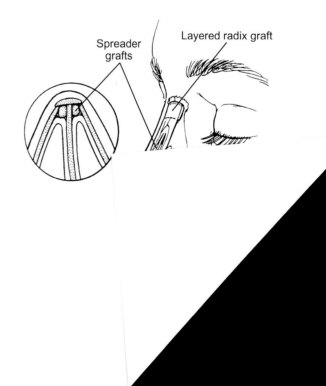

Spreader grafts

Layered radix graft

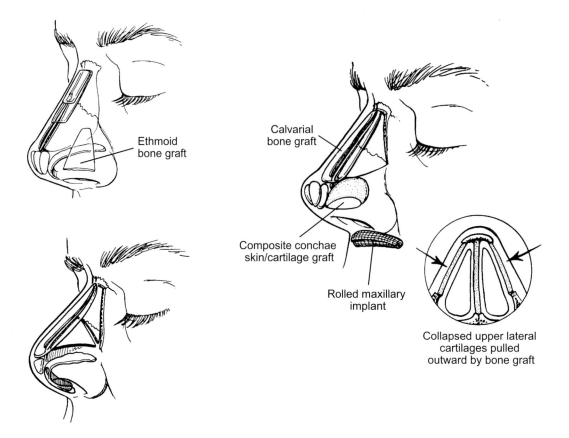

Ethmoid bone graft

Calvarial bone graft

Composite conchae skin/cartilage graft

Rolled maxillary implant

Collapsed upper lateral cartilages pulled outward by bone graft

2. External valvular reconstruction can be accomplished by using battens of cartilage or bone that span the area of rim collapse or the alar crease[6,7] or by composite skin/conchal cartilage grafts.[7] Mean nasal airflow doubles with external valvular reconstruction alone using either method (n = 7, mean airflow 343 ± 183 ml/14 sec [preoperatively], 1022 ± 533 ml/14 sec [postoperatively], $p < 0.07$).[6,7,13,14]

3. Tip reconstruction may be accomplished in some cases by selectively grafting the skeletally deficient lobular parts using small crushed grafts in limited pockets. This technique is particularly useful when the tip lobule itself is large enough and needs recontouring rather than additional projection.

4. Whether in primary or secondary cases, the thicker the skin, the more critical it is for the surgeon to resist the temptation to only reduce the nose and plan a strategy that includes augmentation of skeletally deficient parts instead so that skeletal volume is only redistributed, soft tissue support is maintained, and contraction of skeletal and soft tissues will not occur.[1,2,5,8,15]

5. Single-unit dorsal grafts will still be needed for substantial bridge defects in thin-skinned patients; not all patients can be treated with minimal donor material.

6. However, multiple staggered grafts (even using tangentially split crushed ear cartilage) can form a smooth dorsum in patients with adequately thick soft tissue cover.

CASE ANALYSES

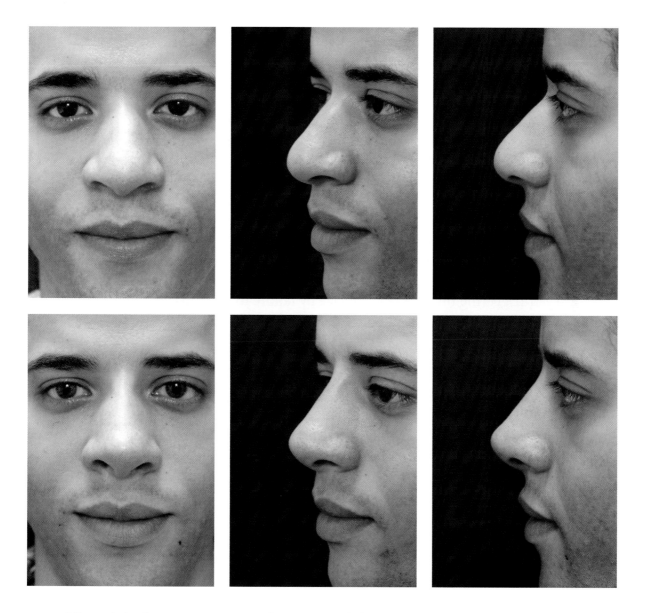

The original preoperative configuration of this patient closely resembled that of the patient shown on p. 716. Note the low root, high dorsum, and blunt, poorly defined tip with medium-thickness soft tissue cover. Despite a substantial skeletal reduction, skin sleeve volume changed very little, but contraction of the unsupported soft tissues produced the typical appearance of supratip deformity. Augmentation with dorsal and tip grafts without further skeletal reduction was needed to create the skeletal contours that could not be achieved by reduction alone.

Part of the difficulty in rhinoplasty stems from two false assumptions. First, it is assumed that the skin sleeve is a passive structure that will always contract to reveal the shape of a reduced underlying skeleton (true only to a limited degree in many noses and less true as the soft tissue cover thickens). Second, it is assumed that changes in each nasal area are regional, not global, so that each nasal area functions independently rather than interdependently. The prior cases illustrate the fallacy of both assumptions. If soft tissues had the infinite ability to contract to a reduced underlying skeleton, the secondary supratip deformity seen in the following case could not have occurred and augmentation would not have corrected it. If each nasal region functioned independently, skeletal reduction in this case would not have produced an apparent increase in nasal base size, loss of support to the internal valves, and an alteration in nostril contour and columellar position. The surgeon must be wary of triggering unexpected sequelae by failure to recognize the limitations of two classic assumptions about reduction rhinoplasty.

As the thickness of the soft tissue envelope increases, its capacity to redrape, contract, and reveal the shape of the underlying framework is diminished.

Structural alterations created in one anatomic region of the nose will necessarily affect the structure and function of adjacent anatomic areas.

The large nasal base is not a size problem but rather a balance problem. Thus the large base should be approached with the goal of creating harmony by augmenting the dorsum to match the lower third of the nose.

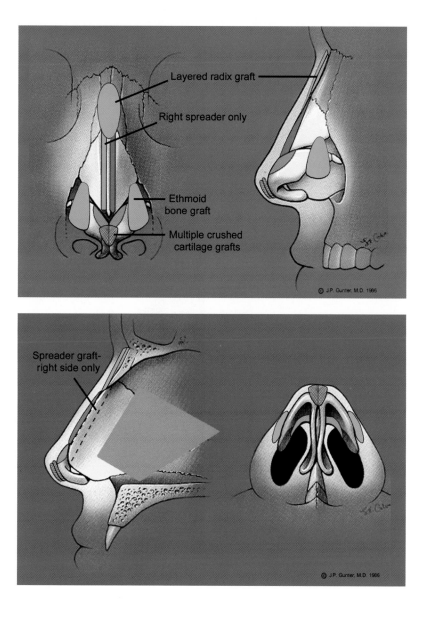

Layered radix graft

Right spreader only

Ethmoid bone graft

Multiple crushed cartilage grafts

© J.P. Gunter, M.D. 1986

Spreader graft- right side only

© J.P. Gunter, M.D. 1986

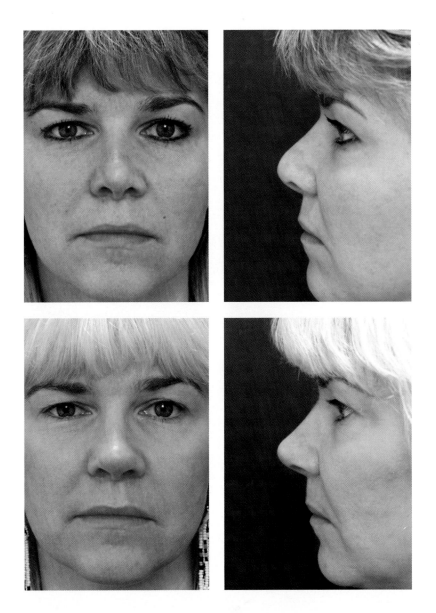

This young secondary rhinoplasty patient brought with her a photograph of her unoperated nose. Her original aesthetic goal had been to reduce the size of a nasal tip that she perceived as bulbous. Three rhinoplasties and insertion of a dorsal silicone prosthesis left her graft depleted because 90% of the nasal septum and cartilage from one concha has been removed. Airway obstruction existed from internal valvular incompetence and loss of support to the external valves following alar cartilage reduction. The patient's aesthetic and surgical goals were to remove the cold-sensitive, movable prosthesis that threatened to extrude, correct airway obstruction, and restore the preoperative retroussé and convex lateral crural configuration. The surgical plan consisted of maxillary augmentation; removal of the silicone implant; and placement of a dorsal graft of calvarial bone and composite skin/conchal cartilage grafts,[13] in which the cartilaginous segment replaced the convex lateral crura

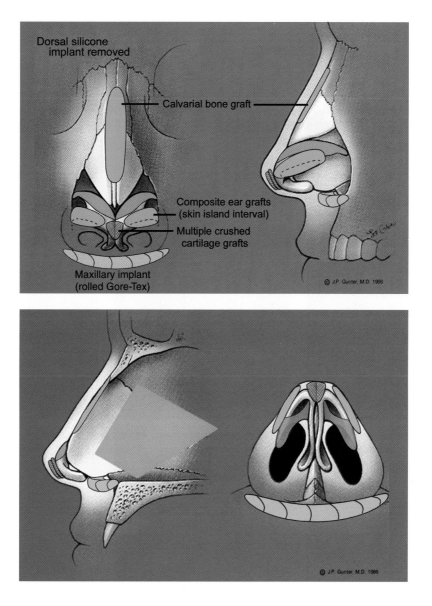

and supported the external valves and the skin island replaced the vestibular skin deficiency, and multiple ear cartilage tip grafts. Postoperative views show an improved contour of the maxillary arch, support of the lateral alar walls, and restoration of the patient's convex preoperative tip lobular configuration. The calvarial graft has solidly united to the bony arch.

> *In graft-depleted patients significant changes in the shape of the nasal tip can be created by placing even small amounts of graft material high in the tip lobule. It is critical in such patients to limit the caudal dissection of the pocket and to ensure a smooth surface contour; the dissection of such limited pockets is facilitated by the use of the closed rhinoplasty technique.*

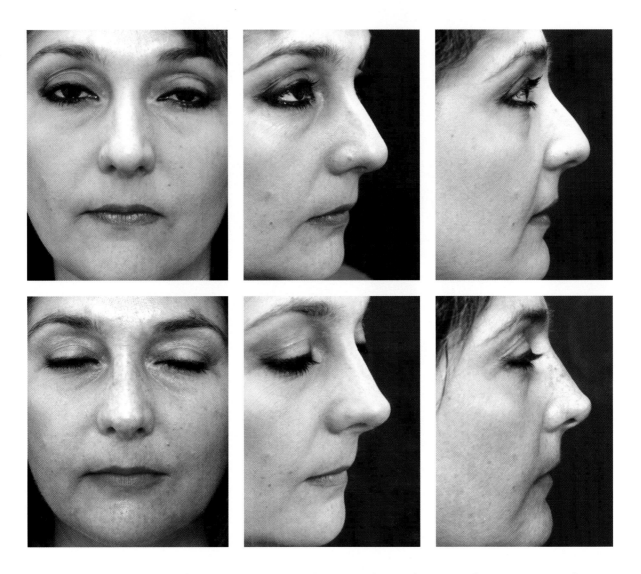

This patient had four prior open reduction rhinoplasties. The septum and portions of both ears had previously been harvested. Fortunately her soft tissue cover was thick enough that tangentially split crushed ear cartilage and its surrounding fibrous tissue placed in the cephalic portion of the dorsum and tip lobule improved overall nasal balance and obtained the tip lobular shape that the patient desired.

Crushed ear cartilage is not a prime donor material and is not recommended in patients with medium-thickness or thin soft tissue cover. However, the surgeon must always choose among the available alternatives. This patient re-

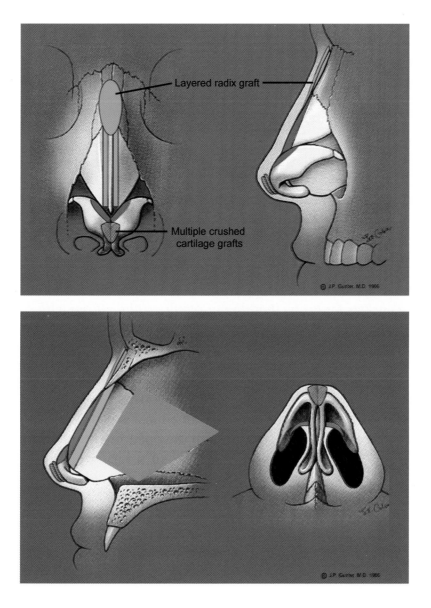

quired only 2 mm of dorsal augmentation and some tip refinement; rib grafts were unwarranted and calvarial grafts were unnecessarily risky in a 60-year-old patient and would supply too much donor material. In some cases the desired improvement can be obtained with minimal graft material if the soft tissue cover is adequately thick and the surgeon is fortunate enough (as I was in this case) to obtain sufficient amounts of usable autologous tissue.

To obtain minimal dorsal augmentation, crushed auricular cartilage may be used as a compromise in the graft-depleted patient provided there is adequate thickness of the soft tissue envelope.

DISCUSSION

A few technical points should be emphasized. I do not perform open rhinoplasty and make external incisions only to reduce skin volume (as in dorsal skin resection for intractable supratip deformity or in alar wedge resection), never for access alone. I do not fault surgeons who prefer the open rhinoplasty method. For many of these techniques, nevertheless, open rhinoplasty would not make the surgery easier but on the contrary more difficult. For example, with open rhinoplasty the surgeon not only has the opportunity to fix all grafts, but he *must* fix all grafts. With the closed approach, however, dorsal grafts, radix grafts, spreader grafts, lateral wall grafts, and (particularly) tip grafts can be placed in separate pockets that maintain their position and limit displacement.

The closed approach to rhinoplasty facilitates the dissection of limited, discrete pockets for grafts that do not require stabilization with sutures.

For this reason it would be difficult to use many of the techniques described here and elsewhere through the open approach[1,2,7,8,15] because donor materials are deficient or inadequate for the usual reconstructive techniques. Many of the grafts are crushed or otherwise modified in a way that makes them very difficult to suture, which is necessary with the open method but unnecessary with the closed method. Second, the degree of scarring present in patients who have undergone one or more open or closed rhinoplasties can make an open rhinoplasty dissection tedious and bloody, and grafts placed under tension may compromise columellar circulation. Whether performed open or closed, the surgeon using these techniques must be wary of placing the grafts under excessive tension or forcing oversized grafts into inadequate pockets and beneath insufficient soft tissue cover. Although it may be entirely possible and safe for the surgeon skilled in open rhinoplasty to use many of these techniques in that medium, I do not believe that it would be simpler to do so.

Many of the techniques using small amounts of graft material described here would be difficult to execute via the open rhinoplasty approach given the wide dissection and subsequent need for graft fixation with that method.

Cartilage grafts in the graft-depleted patient are often small and crushed or otherwise modified so that fixation with sutures would be quite difficult.

The alar cartilages may be modified either by delivery as a bipedicle flap or retrograde through an intercartilaginous incision. I use the former when more substantial modification of the alar cartilages is necessary and the latter when only a modest cephalic trim of the lateral crura is needed. In general, I use Sheen's methods[2] without modifications. The sequence of the procedures is similar in every case: Skeletal reductions are performed first followed by harvesting of graft materials, placement of grafts, and wound closure as the grafts are positioned so that they will not be dislodged.[2,5]

Although I have described some grafts as crushed, there is clearly a difference between grafts that have been crushed so they are pliable and grafts that have been pulverized. The difference is not an academic one. The greater the degree of crushing, the greater the loss of graft viability, as observed both clinically and in an experimental model.[16,17] Grafts should be crushed only enough to suit the soft tissue cover; the surgeon must remember that he or she is dealing with living tissue that is supposed to last for the patient's lifetime.

Crushing of grafts should be limited to the degree necessary to create the desired soft tissue contour; excess crushing diminishes graft viability.

Infection is always a surgical concern, even in an area as well vascularized as the nose. Postoperative infection in the tertiary rhinoplasty patient or around multiple grafts (particularly in the graft-depleted patient in whom donor materials are so hard to recover) can be particularly disastrous. The surgeon should use meticulous technique, changing gloves and instruments after harvesting ear cartilage and before proceeding to the nose,[2] rinse the grafts in saline and/or antibiotic solution before placement, and insert and remove the grafts as few times as possible. Although I do not believe that a narrow margin of error is the prime reason rhinoplasty is so difficult, there are many technical points in the surgery that can make substantial differences in outcome.

Meticulous sterile technique is especially critical in the secondary rhinoplasty patient who is graft depleted; infection in this situation can be disastrous.

Finally, the importance of valvular reconstruction should not be underestimated; in fact, preliminary evidence in the current series of 340 patients indicates that valvular incompetence may be more important than septal deviation as the primary cause of nasal airway obstruction.[13,14] This conclusion was supported by three pieces of evidence from the initial report on 160 patients: (1) Improvement in total nasal airflow following valvular surgery was the same whether or not a simultaneous septal obstruction was also corrected. (2) In patients with lateralized obstructions the septum was ipsilateral to the subjective obstruction in only 52%; in the other 48% of patients the septal deviation was contralateral to the symptomatically obstructed side. (3) Finally, in 58 secondary rhinoplasty patients who had previously undergone submucous septal resection but still had uncorrected airway obstruction, valvular reconstruction alone corrected the airway in 54 patients (93%).[13]

Valvular reconstruction is essential in many secondary rhinoplasty patients in whom collapse of the external or internal nasal valves contributes significantly to nasal airway obstruction.

As surgeons and patients become more sophisticated about aesthetic and functional goals and as autologous augmentation becomes a more common component of routine nasal surgery, the number of graft-depleted patients will surely increase. By altering the technical rules and strategies of repair, however, it is nevertheless possible to obtain satisfactory aesthetic and functional nasal reconstructions in this more difficult group of rhinoplasty patients.

■ KEY POINTS

■ Internal valvular reconstruction can be accomplished using either spreader grafts or dorsal grafts with equivalent functional effects. Geometric mean nasal airflow doubles with either graft type.

■ External valvular reconstruction can be accomplished with battens of cartilage or bone that span the area of rim collapse or the alar crease or by composite skin/conchal cartilage grafts. Mean nasal airflow doubles with external valvular reconstruction alone with either method.

■ Tip reconstruction may be accomplished in some cases by selective grafting of the skeletally deficient lobular parts using small crushed grafts in limited pockets. This technique is particularly useful when the tip lobule itself is large enough and needs recontouring rather than additional projection.

- Whether in primary or secondary cases, the thicker the skin, the more critical it is for the surgeon to resist the temptation to only reduce the nose and plan a strategy that includes augmentation of skeletally deficient parts instead so that skeletal volume is only redistributed, soft tissue support is maintained, and contraction of skeletal and soft tissues will not occur.

- Single-unit dorsal grafts will still be needed for substantial bridge defects in thin-skinned patients; not all patients can be treated with minimal donor material.

- However, multiple staggered grafts (even using tangentially split, crushed ear cartilage) can form a smooth dorsum in patients with adequately thick soft tissue cover.

REFERENCES

1. Sheen JH. Aesthetic Rhinoplasty, 1st ed. St. Louis: CV Mosby, 1978.
2. Sheen JH, Sheen AP. Aesthetic Rhinoplasty, 2nd ed. St. Louis: Quality Medical Publishing, 1998 (reprint of 1987 ed.).
3. Peck GC. Techniques in Aesthetic Rhinoplasty, 2nd ed. Philadelphia: JB Lippincott, 1990.
4. Rees TD. Aesthetic Plastic Surgery. Philadelphia: WB Saunders, 1980.
5. Constantian MB. Primary rhinoplasty: Basic techniques. In Cohen M, ed. Mastery of Plastic and Reconstructive Surgery, vol 3. Boston: Little, Brown, 1994, pp 1999-2020.
6. Constantian MB. The incompetent external nasal valve: Pathophysiology and treatment in primary and secondary rhinoplasty. Plast Reconstr Surg 93:919, 1994.
7. Constantian MB. Functional effects of alar cartilage malposition. Ann Plast Surg 30:487, 1993.
8. Constantian MB. Experience with a three-point method for planning rhinoplasty. Ann Plast Surg 30:1, 1993.
9. Constantian MB. An alternate strategy for reducing the large nasal base. Plast Reconstr Surg 83:41, 1989.
10. Kern EB. Evaluation of nasal breathing: An objective method. In Rees TD, ed. Rhinoplasty: Problems and Controversies. St. Louis: CV Mosby, 1988, pp 209-222.
11. Sheen JH. Spreader graft: A method of reconstructing the roof of the middle nasal vault following rhinoplasty. Plast Reconstr Surg 73:230, 1984.
12. Sheen JH, Sheen AP. Aesthetic Rhinoplasty, 2nd ed. St. Louis: Quality Medical Publishing, 1998, pp 1044-1055 (reprint of 1987 ed.).
13. Constantian MB, Clardy RB. The relative importance of septal and valvular surgery in correcting nasal airway obstruction. Presented at the American Association of Plastic Surgeons Annual Meeting, St. Louis, May, 1994.
14. Constantian MB, Clardy RB. The relative importance of nasal valvular surgery in correcting airway obstruction in primary and secondary rhinoplasty. Plast Reconstr Surg 98:38, 1996.
15. Sheen JH, Constantian MB. Primary rhinoplasty. In Smith JW, Aston SJ, eds. Grabb and Smith Plastic Surgery. Boston: Little, Brown, 1991.
16. Guyuron B, Friedman A. The role of preserved autogenous graft in septorhinoplasty. Ann Plast Surg 32:255, 1994.
17. Bujia J. Determination of the viability of crushed cartilage grafts: Clinical implications for wound healing in nasal surgery. Ann Plast Surg 32:26, 1994.

40

External Approach
in Secondary Rhinoplasty*

Jack P. Gunter, M.D. ▪ Rod J. Rohrich, M.D. ▪ Fred. L. Hackney, M.D., D.D.S.

*C*onsistent functional and aesthetic results following the correction of secondary rhinoplasty deformities continue to elude the plastic and reconstructive surgeon. The incidence of postoperative nasal deformities requiring secondary rhinoplasty varies from 5% to 12%.[1-2] In the past there has been no consistent prescription for the treatment of secondary nasal deformities.[3-7] However, a systematic approach using the external rhinoplasty technique can ensure more consistent aesthetic and functional results in patients with major postoperative nasal deformities.

THE PROBLEM

The primary problem in secondary rhinoplasty is scarring of the subcutaneous tissue, causing adherence and distortion of the underlying nasal framework. Management of these complex problems has usually been attempted through the standard endonasal approach with limited dissection and placement of grafts in small, tight pockets to avoid displacement.[8-11] The limited dissection and exposure offered by the endonasal approach do not permit accurate assessment and appropriate treatment of the anatomic problem. Adequate results have been attained with this technique, but they have not been consistent, and multiple operations have often been required.

*Adapted from Gunter JP, Rohrich RJ. The external approach to secondary rhinoplasty. Plast Reconstr Surg 80:161, 1987.

The most significant obstacle to overcome in secondary rhinoplasty is scarring of the subcutaneous tissue that causes adherence and distortion of the underlying nasal framework. The limited dissection afforded by the endonasal approach does not allow accurate assessment and subsequent correction of the anatomic abnormalities associated with secondary rhinoplasty.

Skin covering and nasal lining problems may occasionally have to be addressed in patients who have had rhinoplasty,[12-14] but most of the surgery is directed toward the nasal framework.[15,16] It must be reconstructed to provide patent nasal airways and a correct anatomic foundation for skin redraping. The external approach eliminates the restrictions imposed by the standard endonasal approach and has proved to be a major advance in obtaining consistent results in the management of these complex problems.[17]

ADVANTAGES AND DISADVANTAGES

The major advantage of the external approach is complete anatomic exposure.[18] It allows a direct view of the nasal framework deformity without distortion from retraction. If there is adequate skin covering and lining and the surgeon is familiar with the influence the supporting framework has on the shape of the nose, the task of reconstructing the desired framework is simplified.

Advantages and Disadvantages of the External Rhinoplasty Approach

Advantages	Disadvantages
Binocular visualization	External nasal incision (transcolumellar scar)
Evaluation of complete deformity without distortion	Prolonged operative time
Precise diagnosis and correction of deformities	Protracted nasal tip edema
Allows use of both hands	Columellar incision separation and delayed wound healing
More options with original tissues and cartilage grafts	Suture stabilization of grafts often required
Direct control of bleeding with electrocautery	

> *The open rhinoplasty approach allows complete anatomic exposure and accurate diagnosis of the underlying nasal framework deformity.*

With complete visualization the deformed nasal framework structures can be dissected and stabilized in their correct anatomic positions. If cartilage grafting is required, the graft can be accurately shaped and stabilized. Furthermore, in a teaching situation, the entire operation can be done under direct vision.

After the framework is reconstructed, its final position and shape can be completely evaluated and any discrepancies corrected. The skin is redraped to assess the effect of the reconstructed framework on the external appearance. If the shape is not satisfactory, the skin is retracted and further adjustments made prior to closure of the transcolumellar incision.

The main objection to the external approach is the transcolumellar scar.[19,20] However, in our series the scar has proved to be of little concern to the patients and no external incisions have had to be revised. Potential disadvantages of wound separation and delayed secondary healing have not occurred.

> *Extensive experience with the open approach has failed to reveal any significant concerns over the quality of the transcolumellar scar from the patient's or surgeon's perspective.*

The external approach may increase the operative time and prolong tip edema. The increased operating time is necessary for the suture stabilization required for any grafting and/or repositioning of the anatomic structures and accurate closure of the transcolumellar incision. Prolonged tip edema has not been a problem in our series.

> *The open rhinoplasty approach may increase operative time, but prolonged tip edema is difficult to evaluate.*

From a practical viewpoint the advantages provided by the 6 to 8 mm skin incision traversing the columella far outweigh the potential disadvantages in the management of these patients with major postoperative nasal deformities.

PREOPERATIVE ASSESSMENT AND PLANNING

The evaluation begins by defining the deformity, which is accomplished by a detailed history and complete aesthetic facial and nasal analysis. This leads to a precise anatomic diagnosis, which is the key to achieving an optimal functional and aesthetic result.[21-23] A systematic examination of the nose to define the deformity includes:

Nasofrontal angle position
Bony pyramid
Upper lateral cartilages
Supratip area
Nasal tip
    Projection
    Rotation
    Symmetry
    Position of tip-defining points

Alae
    Width
    Collapse
    Retraction
Columella
    Degree of show
Columellar-labial angle
Internal nasal examination
    Internal nasal valves
    Septum
    Turbinates

Starting superiorly, the nasofrontal angle height and depth are noted. The bony pyramid, upper lateral cartilages, and supratip are evaluated for their length, height, width, and symmetry. The nasal tip is evaluated in terms of its projection, rotation, symmetry, and position of the tip-defining points. The alae are inspected for increased width, collapse, or retraction. The columella is examined for increased or decreased show. The columellar-lobular and columellar-labial angles are evaluated to ascertain the desired angulation. The internal nasal examination evaluates patency of the nasal valves, position of the septum, and state of the turbinates.

Systematic Evaluation of Postoperative Surgical Nasal Deformities

Define the deformity
    Detailed history
    Facial analysis
    Nasal analysis
Determine the etiology
    Displaced anatomic structures
    Underresection
    Overresection
    Combination of above

Establish surgical goals
Formulate the treatment plan
    Repositioning of displaced anatomic
        structures
    Amount and location of further resection
    Location and type of tissue replacement
    External vs. endonasal approach

The etiology of a postoperative nasal deformity is usually one or a combination of three problems:

1. Displaced anatomic structures
2. Underresection due to incomplete surgery
3. Overresection due to overzealous surgery

After the diagnosis is determined, the goals of the surgery are established and a treatment plan is formulated. The goals are individualized for each patient according to the deformity. The goals may be to augment the nasofrontal angle, straighten the nasal dorsum, lower the supratip area, correct tip asymmetry and alar collapse, decrease columellar show, etc. Formulation of the treatment plan includes repositioning displaced anatomic structures. If there is underresection, the amount and location of further resection are determined. If there is overresection, it is determined what tissues are missing and where replacement is needed. Autologous cartilage is preferred for any nasal framework replacement.

Secondary rhinoplasty is usually associated with a diagnosis of displaced anatomic structures or underresection or overresection during previous rhinoplasty. A treatment plan can be formulated to address each of these problems.

Finally, it is decided whether the endonasal or external approach should be used. For simple deformities the standard endonasal approach is often adequate, but for complex postoperative nasal deformities the external approach is preferred. All secondary surgery is deferred until 12 months after the last rhinoplasty.

OPERATIVE TECHNIQUE

An organized approach to the external rhinoplasty technique is carried out in the following sequence.

Anesthesia
Incisions
Skin elevation
Intraoperative diagnosis
Dissection of displaced tip cartilages
Assessment of tip projection
Dorsal reduction if indicated
Septal and/or turbinate surgery if indicated
Osteotomies

Establishment of final tip projection
Dorsal augmentation if indicated
Final tip cartilage positioning
Final inspection
Wound closure
Application of splints and dressings

With the patient under general anesthesia the external nose and septum are injected with 0.5% lidocaine with 1:100,000 epinephrine, and the internal nose is packed with gauze soaked with a vasoconstricting medication.

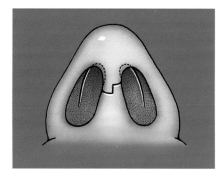

Bilateral marginal incisions along the caudal edge of the lower lateral cartilages are terminated medially at the narrowest part of the columella and connected with a transcolumellar incision. A straight-line incision is avoided by placing a broken-line incision across the columella, which allows precise wound closure. A broken-line incision can have various designs. A stair-step design is shown above. The broken-line incision along with the splinting supplied by the underlying cartilages aids in preventing scar contracture that could deform the columella. Some surgeons prefer to place the incision more posteriorly where the feet of the medial crura start to flare.

The columellar incision is usually designed as a broken line to allow precise wound closure and to camouflage the scar.

Before the skin is elevated, crosshatches are made with a scalpel to allow for more accurate wound approximation when the incisions are closed. The skin elevation is begun by dissection of the thin columellar skin off the caudal edges of the medial crura and the intervening subcutaneous tissues.

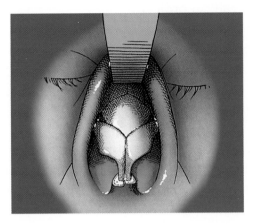

The dissection continues over the lateral crura and cartilaginous-bony dorsum up to the root of the nose. Retraction of the undermined area exposes the entire nasal framework.

A crosshatch can be made across the marginal incision site before the incision is made to allow for accurate alignment of the incision during closure.

After the soft tissues are elevated from the nasal framework, the tip cartilages are evaluated and correlated with the preoperative diagnosis. The extent of the nasal tip deformity is determined, and any cartilages displaced or distorted by scar tissue are dissected free, but final correction is delayed. Next it is determined if tip projection needs to be altered since this will determine the height at which the dorsal profile line should be set. Any alteration of the dorsum should be performed with the final tip projection in mind.

After the skin is reflected from the nose, the scar tissue is dissected free from the cartilages to help define the deformity.

After the desired tip projection is determined, the cartilaginous-bony dorsum is evaluated and any needed reduction of the dorsum performed. Reduction of the bony dorsum is usually performed with a rasp, and the cartilaginous dorsum is lowered with a No. 15 blade. The mucosa at the junction of the septum with the upper lateral cartilages is freed from the cartilages by developing submucosal tunnels bilaterally. This allows the septum to be separated from the upper lateral cartilages without transecting the mucosa. Maintaining the integrity of the mucosa helps stabilize the septum during its alteration. It also forms a trough so that a spreader graft can be placed to move the upper lateral cartilages laterally if there is collapse of the upper lateral cartilages and/or narrowing of the internal nasal valves. When augmentation is indicated, it is delayed until osteotomies are performed.

After the desired tip projection has been determined, the dorsum can be augmented or reduced with the planned tip projection in mind.

If septal work is required, the septum can be approached from the septal angle or through a separate transfixion incision. The mucoperichondrium is elevated on one side only, and the appropriate septal modification is performed. If there are problems at the junction of the caudal septum and the anterior maxillary crest area and a transfixion incision is not used, it may be necessary to separate the medial crura to gain better exposure. There should be no hesitancy in doing this, but their attachment to each other, which aids in support of the tip, must be reestablished by suturing the crura back together after the septal work and any turbinate manipulation are completed.

If a septoplasty is required, the septum can be approached from the anterior septal angle or through a separate transfixion incision.

When the septal work is completed, attention is directed to the tip, where final modification of the tip cartilages is performed and tip projection is established. If increased tip projection is desired, it is usually accomplished with an autologous cartilage strut placed in a soft tissue pocket extending from the anterior surface of the maxilla to between the feet of the medial crura. The soft tissue pocket is stopped short of the anterior nasal spine to leave a soft tissue pad between the base of the strut and the nasal spine. The strut is placed and the medial crura are advanced on the strut until the desired tip projection is accomplished. The medial crura are secured to the strut with 5-0 PDS.

Indicated osteotomies are performed next to properly align the nasal foundation before dorsal augmentation. With the foundation aligned the septum is reexamined to confirm its midline position. When the tip projection is established, any indicated dorsal augmentation is performed. In most instances the dorsal onlay grafts are stabilized with sutures, but cutaneous Kirscher wires may be used in the glabellar area. Final positioning of the tip cartilages is accomplished with suture stabilization. Onlay tip grafts are placed and secured if needed.

The skin is redraped after a final inspection of the nasal framework. The external appearance is evaluated, and the incisions are closed. After closing the marginal incisions with interrupted 4-0 chromic catgut sutures, the transcolumellar incision is meticulously closed with interrupted 6-0 nylon sutures. If septal work has been performed, bilateral septal splints are placed and sutured in place with through-and-through 3-0 nylon sutures. Nasal packing is avoided if hemostasis is adequate. Steri-Strips and an aluminum cast are placed on the nose and remain for 1 week.

Autologous Cartilage Grafting

When augmentation is needed, autologous cartilage is preferred. Septal cartilage is the graft of choice when it is available. A large amount can be harvested from the same operative field, and it is more rigid, provides better support, and does not have the convolutions found in auricular cartilage. It works as a dorsal onlay graft, columellar strut, or spreader grafts between the upper lateral cartilages and the septum. It can also be used to support or replace parts of the lower lateral cartilage complex.

Septal cartilage is the first choice for autologous cartilage grafting because it is rigid, relatively straight, and can be used in a variety of grafting situations.

The auricle can provide a large amount of cartilage for nasal reconstruction. Because of its flaccidity and convolutions, it is best used when these characteristics are desired. It is best for reconstructing the lower lateral cartilage complex and placement in the columella to provide tip support. However, it is a second choice to septal cartilage because of the inherent difficulty in obtaining and maintaining the desired shape.

Ear cartilage is limited by its flaccidity and convolutions; however, a large amount is available. In particular, it is useful for lower lateral cartilage reconstructions.

When septal cartilage is not available and support is the main consideration, autologous rib cartilage is used. If a limited amount of cartilage is needed, a small incision is made over the anterior end of the first floating rib and the cartilaginous portion removed. It is ideal for a columellar graft in that it is tapered, has a slight curve, and is strong enough to increase and maintain tip projection. If a large amount of cartilage is needed, the incision is made over the fifth rib, where sufficient rib cartilage can be harvested for dorsal augmentation and columellar grafts from the fifth rib and possibly the fourth or sixth ribs. According to the principles of Gibson and Davis[24] and Fry,[25] the cartilage must be carved so that equal amounts are removed from both sides to prevent warping or bending. However, even with judicious carving there is still a tendency for warping. Our technique of internal stabilization has limited such warping. The details of this are presented in Chapter 28. End slices of rib cartilage, which have a tendency to curl, can be used for lateral crural replacement and selective onlay grafts.

Costal cartilage is indicated when the amount of septal cartilage is inadequate and/or when rigid support of the osseocartilaginous framework or soft tissue is a necessity.

CASE ANALYSES
Augmenting the Nasal Dorsum and Increasing Tip Projection With Autologous Septal Cartilage Grafts

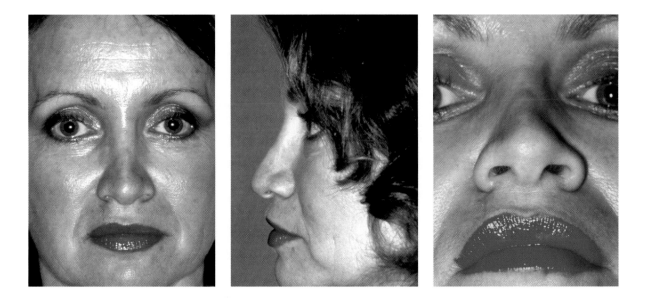

This 42-year-old woman had a rhinoplasty 20 years previously. She had difficulty with nasal breathing, especially through the left nostril, and felt her nose was getting wider. On the frontal view narrowing of the middle third of the nose due to collapse of the upper lateral cartilages, asymmetry of the supratip area, and a wide alar base were apparent. The profile view revealed a low nasal dorsum with decreased tip projection, fullness in the supratip area, and a very acute columellar-labial angle. The basal view confirmed lack of tip projection and asymmetry of the nostrils. The internal examination revealed deviation of the septum and bilateral collapse of the valve areas.

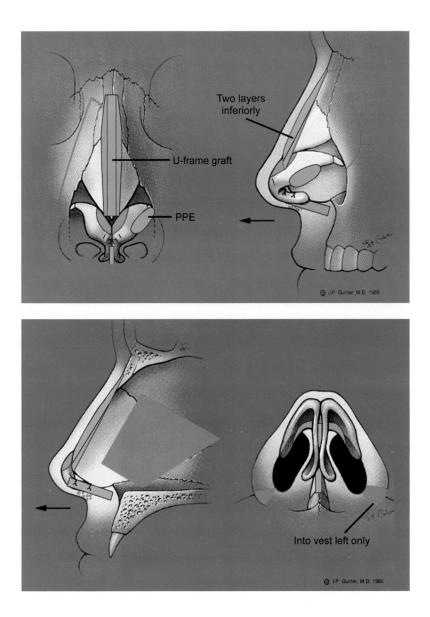

The osseocartilaginous framework was exposed through transcolumellar and marginal incisions. A septoplasty was performed to correct the deviated septum and harvest as much septal cartilage as possible, leaving an 8 mm L-shaped strut. A 28 mm inverted U-frame graft of septal cartilage with two layers placed caudally to increase the thickness in that area was used to augment the dorsum and correct the upper lateral cartilage collapse. A septal cartilage strut was placed in a pocket dissected between the medial crura, leaving a soft tissue pad between the base of the pocket and the nasal spine so the base of the strut would not rest directly on the spine. The crura were advanced on the strut and sutured to increase tip projection. Pieces of morselized cartilage were placed subcutaneously at the columellar-labial angle to fill out the angle. The lateral crura were trimmed, leaving symmetric 6 mm rim strips. Horizontal transdomal sutures were used to angulate the domes to accentuate the tip-defining points and tied together to decrease the interdomal distance.

A thin piece of perpendicular plate of the ethmoid was placed in the left alar groove area to correct a depression in that area due to lack of support of the crus. Bilateral alar base resections were performed extending into the vestibule on the left side but not the right in an attempt to make the nostrils more symmetric.

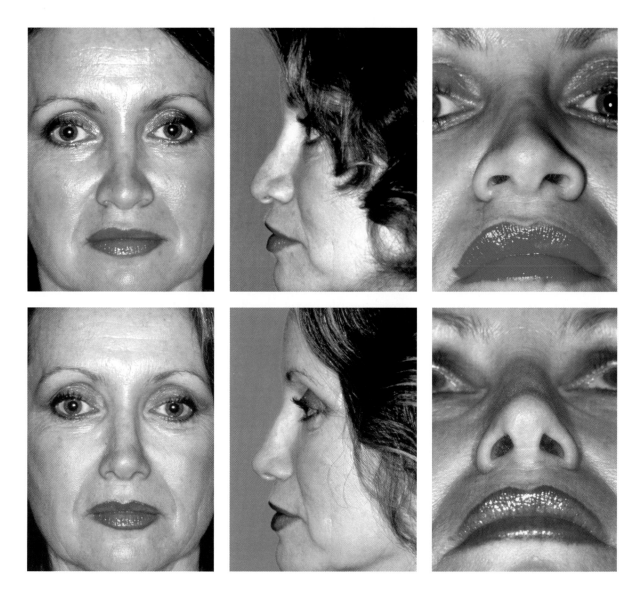

The 1-year postoperative photographs show correction of the dorsal deformity with the inverted U-frame dorsal onlay graft, improvement of tip symmetry using cartilage trimming, and suture repositioning and reshaping along with an onlay graft of the perpendicular plate of the ethmoid in the left alar groove area. Tip projection was increased with the columellar strut, which along with the morselized cartilage grafts helped to open the acute columellar-labial angle. Nostril symmetry was improved by asymmetric alar basal resections.

Correction of Marked Loss of Tip Projection and Dorsal Height With Autologous Rib Cartilage Grafts

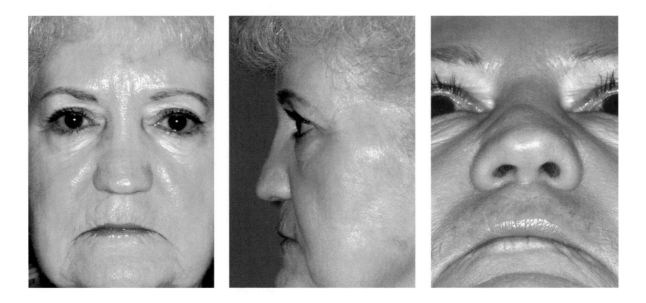

This 61-year-old woman had an accident as a child and had surgery at age 18 to correct a nasal deformity. As she aged, nasal breathing became more difficult and was causing her considerable problems. The frontal view revealed a wide bony as well as a wide alar base. The nasal dorsum appeared flat and there was no columellar show. On the profile view decreased tip projection was noted with decreased dorsal height and a retracted columellar-labial angle with decreased columellar show. A wide alar base, lack of tip support, and nostril asymmetry were seen on the basal view. The internal examination revealed a slightly deviated nasal septum with a small central perforation. There was collapse of the nasal valves and no caudal septal support.

The infrastructure of the nose was visualized through an open approach. A small piece of an ossified rib graft was removed from the dorsum and the dorsum smoothed by rasping the bone and trimming the cartilaginous dorsum with scissors. A pocket was dissected between the medial crura to the nasal spine from which the soft tissue attachments were elevated. Cartilage grafts from the ninth and tenth ribs were carved for dorsal onlay and columellar strut grafts. The dorsal graft measured 40 mm in length, the widest width was 8 mm, and the height was 10 mm at the caudal end and 2 mm at the cephalic end. It was placed on the dorsum and the distal ends of the upper lateral cartilages sutured to the inferior edges of the graft to open the valve areas and stabilize the graft. The 32 × 2 × 3 mm columellar strut graft, notched at the base so it would fit over the nasal spine like a saddle on a horse, was placed astride the spine. The medial crura were advanced on the strut and sutured to increase tip projection and move the columellar-labial angle forward. This also narrowed the alar base and elongated the round nostrils. Horizontal mattress sutures in the dome areas were used to angulate the domes and bring the tip-defining points closer together. A thin onlay graft of rib cartilage was placed over a slight convexity of the right lateral crus. Lateral osteotomies were performed to narrow the bony base. The transcolumellar incision was closed in a single layer under considerable tension because of the amount of tip projection that was gained with these maneuvers, but there were no problems with healing postoperatively.

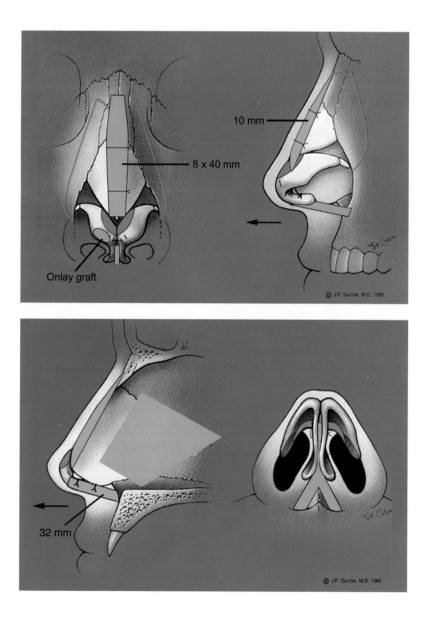

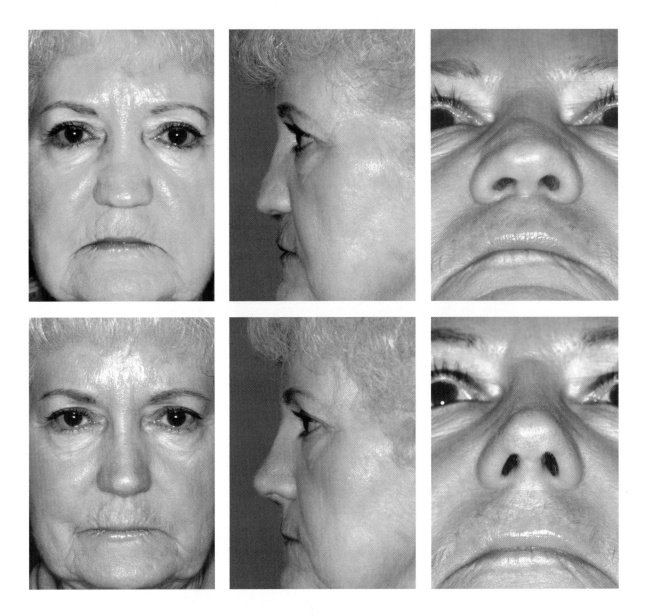

Fourteen months postoperatively the intercanthal distance appears to be less and the dorsum narrower due to placement of the dorsal onlay graft and the lateral osteotomies. The increased tip projection gained from advancing the medial crura on the columellar strut has resulted in a decrease of the alar base width, an oval appearance of the nostrils, increased columellar show, and a more obtuse columellar-labial angle. Trimming the lateral crura and reshaping the dome areas with sutures along with the onlay graft have resulted in a more sculpted, symmetric tip.

Correction of Severe Nasal Tip Deformity With Autologous Septal Cartilage

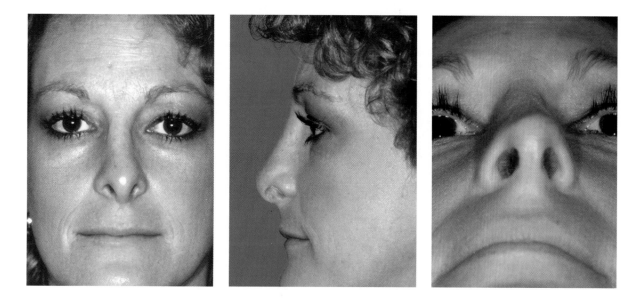

This 31-year-old woman had her nose broken at 13 years of age and had two nasal surgeries to correct the problem. The last surgery was performed 8 years previously. The patient stated she was still having problems breathing and did not like the appearance of her nose, especially the nostrils. On the frontal view the dorsum appeared "tubed," deviated to the right, and the upper lateral cartilage area narrowed. Increased infratip lobular show was the result of severely retracted alae and a hanging columella. A shallow nasofrontal angle was seen on the profile view with a slightly high bridge and inadequate infratip lobular projection. Marked increased columellar show was caused by the hanging columella and retracted alae. The basal view revealed asymmetry of the nostrils with a slightly widened distance between the tip-defining points, and the left dome appeared more projected than the right.

An open approach was used to expose the osseocartilaginous framework. Distorted, retracted lateral crura were observed intraoperatively, although most of the body of each crus remained intact. There was irregularity of the bony and cartilaginous dorsum as well as collapse of the upper lateral cartilages with persistent deviation of the septum.

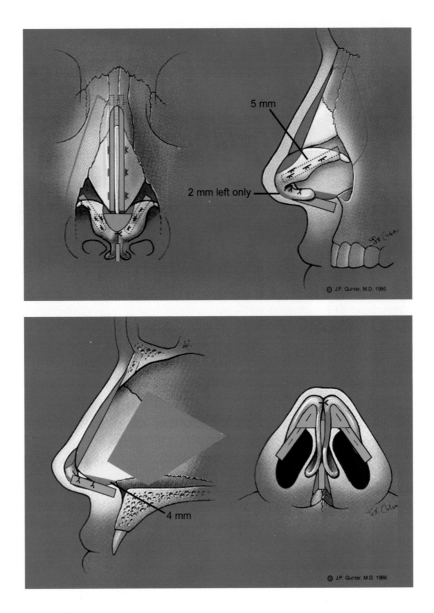

The dorsum was smoothed by rasping the nasal bones and trimming the dorsal septum. Four millimeters of the caudal septum was resected with the mucoperichondrium to raise the columella and recess the columellar-labial angle. The mucoperichondrium was elevated off the intact nasal septum. Leaving an 8 mm L-shaped septal cartilage strut, the rest of the septal cartilage and part of the perpendicular plate were harvested for grafting. This corrected the deviated septum. Dorsal spreader grafts were placed to correct the upper lateral cartilage collapse. A columella strut was placed in an undermined pocket between the medial crura. The crura were differentially advanced and sutured in place to achieve the same height for both domes and to stabilize the medial crura. Two millimeters of caudal margin was resected from the left medial crus to mirror the right crus. The lateral crura were trimmed to a 5 mm width, and double-layer grafts were sutured to the underneath surface in a pocket made by undermining the vestibular skin off the deep surface of the cartilage. The lateral crura were repositioned outward and downward with these grafts by suturing them to the distal end of the upper lateral cartilages. To increase infratip lobular projection, a triangular graft was wedged between the septal angle and the domes and sutured in place. Lateral osteotomies were performed to move the nasal bones to the midline.

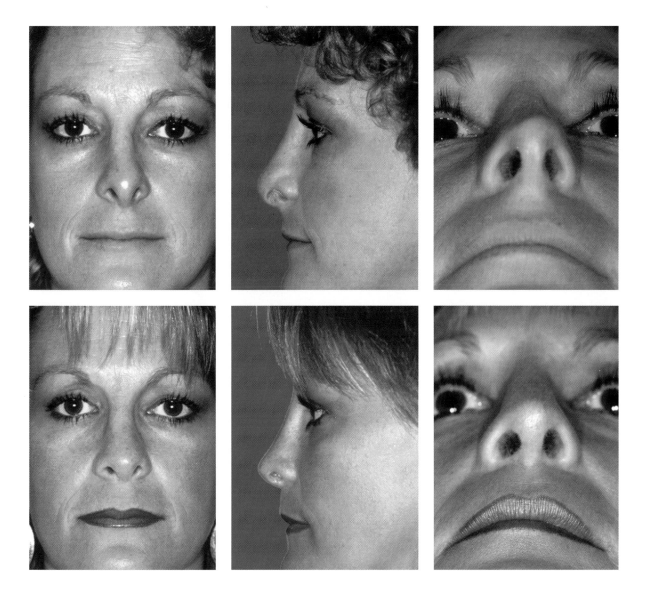

Seventeen months postoperatively the osteotomies and spreader grafts have straightened the nose and corrected the collapse of the upper lateral cartilages. There is less infratip lobular show after raising the columella, trimming the medial crura, and lowering the alar rims with the double-layer cartilage grafts wedged and sutured between the underneath surface of the lateral crura and the upper lateral cartilages. These grafts also widened the alar rims, creating a more aesthetic appearance. A straighter dorsum with a slight supratip break and an improved alar-columellar relationship are seen on the profile view. Advancement of the medial crura on the columellar strut equalized the height of the domes, as seen on the basal view.

DISCUSSION

The concept of using a transcolumellar incision for complete exposure of the nasal tip cartilages was initially described by Rethi in 1934.[26] Sercer (1958)[27] and Padovan (1966)[28] extended this concept to include exposure of the middle third and nasal dorsum. The technique was further developed and indications were broadened by Goodman and co-workers[29-32] and others.[33-37]

The major advantage of the external approach in the management of secondary nasal deformities lies in the complete, undistorted anatomic exposure of the nasal framework. This allows for a precise anatomic diagnosis and correction of the deformity with original tissues and/or supplemental cartilage grafts. The bony and cartilaginous structure can be continuously assessed intraoperatively. The final anatomic alignment and symmetry of the nasal framework become predictable.

Despite all the advantages of the external approach, it is not indicated for every secondary nasal deformity. Patients with a combination of displacement, underresection, and/or overresection of the nasal framework represent postoperative problems ideal for external rhinoplasty.

The major potential disadvantage of the external rhinoplasty technique is the transcolumellar scar. Using the stair-step incision over the middle columella with strict attention to operative technique in over 100 patients, we have had few patient complaints and have performed no revisions on the external rhinoplasty scar.

Major postoperative nasal deformities present a difficult challenge in that the patient is already dissatisfied with the previous rhinoplasty(ies) and has a distorted nasal framework with aesthetic and/or functional compromise. The complexity of secondary nasal deformities requires strict adherence to the basic principles as outlined, an understanding of the individual's aesthetic nasal analysis, and a predetermined goal-oriented treatment plan. Use of the external approach for major postoperative nasal deformities has produced more consistent aesthetic and functional results in the management of these multifaceted problems.

41

Endonasal Vs. External Approach in Secondary Rhinoplasty*

Rod J. Rohrich, M.D. • Jack H. Sheen, M.D.

*W*e are all aware of the potential consequences of primary rhinoplasty that resurface in the secondary rhinoplasty patient. A magnitude of problems can occur. Dorsal support may be lost, nasal bones can be broken and moved medially following bony arch removal, septal support may be compromised following septoplasty, soft tissues may not drape aesthetically over the new skeleton, airways can be compromised subsequent to mucosal trim or collapsed alar walls, and relationships of anatomic structures may be abnormal. The choice as to whether to proceed endonasally or through a transcolumellar incision depends on the surgeon's skill and experience with each technique and the complexity and seriousness of the secondary deformity. Rohrich is an enthusiastic advocate of the external approach; Sheen is equally committed to the endonasal approach. *However, both agree that in the severely scarred, tethered nose with diminished vascularity, the endonasal approach is always indicated.* Rohrich and Sheen describe the potential advantages and disadvantages of these two approaches.

*Reprinted from Grotting JC, ed. Reoperative Aesthetic and Reconstructive Plastic Surgery, vol 1. St. Louis: Quality Medical Publishing, 1995, pp 417-429.

External Approach

Rod J. Rohrich, M.D.

The 6 mm transcolumellar scar, which is minimal in most instances, is well worth the increased visualization the open approach affords. The access provided by this approach permits direct visualization of the deformity without distortion and allows correction of the deformity by suture repositioning as opposed to graft stabilization. With the external approach it is possible to execute techniques that in many cases are less accurate with the endonasal approach.

My review of over 200 cases in which an external approach via a stair-step transcolumellar incision was performed revealed only one instance in which an incision required revision due to a step-off as the result of a technical error during the initial closure at the lateral columellar rim. Furthermore, my experience with the external approach indicates that this technique does not prolong operative time and does not increase tip edema any more than some endonasal cartilage delivery techniques. Delayed healing and wound separation have not been problems in my experience with the external approach. However, it must be emphasized that the open approach is not merely an approach to explore and expose the nose; rather it is another technique in our armamentarium through which the operative principles of rhinoplasty are applied.

External Approach

Advantages
Provides binocular visualization
Permits complete evaluation of deformities without distortion
Allows precise diagnosis and correction of deformities
Allows bimanual use of hands
Provides a wide range of reconstructive options with original tissues and
  cartilage grafts
Allows direct control of bleeding with electrocautery
Permits suture stabilization of grafts
Allows optimal control in repositioning/suturing lower lateral cartilages and
  grafts

Disadvantages
Leaves transcolumellar scar
Prolongs operative time
May result in slightly protracted nasal tip edema
May cause columellar incision separation and delayed wound healing (rare)

If one violates the principles of rhinoplasty by failure to follow proper techniques, significant scarring, asymmetry, and even loss of nasal skin can result. The key to performing proper meticulous surgical technique is a knowledge of nasal anatomy and vasculature. Specifically, when one transects the columellar arterial branches to the nasal tip, the blood is now supplied from the lateral nasal vessels, which arise 2 mm above the alar groove and off the angular vessels bilaterally. One must stay close to the perichondrium of the lower lateral cartilages as one proceeds medial to lateral with both endonasal and external approaches to maintain the integrity of these vessels. If one is aggressive in undermining, dissects in the wrong plane, and transects these vessels concomitant with alar base resection and tension on closure of the nasal tip, disastrous consequences will result. These problems are related to improper technique and inadequate knowledge of nasal anatomy and can occur with both the external and endonasal approaches.

Furthermore, the improper placement of the incision either at the base or near the tip will guarantee a poor result. I must stress that an accurate preoperative anatomic diagnosis in the clinical aesthetic nasal analysis must be made before proceeding with the approach described.

OVERVIEW OF OPERATIVE TECHNIQUE

A logical, carefully executed surgical plan is essential in performing external rhinoplasty.

Surgical Plan
- Anesthesia
- Incisions
- Skin elevation (dissection of tip cartilages and dorsum)
- Intraoperative diagnosis
- Initial tip projection assessment/correction
- Septal and/or turbinate surgery and septal graft harvest (if indicated)
- Dorsal reduction/augmentation and lateral wall support (if indicated)
- Final tip projection/refinement/positioning
- External percutaneous osteotomies (if needed)
- Final inspection
- Wound closure
- Alar base/nasal site correction with composite grafts (if indicated)
- Splints and dressing

With the patient under general anesthesia, the external nose and septum are injected with 8 ml of 1% lidocaine (Xylocaine) with 1:200,000 epinephrine, and the nose is packed internally with ¼-inch cotton pledgets soaked with oxymetazoline hydrochloride (three pledgets per side).

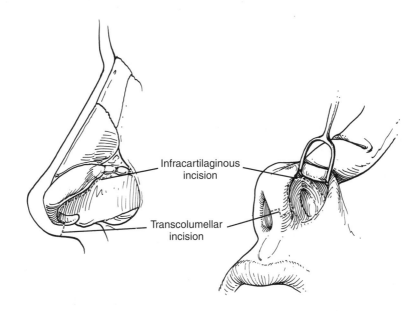

Bilateral infracartilaginous incisions are made along the caudal edges of the lower lateral cartilages. Medially the incision ends at the narrowest part of the columella and is connected with a stair-step transcolumellar incision. The stair-step incision is made in the midportion of the columella and allows for precise wound closure.

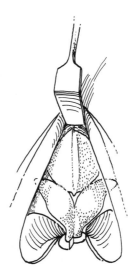

Skin elevation is begun by dissecting the columellar skin off the caudal edges of the medial crura superiorly to the middle crura. The dissection continues lateral to medial along an intracartilaginous incision, hugging the lower lateral cartilages and then exposing the domes at the nasal tip area. The dissection is continued along the upper lateral cartilages and onto the bony dorsum up to the radix. Retraction of the undermined area exposes the entire nasal framework. If tip projection must be altered, the new tip configuration will determine the height at which the final dorsal profile line is set. Any changes in the dorsum must be performed in concert with the final tip projection.

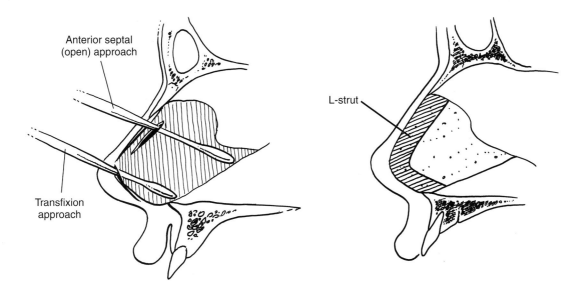

If septal cartilage grafts are required or if the septum needs correction for obstruction, the septum is approached from the septal angle or through a separate transfixion incision. The mucoperichondrial hemiflaps are elevated, and the appropriate septal modification and/or septal cartilage harvest is performed. One must leave at least an 8 mm dorsal and caudal L-strut.

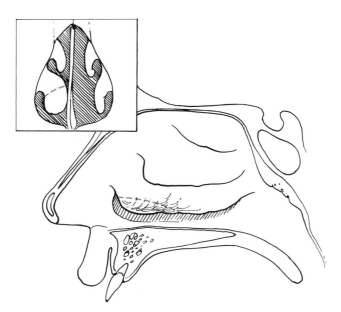

If the caudal septum is deviated, the medial crura are separated to gain better exposure and to correct the caudal septal deviation. The medial crural support is reestablished once the medial crura are sutured back together after the septal correction is completed. If indicated, partial resection of hypertrophied anterior/inferior turbinates is performed at this time. If donor material is needed (rib or ear), these grafts are harvested after the nasal framework has been exposed and the deformities and deficiencies have been confirmed.

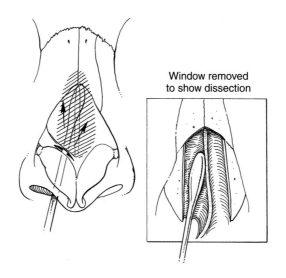

Next the cartilaginous-bony dorsum is evaluated, and any needed dorsal reduction/augmentation is performed. The bony dorsum is usually reduced obliquely with a sharp, down-biting rasp, and the height of the cartilaginous dorsum is lowered incrementally with a No. 15 Bard-Parker blade. The mucosa at the junction of the septum and the lateral cartilages is freed from the cartilages to form submucosal tunnels bilaterally so that the septum can be separated from the upper lateral cartilages without transecting the mucosa.

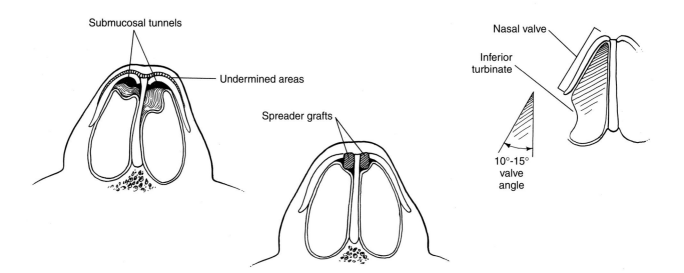

Maintaining the integrity of the mucosa helps to stabilize the septum. The intact mucosa also forms a trough so that spreader grafts can be placed to move the upper lateral cartilages laterally in the event of the collapse of the upper lateral cartilages and/or the pinching of the internal nasal valves. The goal is to preserve or reconstitute the internal nasal valves at an angle of 10 to 15 degrees.

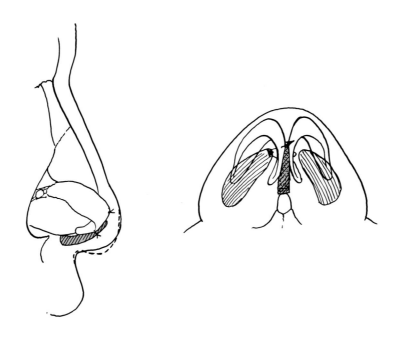

Attention is then directed to final tip cartilage modifications. If increased tip projection and/or refinement is desired, it is usually initiated with the placement of an autologous cartilage strut in a pocket extending from between the feet of the medial crura, which unifies the lower lateral cartilages. The strut is placed and medial crura arc advanced on the strut until the desired tip projection is achieved. The medial crura are secured to the strut with 5-0 PDS sutures.

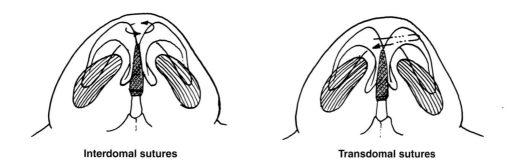

Interdomal sutures   **Transdomal sutures**

Further increase in tip projection and refinement is obtained with interdomal and/or transdomal sutures. These maneuvers will increase tip projection 2 to 3 mm. If more tip projection is needed, the unified tip complex can be hinged off the anterior septal angle.

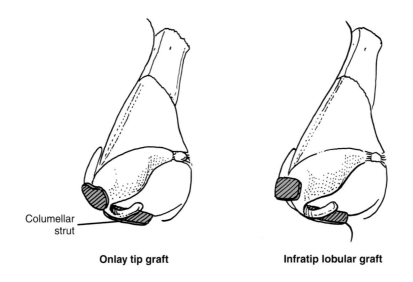

Onlay tip graft   **Infratip lobular graft**

Columellar
strut

Once satisfactory tip projection has been attained, any needed dorsal augmentation is performed. Our graft preference is septum, if available. In most instances dorsal onlay grafts are stabilized with 5-0 PDS sutures at the osseocartilaginous junction and near the anterior septal angle. Final positioning of the tip cartilages is accomplished with suture stabilization. If indicated, onlay tip grafts are placed and secured. A Peck graft placed on the domal area increases tip projection, whereas an infratip lobular graft described by Sheen is more versatile by increasing definition and projection and giving the illusion of increased nasal length.

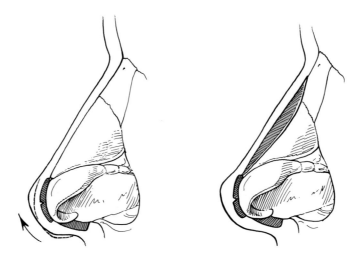

A combination tip/infratip graft provides further versatility by increasing tip projection, definition, and refinement. If further dorsal augmentation is indicated, a dorsal onlay graft is contoured and secured in place.

The skin is redraped after final inspection of the nasal framework. The infra-cartilaginous incisions are closed with interrupted 5-0 chromic catgut sutures, and the transcolumellar incision is meticulously closed with interrupted 6-0 nylon sutures. If septal surgery has been performed, bilateral septal splints are placed and sutured in place with through-and-through 3-0 nylon sutures. Alar base or nostril site correction and/or composite graft placement are performed next. Nasal packing is avoided if hemostasis is adequate. An external dressing of ½-inch Steri-Strips from the radix to supratip area and a metal splint (Denver) to mold the lateral walls are applied on the nose and worn for 1 week.

Endonasal Approach

Jack H. Sheen, M.D.

Any surgical approach is technique dependent. With regard to secondary rhinoplasty it is my belief that in comparison to the external approach, the endonasal approach, in general, is more forgiving, less traumatic, and less time consuming and produces a better result because the dissection is limited to the area of correction. The endonasal approach has served me well during my 30-year fascination with secondary rhinoplasty. I have never believed that the exposure provided by the external approach was of sufficient benefit to offset its disadvantages. I simply do not agree with the advocates of the open approach who argue that only a few exceptional surgeons can truly master the endonasal approach. With some effort and practice most rhinoplasty surgeons can become proficient using the closed technique with obvious benefit to the patient. The trend today is toward limiting incisions; minimally invasive surgery has revolutionized the practice of general surgery and is beginning to have a similar impact on aesthetic and reconstructive surgery. It makes little sense to embrace a surgical approach that creates an external incision in an aesthetic procedure when it is possible to perform the same operation successfully with no visible scars. Proponents of the open approach maintain that an invisible scar that crosses the columella is the only residual effect. However, I have witnessed complications far more serious—everything from severely notched columellar scars to sloughs of the base of the nose. The novice is well advised to take heed of these complications.

Other attributes of the external approach have been highly overrated, and the merits of the endonasal approach have been too often overlooked. The endonasal technique offers limited dissection and preservation of vascularity, whereas all too often the sequela of the open technique is decreased vascularity subsequent to wide skeletonization. The endonasal approach eliminates

---

Endonasal Approach

Advantages

Leaves no external scar

Limits dissection to areas needing modification

Permits creation of precise pocket so graft material fits exactly without need for fixation

Allows percutaneous fixation when large pockets are made

Promotes healing by maintaining vascular bridges

Encourages accurate preoperative diagnosis and planning

Produces minimal postsurgical edema

Reduces operating time

Results in fast patient recovery

Creates intact tip graft pocket

Allows composite grafting to alar rims

Disadvantages

Requires experience and great reliance on accurate preoperative diagnosis

Prohibits simultaneous visualization of surgical field by teaching surgeon and students

Does not allow direct visualization of nasal anatomy

Makes dissection of alar cartilages difficult, particularly in cases of malposition

---

the need for graft fixation by creating a pocket just large enough to accept the graft. If the pocket is oversized, a transcutaneous suture is a simple remedy. In addition, a closed pocket supports tip grafts. Stabilization can be achieved as simply endonasally as with the open technique because graft stabilization is more dependent on bed preparation than on suture fixation. Diagnosis of a problem does not depend on surgical exposure. Contour is an external manifestation of the underlying skeleton. If alar cartilages are deficient, the notch or collapse is visible externally. The same is true of the middle vault where the position, size, and condition of the upper lateral cartilages and their relationship to the caudal bony arch are visible through the skin as is the dorsal edge of the septum. With very short nasal bones an inverted V is prominent; the position of the fractured bony arch and the relationship of the two sides to each other are readily assessed on a frontal view of the nose. The condition and presence of septal cartilage, need for turbinate reduction, and presence of internasal synechiae or stenosis can be determined with a good headlight, speculum, and cotton swab. The idea that anatomy is somehow distorted using the endonasal technique is also inaccurate. The middle vault, bony arch, and root can be effectively visualized through a single intracartilaginous incision using an Aufricht retractor and a headlight.

I find it puzzling that proponents of the external approach cite the use of two hands as a benefit of the open technique. It is hard to imagine operating open or closed without the use of two hands. The nondominant hand, specifically the index and middle fingers, is essential for determining the position and depth of the dissecting instrument.

The value of the open technique as a teaching tool is questionable. The anatomy laboratory is a more appropriate setting for learning anatomy and technique than the operating room.

OVERVIEW OF OPERATIVE TECHNIQUE

Careful planning is key to secondary rhinoplasty using the endonasal approach.

Surgical Plan
- Anesthesia
- Incisions
- Pocket dissection and bed preparation (dorsal alignment)
- Intranasal surgery (functional correction if necessary including treatment of turbinate and bony problems)
- Dorsal augmentation
- Lateral wall support/augmentation or reduction
- Tip exposure and preliminary positioning
- Alar wedges, composite grafts, etc. with complete closure of all wounds
- Final tip graft placement and closure
- Packs, splints, and dressing

My anesthesiologist uses propofol (Diprivan) to induce general anesthesia and maintains the level of anesthesia with desflurane (Suprane). Neither a narcotic nor amnestic is used preoperatively. For local anesthesia I have found that 0.75% bupivacaine hydrochloride (Marcaine) with 1:100,000 epinephrine produces a longer lasting effect than lidocaine, decreasing the need for pain medication in the immediate postoperative period. Although some believe there is little difference, I believe the high concentration of epinephrine has a superior hemostatic effect. In my experience the low concentration is associated with more intraoperative bleeding. In my first 15 years of practice I used only local anesthetics because the effect of early anesthetics (before the introduction of enflurane) was an increase in operative bleeding. During that time I used lidocaine with 1:50,000 epinephrine and the field was definitely less bloody than it is today using 1:100,000 epinephrine.

The exact areas to be augmented or reduced are marked before the tissues are injected. These marks are excellent guides when the pocket is being formed.

Accurate anatomic diagnosis is essential since separate incisions must be made for each deformity. For instance, if the dorsum is deficient and there is a collapsed ala on the left side as well, the opening incision will begin at the left nostril rim, penetrate the lateral wall to the dorsum, and then extend to the root. This one incision not only elevates a good pocket for augmenting the deficient dorsum but also allows for the placement of a support graft along the rim.

The guiding principle is to limit the dissection. Incisions and dissections are customized. If alar wedges are planned, the dorsal incision is made approximately 1.5 cm cephalad to the rim. An alar rim pocket is then formed through the opened alar lobule. A narrow pocket can be fashioned to support a collapsed ala or a broad pocket may be created to elevate a deepened alar groove. The pocket thus can be designed to precisely fit the deformity. The support graft may be inserted through the open alar incision with confidence since the pocket is closed. If lateral wall augmentation on the opposite side is needed, a very short (1 to 1.5 cm) incision on the opposite side at the intercartilaginous area is made, and dissection is limited to the area to be augmented. This allows for precise placement of a suitable graft.

The graft material—whether septal cartilage and bone, ear cartilage, cranial bone, or rib—is usually harvested after the initial incisions and dissections have been made. A separate setup is used for each donor site, and instruments and gloves are changed after the material has been obtained. The choice of graft material is made before surgery. Occasionally the harvest of poor-quality material from a primary site will force the use of a secondary donor area.

I perform tip graft placement last because the tip is the nasal structure that is the most sensitive to manipulation, and by establishing the dorsal height first, I can determine tip position and contour in relation to the new position of the dorsum. Although I may prepare the tip graft pocket before complete closure of all the wounds, the tip graft is placed last to avoid graft displacement. The one exception to this rule is alar wedges. Nostril size and shape are dependent on the anterior position of the tip lobule, and so a preliminary tip graft is placed to better judge the size and placement of the alar resection.

To prepare for a tip graft, the tip lobule is approached through an incision along the border of the middle crus beginning at the columellar-lobular junction and extending approximately 1 cm anteriorly. It is here the closed pocket can be most useful in obtaining anterior projection. With a closed pocket the graft is fixed at the posterior limit of the pocket and the tissue of the tip has to be forced anteriorly. After dissection of the tip graft pocket is completed, tip grafts are inserted, extending the tip lobule into its anterior position. The quality, size, and character of the graft material determine the contour and position of the tip lobule. The alar wedges are completed, and then the definitive tip grafts are placed. Surface definition is obtained as the grafts are inserted. The grafts are placed only after all of the incisions have been closed and no further manipulation is anticipated. Tip grafts must always be rinsed in saline solution before dipping into an antibiotic solution (lincomycin hydrochloride [Lincocin]), and they must not be touched with the gloved hand before insertion. The most common problem after tip grafting is infection, a complication that is completely related to technique and is thus preventable.

After all of the incisions have been closed, intranasal packs are placed over a No. 14 catheter if septal surgery has been performed. The use of splints sutured across the septal partition is appealing and feasible if the dissection is limited and the mucoperichondrial flaps are intact on both sides. The nostrils limit the size of the splints. In my experience most septoplasties involve some bony resection and extend quite far posteriorly, which precludes the usual intranasal splint. For that reason I believe that total packing will guard against postoperative bleeding. I leave the packing in place for 1 week.

The first strip of ½-inch paper tape is placed on the nose with a notch that fits over the lobule and onto the lateral nasal walls to support the lobule. The second strip is taped just cephalad to the tip and perpendicular to the first piece to secure the grafts. Subsequent strips of tape extend to the root. Final adjustments are made during taping to ensure proper position of the dorsal graft. Fast-setting plaster (two layers) is placed over the dorsum, folding the distal edge over 4 to 8 mm to make the distal part more substantial. This plaster is molded into the tape for good fixation, and two more strips of tape fix its position and complete the dressing. A small 2 × 2 gauze pad is then placed under the nose and held in position with a strip of ½-inch paper tape (mustache dressing).

42

Correction of the Pinched Nasal Tip With Alar Spreader Grafts*

Jack P. Gunter, M.D. • Rod J. Rohrich, M.D. • Fred L. Hackney, M.D., D.D.S.

*T*he pinched nasal tip deformity is secondary to collapse of the alar rims subsequent to loss of lateral crural support from either congenital or acquired causes. A pinched nasal tip detracts from nasal aesthetics and, if severe, impedes nasal airflow during inspiration.[1] To correct the aesthetic and functional deformity of a pinched nasal tip, we developed a technique that consists of grafts of autologous septal or auricular cartilage placed in such a manner that they spread the collapsed lateral crura and buttress them from beneath.

ALAR RIM ANATOMY AND AESTHETICS

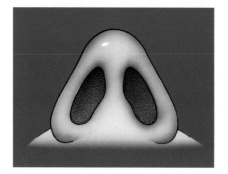

Viewed from below, the ideal nasal base resembles an equilateral triangle with an outward bowing of the posterior alar rims and a rounding of the nasal tip. Although the resilience of the alar rims is influenced by the thickness of the skin and the action of the nasal dilator muscles, ultimately it is the strength and position of the lateral crura of the lower lateral cartilages that determine the condition of the alae.[2,3]

*Adapted from Gunter JP, Rohrich RJ. Correction of the pinched nasal tip with alar spreader grafts. Plast Reconstr Surg 90:821, 1992.

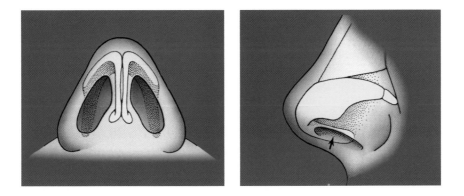

The caudal margin of the lateral crus runs posteriorly from the dome area parallel to the alar rim up to one half its length before it curves cephalad.[2,4] When the lateral crus is weak, the anterior and midportion of the rim may collapse since these areas are directly supported by the lateral crus, whereas posteriorly the rim has no cartilage support but is held in position by the thick alar skin.[3,5,6]

A weak lateral crus may result in rim collapse.

OPERATIVE TECHNIQUE

The external approach is used exclusively for this technique. The medial ends of bilateral marginal incisions are connected by a staggered transcolumellar incision at the narrowest portion of the columella, and the skin is undermined and retracted off the osseocartilaginous framework of the nose. The cause of the external deformity can then be visualized.[7]

If one crus is missing or cannot be used for reconstruction, we prefer to replace the crus with a piece of auricular cartilage carved to the shape and contour of a normal crus. An extension is maintained on the medial end of the graft and sutured to the remaining intact anterior end of the medial crus. The graft is then bent at the area of the dome and suture stabilized at the desired angle with a horizontal mattress suture. If reconstruction of both crura is required, the above procedure can be performed bilaterally or an "anchor graft" of autologous cartilage, as described by Juri et al.,[10] can be used.

In patients in whom the lateral crura have been completely resected or are so distorted they cannot be used for reconstruction, the crura must be reconstructed.

When strips of lateral crura 2 mm or more in width are still present bilaterally, an alar spreader cartilage graft is used to bridge the space between them and to push these remnants laterally to correct the collapse. Septal cartilage is our first choice of graft material because it is in the same surgical area,[8] but the concha can be used if septal cartilage is not available.

In patients with 2 mm or more lateral crural width, an autologous cartilage graft is used to spread the remaining strips of lateral crura laterally.

The shape of the graft depends on the severity of the collapse and other factors related to the tip. The exact dimensions of the graft also vary from patient to patient, keeping in mind that the graft is to extend horizontally across the tip to push out the existing concavities in the crura.

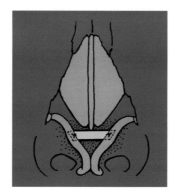

A single bar graft is usually sufficient for correction of bilateral collapse in the midportion of the crura. To prepare the recipient sites to accept the ends of the graft, bilateral pockets are undermined between the areas of greatest collapse of the cartilage and the vestibular skin. Undermining begins at the cephalic margin of each crus and stops just short of the caudal margin. A 1½-inch 25-gauge needle is passed across the septal angle through the collapsed segments of the crura. The skewered crura are pushed laterally on the needle until they begin to bow outward. The distance between the cartilage is then measured along the needle, and the cartilage graft is carved to the same length. The graft ends are inserted in the pockets deep to the collapsed crura and are sutured to the crura with horizontal sutures of 5-0 Vicryl, taking care not to penetrate the vestibular skin.

The skin is redraped over the nasal tip to assess the effect. If the graft is too long, the tip will be too broad and the nostrils will flare, in which case the graft must be removed and trimmed until the desired length is reached. If the graft is too short, the tip will still look somewhat pinched, and a longer graft is indicated. In all cases the goal of grafting is to separate the lateral crura so that the alar collapse is corrected but not so much as to cause nostril flare.

If the graft is too long, the tip will be too broad and the nostrils will flare.

If the distance between the alar rims appears to be correct but the tip is leaning to one side, the tip can be restored to the midline by shifting the graft so that the length of the graft is shorter on the side to which the tip is leaning. This asymmetric placement of the alar spreader graft is anchored to the septal angle with 5-0 Vicryl suture. Unilateral alar rim collapse is corrected with an alar spreader graft that pushes the collapsed lateral crus outward and is suture stabilized to the septal angle to prevent the collapsed crus from returning to its original position and displacing the normal crus.

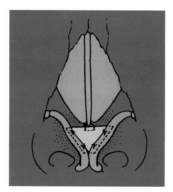

When additional support is needed for better tip definition or to increase projection of the tip, a triangular graft is used. In such cases the graft pockets are undermined from the collapsed portions of the crura caudally to the domes so that the remaining strips of alar cartilage overlap the lateral edges of the triangular graft. The graft should be carved so that the base is wide enough to push the collapsed crural strips outward into their desired positions. The apex of the graft extends to the undersurface of the domes. The lateral crura strips are sutured to the lateral edges of the graft just short of the dome areas. This aids in stabilizing the domes for suture positioning and shaping.

To accentuate the tip-defining points, the angulation at the domes is increased by passing a horizontal mattress suture of 5-0 clear nylon through the medial and lateral surface of each dome so that the knot is tied on the medial surface and tightened until the desired angulation is achieved. To decrease the distance between the tip-defining points, one end of each knot is tied and tightened until the desired distance is reached.

If tip projection is short of ideal, the length of the triangular graft is increased to elongate the lateral edges of the graft. The rim strips are advanced on the edges and sutured to increase the projection. The domes are then shaped with sutures.

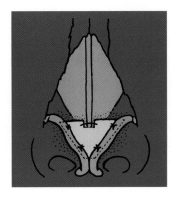

If the problem is collapse of the posterior alar rim, the triangular alar spreader graft can be designed with posterolateral extensions sufficiently wide to push the caved-in posterior alar rims outward.

If an alar retraction component is present in addition to alar rim collapse, a triangular graft slightly wider than needed is sutured to the collapsed rim strips and a partial-thickness incision made along the midline. The halves are squeezed to create a hinged fracture along the incision line to force the caudal edges of the graft inferomedially. The angular prominence of the hinge at the base of the graft is excised with a No. 15 blade. The base is sutured to the septal angle with a horizontal mattress suture of 5-0 Vicryl to ensure that the graft remains bent, pushing the alar rims downward.

An additional benefit of alar spreader grafts is that they can sometimes assist in correcting collapsed internal valves. This occurs when the scar tissue between the resected cephalic margin of the lateral crura and the caudal end of the upper lateral cartilages created by previous surgery is left intact.

Alar spreader grafts may help correct collapsed internal nasal valves.

Placement of the graft displaces the lateral crura outward and simultaneously pulls the caudal end of the upper lateral cartilages laterally by virtue of the scar-tissue attachment. The lateral movement of the upper lateral cartilages increases the opening of the internal valves.

CASE ANALYSES
Pinched Nasal Tip Following Primary Rhinoplasty

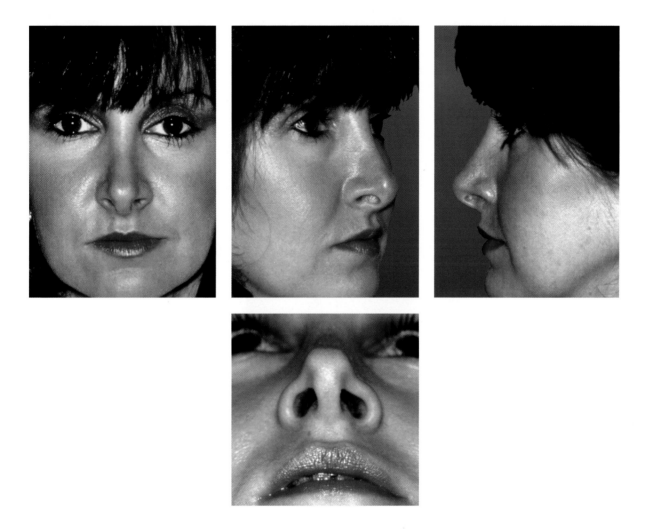

This 32-year-old woman had a rhinoplasty 8 years before and was dissatisfied with the aesthetic result. She also complained of mild difficulty breathing through her nose. On the frontal view the midportion of the nasal dorsum was seen to be narrowed, the tip pinched, and the infratip lobular height increased. The lateral view revealed increased columellar show and increased infratip lobular height. The oblique view confirmed the frontal and lateral findings. The basal view showed bilateral collapse of the anterior alae with a clover-leaf appearance and increased distance between the tip-defining points.

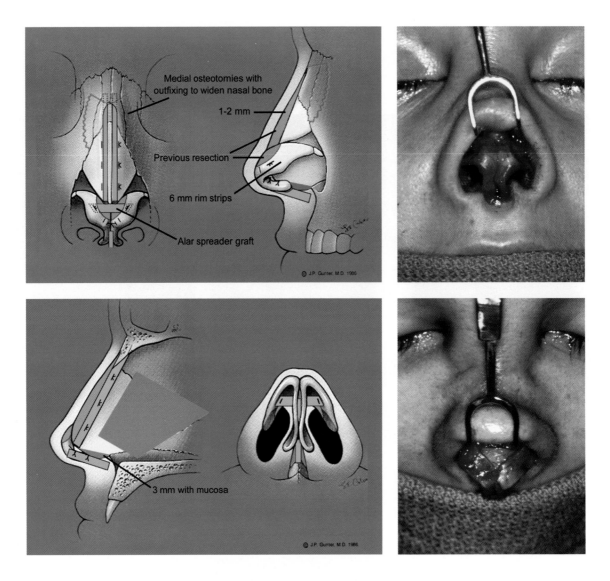

Bilateral marginal incisions were connected by a transcolumellar incision, and the skin was undermined off the tip cartilages and dorsum under loupe magnification. The skin was reflected backward off the nose, and the remaining lateral crural strips were seen to be collapsed bilaterally. The dorsum had been overresected, and there was bilateral collapse of the upper lateral cartilages. Cartilage was harvested from the remaining septum, and dorsal spreader grafts were placed between the dorsal edges of the upper lateral cartilages and the dorsal septum to reconstruct the dorsum. A bar graft was used to spread the alae and correct the alar collapse. It was sutured to the undersurface of the remaining strips of lateral crura. The tip-defining points were accentuated with horizontal mattress sutures of 5-0 nylon passed subcutaneously to the vestibular skin through the medial and lateral walls of the domes and tied on the medial surface of each dome. The ends of one of the sutures on each side were then tied together and tightened to decrease the distance between the tip-defining points. A 3 mm strip of caudal septum with mucosa was resected to raise the columella and decrease the infratip lobular show.

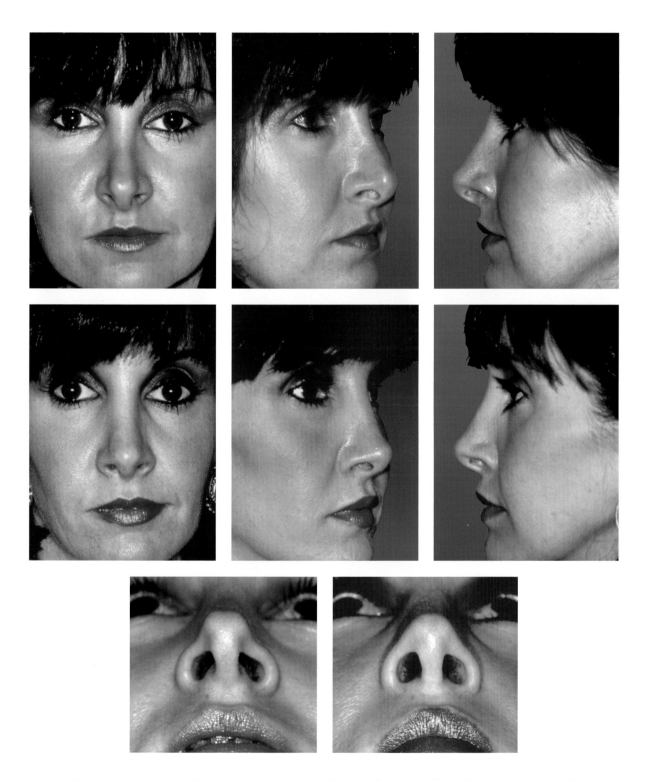

Twenty-three months postoperatively the tip looks fuller, there is a smooth gradient down to the alar base, and the infratip lobular height is decreased. The lateral and oblique views show correction of the increased columellar show and the increased infratip lobular height. On the basal view the nose presents a more aesthetic triangular outline with minimal scarring from the transcolumellar incision. The patient has no difficulty breathing through her nose.

Congenital Asymmetric Pinched Nasal Tip

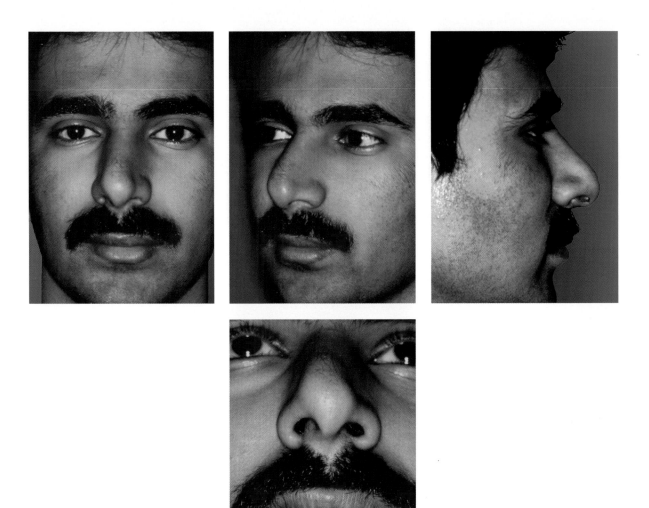

This 24-year-old man complained that his nose had been crooked for as long as he could remember but denied breathing difficulties. There was a history of possible trauma as a young child. On the frontal view the nasal dorsum and tip appeared deviated to the right with collapse of the left upper lateral cartilage. The nasal tip was asymmetric with obvious collapse of the left alar rim and increased distance between the tip-defining points. The infratip lobular show was slightly exaggerated. The lateral view revealed weak projection of the tip and a supratip fullness. The oblique view substantiated the frontal and lateral findings. On the basal view the caudal septal deviation into the right nostril and collapse of the left upper lateral cartilage were clearly seen, and the left alar rim was obviously concave. The increased distance between the tip-defining points was also verified.

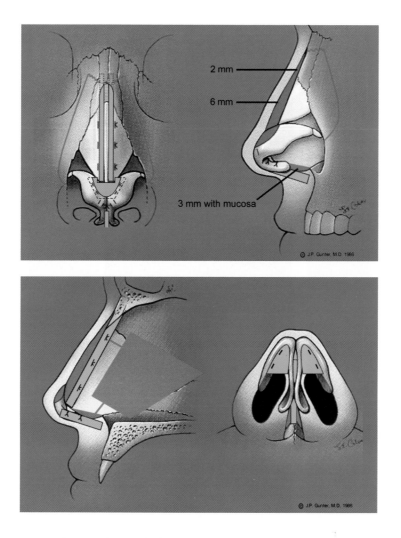

An open approach confirmed the preoperative diagnosis. The nasal hump was removed. A septoplasty and lateral osteotomies corrected the dorsal deviation and placed the caudal septum back in the midline. Dorsal spreader grafts were secured between the dorsal septum and the edge of each upper lateral cartilage to correct the collapsed cartilage on the left and prevent collapse on the right. The cephalic margins of the lateral crura were trimmed, leaving 6 mm rim strips bilaterally. Bilateral pockets were fashioned by undermining between the vestibular skin and the undersurface of the crural strips. The lateral edges of a triangular graft of septal cartilages were inserted into the pockets. The crural strips were advanced on the lateral edges of the graft and sutured to it. The advancement moved the tip-defining points downward and anteriorly to decrease infratip lobular show and enhance tip projection. The base of the graft was positioned in the midline and sutured to the septal angle. The tip-defining points were accentuated with horizontal mattress sutures tied on the medial surfaces. They were moved closer together by tying one end of each suture together and tightening the knot until they were the desired distance apart. A 2 mm strip of caudal septum with mucosa was resected to raise the columella slightly and further reduce infratip lobular show.

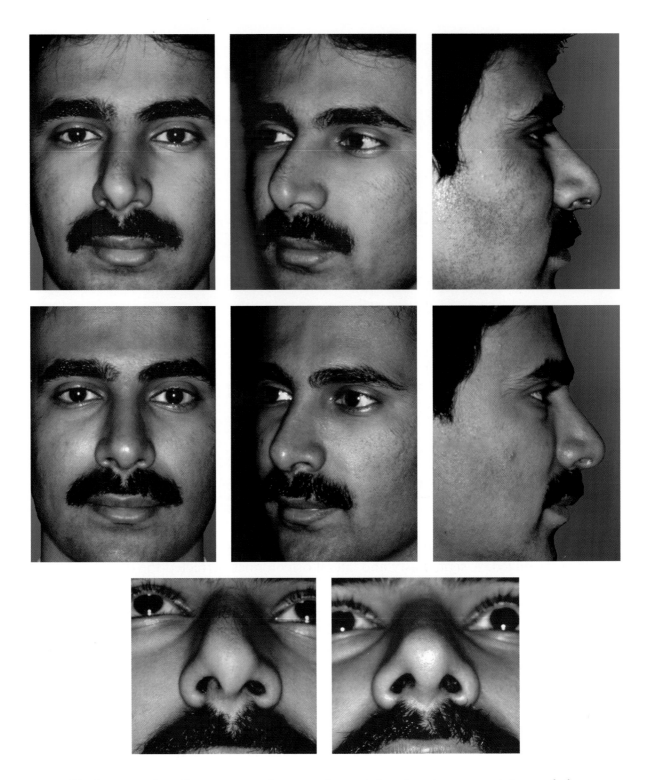

Twelve months after surgery the nose is straight, the tip symmetric, and the excessive infratip lobular show corrected. The lateral and oblique views show better tip projection and correction of the supratip fullness. On the basal view the nostrils are symmetric and the tip has better definition with a decreased distance between the tip-defining points. The left alar rim is no longer concave and the columella does not slant.

DISCUSSION

Alar rim collapse can be congenital or traumatic but most often results from excessive resection of the lateral crus of the lower lateral cartilage during cosmetic rhinoplasty. Inadequately supported by cartilage, the nostril rim caves in under the weight of the skin, and this collapse is often exacerbated by the negative pressure in the nasal vestibule on inspiration. When the collapse is bilateral, the nasal tip looks pinched and on the basal view has a clover-leaf shape. In severe cases the collapsed rims limit the volume of air that can flow through the nose.[1,5,6,9]

Numerous authors have attempted to deal with the problem of alar rim collapse in various ingenious ways. Juri et al.[10] proposed three types of anchor grafts from the concha of the ear that are sutured to the remaining medial crural elements. The wings of the anchor are fashioned to extend into the alar walls to support them. Chait and Fayman[11] used tip grafts of costal cartilage molded like a boomerang to replace the medial and lateral crura on one side. The graft is inserted in such a way that the natural spring of the cartilage pushes the alar rim outward, opening the nostril, and the vertical strut of the graft is affixed to the medial crus on the opposite side. The authors recommend this technique in cases of postreconstructive deformity when the bulky flap used for the reconstruction obstructs the airway. Nicolle[12] suggests a comma-shaped tip graft sculpted from septal cartilage to substitute for the missing spring and arch of a tip cartilage. The narrow medial end of the graft overlies the dome area, and the wider base overlies the remnant of the lateral crus. The graft is placed in a small pocket so that it fits snugly and expands the overlying skin. Kamer and McQuown[13] described miniature composite grafts of skin and cartilage from the ear to correct alar retraction/pinching. The miniature composite grafts are harvested from just below the inferior crus of the anthelix and are sutured into a vestibular defect created by releasing the scarified vestibular skin and lateral crus that caused the retraction/pinching deformity.

We have also tried to correct alar rim collapse using strips of septal cartilage running in the direction of and lateral to the remaining lateral crura. The strips were placed so that they overlapped the rim of the piriform aperture posteriorly and the anterior crural remnant at the dome area. We experienced two problems with this method. Often there was not enough septal cartilage available to make the grafts as long and wide as needed, and sometimes the grafts failed to push out the alar rims sufficiently.

Since 1983 we have used grafts of autologous cartilage to correct nasal tip deformities secondary to collapsed lateral crura with remaining crural strips of 2 mm width or greater. These alar spreader grafts are in the shape of a bar or triangle and are placed deep to the collapsed lateral crura to force them apart and prop them up into their correct position.

The most difficult part of this technique to master was accurately predicting the width of the graft that was needed for correction of both the functional and aesthetic deformity before it was carved. The wider the graft, the more likely it was to improve function, but at a certain point it began to detract from the aesthetic appearance. To suture the graft in place, we redraped the skin, and if we found that it did not give the desired correction, we had to remove the graft, modify it, and suture it back in place, which not only was time consuming but sometimes damaged the graft. The problem was solved by passing a needle through the collapsed segments of the crura and sliding the cartilages on the needle until they became slightly convex. The length of the needle between the cartilages is the distance the graft must span, and it is carved accordingly.

The only other problems associated with the alar spreader graft technique have been inadequate correction and/or tip asymmetry postoperatively. These were attributed to the surgeon's inability to carve the graft to the proper dimensions or to stabilize it adequately. There have been no infections or graft losses, and we have not been able to detect any absorption of the grafts after 8 years.

■ KEY POINTS

- ■ Alar rim collapse can be congenital or traumatic but most often results from excessive resection of the lateral crus of the lower lateral cartilage during cosmetic rhinoplasty.

- ■ The alar spreader graft technique offers versatility and durability of results in correcting the pinched nasal tip deformity secondary to collapsed lateral crura.

- ■ Functionally, alar spreader grafts strengthen the vestibular walls and improve nasal respiration by correcting severely collapsed alar rims and by increasing the opening of the internal nasal valves in certain situations.

- ■ Aesthetically, alar spreader grafts improve the contour of the alar rim and nasal tip with autologous semirigid tissues that give long-lasting results.

REFERENCES

1. Cottle MH. Structure and function of the nasal vestibule. Arch Otolaryngol 62:173, 1955.
2. Gunter JP. Anatomical observations of the lower lateral cartilages. Arch Otolaryngol 89:599, 1969.
3. Griesman B. Muscles and cartilages of the nose from the standpoint of a typical rhinoplasty. Arch Otolaryngol 39:334, 1944.
4. Sheen JH, Sheen AP. Aesthetic Rhinoplasty, 2nd ed. St Louis: Quality Medical Publishing, 1998 (reprint of 1987 ed.).
5. DesPrez JD, Kiehn CL. Valvular obstruction of the nasal airway. Plast Reconstr Surg 56:307, 1975.
6. Haight JS, Cole P. The site and function of the nasal valve. Laryngoscope 93:49, 1983.
7. Gunter JP, Rohrich RJ. External approach for secondary rhinoplasty. Plast Reconstr Surg 80: 161, 1987.
8. Gunter JP, Rohrich RJ. Augmentation rhinoplasty: Dorsal onlay grafting using shaped autogenous septal cartilage. Plast Reconstr Surg 86:39, 1990.
9. Courtiss EH, Gargan TJ, Courtiss GB. Nasal physiology. Ann Plast Surg 13:214, 1984.
10. Juri J, Juri C, Grilli DA, Zeaiter MC, Vazquez GD. Correction of the secondary nasal tip and of alar and/or columellar collapse. Plast Reconstr Surg 82:160, 1988.
11. Chait LA, Fayman MS. Treatment of postreconstructive collapsed nasal ala with a costal cartilage graft. Plast Reconstr Surg 82:527, 1988.
12. Nicolle FV. The comma-shaped tip cartilage graft. Aesthetic Plast Surg 12:223, 1988.
13. Kamer FM, McQuown SA. Minicomposite graft for nasal alar revision. Arch Otolaryngol Head Neck Surg 113:943, 1987.

PART SEVEN

Traumatic Deformities and the Deviated Septum

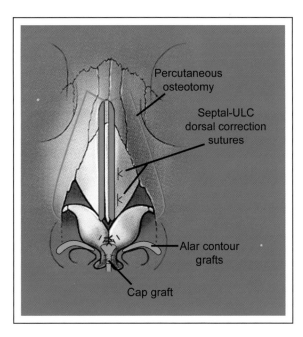

Percutaneous osteotomy

Septal-ULC dorsal correction sutures

Alar contour grafts

Cap graft

43

Acute Nasal Fracture Management: Minimizing Secondary Nasal Deformities*

Rod J. Rohrich, M.D. · William P. Adams, Jr., M.D.

*L*ess force is required to induce nasal pyramid fractures than any other facial bone; considering this as well as the prominence of the nose it is not surprising that nasal fractures are the most commonly seen facial fractures.[1-5] The increasing prevalence of this injury presents challenging treatment options. Nasal fractures are often discussed as minor injuries[6]; however, the incidence of posttraumatic nasal deformity remains alarmingly high (14% to 50%). Since revision rhinoplasty for traumatic nasal deformity can be difficult, guidelines are needed to optimize the management of acute nasal fracture.

Nasal fractures are the most common facial fracture.

Numerous factors contribute to a suboptimal functional and aesthetic result, including timing, edema, undetected preexisting nasal deformity, and occult septal deviation/injury; therefore we have devised a clinical algorithm for acute nasal fracture management that includes a complete evaluation of the nasal deformity (internal and external) and precise anatomic reduction under controlled conditions to improve long-term results and reduce posttraumatic nasal deformities.

Since Malianc[7] published his classic book on management of acute nasal injuries in 1947, there has been considerable debate regarding optimal care of acute nasal fractures. Discrepancies in timing, method, and postoperative management are common in the literature.[1-3,8-10]

---

*Excerpted in part from Rohrich RJ, Adams WP Jr. Nasal fracture management: Minimizing secondary nasal deformities. Plast Reconstr Surg 106:266, 2000.

Table 43-1. Incidence of Secondary Nasal Deformity After Acute Closed Nasal Fracture Reduction

Author	% Secondary Nasal Deformity (No. of Cases)
Watson et al.[16]	29%-50% (29)
Cook et al.[14]	14%-17% (45)
Murray et al.[15]	41% (756)
Waldron et al.[12]	14%-15% (100)
Rohrich and Adams	9% (110)

INCIDENCE OF POSTTRAUMATIC NASAL DEFORMITY

The incidence of postreduction nasal deformities (excluding this study) requiring subsequent rhinoplasty or septorhinoplasty ranges from 14% to 50%,[9,11,12] and several authors report poor results with simple closed manipulation for acute nasal fractures (Table 43-1).[9,12-16]

Fry[17,18] and Mayell[19] described unfavorable structural and aesthetic outcomes following nasal fractures. Waldron et al.[12] conducted a prospective study comparing local vs. general anesthesia for closed reduction and found a 14% to 16% incidence of postreduction deformity (in all groups) at 3 months requiring further surgery. Of those patients with initially identified traumatic septal deviation, 40% to 42% had significant septal deformity at 3 months requiring septorhinoplasty. Cook et al.[14] published a randomized prospective series of 50 patients, again comparing anesthesia for simple reduction of nasal fractures; they found a 14% to 17% incidence of postreduction deformity requiring further surgery. In their prospective series of 756 patients treated with simple reduction Murray and Maran[9] found a 41% incidence of postreduction deformity. They stated quite appropriately, "When outcome of simple manipulation is assessed objectively the technique has a poor success rate; only a proportion of noses are made straight and quite a number left unaltered." In our rhinoplasty analysis of 110 patients treated over the past 11 years by the senior author, we had a 9% (10/110) revision rate.

The incidence of posttraumatic nasal deformity after simple closed reduction in the emergency room ranges from 15% to 42%.

UNRECOGNIZED SEPTAL DEFORMITY

The nasal septum, the single most important structure in determining aesthetic and functional outcome in nasal fractures, must be completely assessed.[4,6] Verwoerd[6] described the pathogenesis of septal fractures, including three septal zones with thicker cartilage: dorsoposteriorly, basally, and caudally. Conversely, the central caudal portion of the septum is thin. The thicker posterior septal cartilage provides the primary support to the nasal dorsum. Trauma to the nasal dorsum leads to lesions in the caudal-basal to cephalo-dorsal supporting cartilage and horizontal fractures of the thinner central region.[6]

Fry[17,18] demonstrated the progressive distortion of fractured septal cartilage caused by the releases of locked internal stresses. Verwoerd[6] and Wexler[20] demonstrated that the septum does not remain straight after manipulation, and the nasal bones tend to unite in the direction of the deviated septum. In our experience the septum is the key structure to align/correct and optimize nasal fracture management and minimize secondary deformity.[21]

Assessment of the extent of septal injury is important to the selection of the proper technique for septal correction. Renner[2] reported that closed reduction with intranasal splints/packs yielded satisfactory results in most simple septal injuries involving the distal portion of the quadrangular cartilage. Pollock[10] advocated a low threshold for open reduction with precise septal correction for moderate to severe septal injuries with complex fracture patterns or involvement of the perpendicular plate of the ethmoid or vomerine groove. In the absence of complete evaluation of the entire septum the mobile anterior portion is reduced, leaving a dislocated rigid posterior septum that results in late functional deformity following closed reduction.[22] In 1968 Adamson et al.[23] advocated acute submucous resection for severely fractured septums. Harrison[22] recognized that low horizontal submucous septal resection removing only the quadrangular cartilage–vomerine groove interface was often not adequate because of the overlapping fractured segment in the perpendicular plate of the ethmoid; he recommended an extended low horizontal and posterior vertical submucous resection to fully address the septal pathology. Murray et al.[15] also attributed the high rate of postreduction nasal deformity requiring salvage septorhinoplasty to an unrecognized septal injury. They found that patients with nasal bones deviated more than half the nasal bridge width had a concomitant C-shaped fracture of the bony and cartilaginous septum. The same authors concluded that acute open reduction with submucous septal resection resulted in an improved long-term cosmetic and functional outcome because of the alleviation of overlapped, interlocking fragments of the septum that usually resulted in the secondary nasal bone deformity.

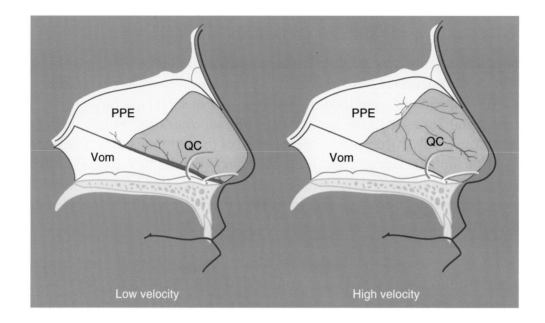

In our experience the most common septal fractures in low-velocity injuries occur inferiorly along the vomerine groove *(Vom)* as fractures or fracture-dislocations. High-velocity injuries or frontal impact result in more extensive septal fractures through the thin central region of the quadrangular cartilage *(QC)* extending posteriorly across the interface with the perpendicular plate of the ethmoid *(PPE)* and inferiorly to the vomer. Aggressive management of these septal injuries is key to successful management of the nasal fracture.

Identification and management of septal fractures are key to successful treatment.

PREOPERATIVE ASSESSMENT

A detailed nasal history and physical examination are essential. A precise account of the mechanism, including injuring agent, direction of blow, and timing of nasal injury, is recorded. A history of epistaxis, sine qua non for a nasal fracture, indicates a laceration of the involved nasal mucosa.[4]

The findings are recorded on the nasal fracture data sheet. Patients may vary in assessment of preinjury nasal shape. Differentiating new and old nasal deformity is sometimes difficult and must be correlated with the history and physical findings. Reviewing old photographs or driver's license photographs is helpful. The standard seven-view nasal photographs are taken (anterior-posterior, right and left lateral, right and left oblique, and low and high basal).

NASAL FRACTURE DATA SHEET

Name: _____ Date: _____ Age: _____

Mode of injury: ☐ Low energy   ☐ High energy

Direction: _____ Appearance: _____

Time since injury: _____

Associated injury: ☐ Soft tissue ☐ Facial fracture

History

Allergies _____

Previous nasal trauma _____

Previous nasal surgery _____

Airway obstruction _____

Medications _____

Pretraumatic photos: ☐ Yes ☐ No

Physical Examination

1. ☐ Unilateral ☐ Bilateral (width of nasal base)

2. Edema: 1+ 2+ 3+

3. Intercanthal distance: _____

4. Ecchymosis: 1+ 2+ 3+

5. Nasal bleeding: ☐ R ☐ L ☐ Bilateral ☐ None

6. Internal nasal examination

   Septal deviation/dislocation/fracture: _____

   Mucosal status: _____

   Septal hematoma: ☐ Yes ☐ No

Nasal Fracture Classification
   I. Simple (unilateral)
   II. Simple (bilateral)
   III. Comminuted unilateral
   IIIA. Comminuted bilateral
   IIIB. Comminuted frontal
   IV. Complex (nasal bone and septal disruption)
   V. Associated naso-orbital ethmoid fracture/midface fracture

The physical examination consists of an integrated systematic approach. The external examination includes inspection for lacerations, wounds, swelling, and deviation and palpation of the proximal nasal skeleton to identify tenderness, crepitus, depression and/or nasal shortening, and widening of the nasal base. Accurate intercanthal measurements are made to rule out a naso-orbital ethmoid fracture, especially noted with severe high-velocity frontal or inferior injuries. The fracture type(s) are defined. Various nasal fracture classifications have been reported.[10,24] We have adopted a practical clinically applicable nasal fracture classification based on the physical examination (see p. 779). The results of the physical examination are recorded on the nasal fracture data sheet. Edema is graded by degree of periorbital edema (1 = minimal/no periorbital edema, 2 = moderate periorbital edema, 3 = severe periorbital edema).

The internal examination requires at a minimum halogen lighting, good suction, a nasal speculum, vasoconstrictive anesthesia, and a 30-degree 3 mm rigid nasal endoscope if the fracture is type III or greater. A complete evaluation of the internal structures, especially the posterior septum, is performed and the deformity and evidence of obstruction recorded on the data sheet. The rigid nasal endoscope may be used to fully evaluate the entire septum, especially the posterior bony septum and vomerine regions in types III, IV, and V nasal fractures. A topical anesthetic consisting of 4% lidocaine and oxymetazoline (Afrin) or phenylephrine hydrochloride (Neo-Synephrine) suffice for a complete examination of the awake patient. Since a complete septal evaluation is central to evaluation of nasal fractures and optimizing results, adequate anesthesia is essential for a complete systematic evaluation.

After adequate vasoconstriction and topical anesthesia of the nasal mucosa, the diagnostic endonasal examination can proceed if desired. The patient is seated in an examining chair with the examiner usually sitting or standing to the right side of the patient. The endoscope is placed in the nasal vestibule and under direct vision is advanced posteriorly. The endoscope is advanced along the floor of the nose and beneath the inferior turbinate. Areas examined include the inferior meatus, turbinates, septum, and posteroinferior septal junction with the perpendicular plate of the ethmoid. Withdrawal of the scope allows for confirmation of fractures and septal disruption. Although the endoscope offers excellent visualization, we usually rely on thorough inspection and examination with a headlight and speculum.

The septal mucosa is inspected for tears and evidence of septal fractures. Prompt diagnosis and treatment of septal hematoma are essential to reduce fibrosis and subsequent septal distortion, abscess, and complete necrosis with resulting saddlenose deformity. Wide dependent drainage followed by packing carefully with antibiotic gauze[8] as well as systemic antibiotic coverage is recommended. Small hematomas may be aspirated[2] with close patient follow-up to determine if reaspiration or drainage is necessary. We prefer incisional drainage over aspiration.

Plain film radiographs are not necessary in the clinical diagnosis of isolated nasal fractures.[2,25] Logan et al.[26] reported a prospective series in which the use of routine x-ray films for the diagnosis of nasal fractures were evaluated and concluded they are not cost effective; however, patients found to have displaced nasal fractures on x-ray films are at higher risk for long-term nasal deformity, and anatomic reduction is highly recommended.

Plain film radiographs are not necessary in the clinical diagnosis of isolated nasal fracture and are not cost effective.

MANAGEMENT AND OPERATIVE TECHNIQUE

Numerous prospective series have been published comparing local vs. general anesthesia for manipulation of nasal fractures.[12,13,16] In most cases these studies prove local anesthesia to be as effective clinically and less expensive than general anesthesia for closed reduction. Wang et al.[4] stated that most adults with uncomplicated fractures may be treated using closed or open techniques with topical/local anesthetics and IV sedation. Cook et al.[14] found externally infiltrative field anesthesia to the nasal dorsum as effective and better tolerated than bilateral specific internal blocks of the infraorbital, infratrochlear, and external nasal nerves. With the external technique the needle is introduced bilaterally at the caudal edge of the nasal bone midway between the nasal bridge and maxilla.

We recommend a brief-acting general anesthetic for complete nasal fracture reduction[2] and find this approach is safe, controls the airway, and allows uncompromised nasal examination, reduction, and manipulation. We reserve local anesthesia with IV sedation for simple type I and II fractures or at the patient's request. We perform nasal reductions in our day-surgery center regardless of the type of anesthesia to maximize the use of superior lighting, nasal fracture/rhinoplasty instruments, and enhanced technical assistance available in that setting. This approach yields more consistent and controlled outcomes with less patient discomfort. Children, however, routinely undergo nasal manipulation under general anesthesia. Similarly, adults with polytrauma require repair of multiple injuries under a general anesthetic. A topical vasoconstrictive agent (Afrin) and 8 to 10 ml of 1% lidocaine with 1:100,000 epinephrine is always used for nasal hemostasis.

Nasal fracture reductions should not be performed in the emergency room, but rather in the controlled setting of an outpatient surgery center with IV sedation or a brief-acting general anesthetic to optimize postreduction results.

Reduction of external nasal bones to an anatomic position is accomplished initially by recreating the fracture. Molding the nasal bones with the fingers is the simplest approach.[10,24,27] Impacted nasal bones require instrumentation for reduction and restoration of nasal length (the most critical dimension to restore). The Walsham forceps are designed for reduction of impacted nasal bones.[2,24] The Asch forceps are designed for reduction of the nasal septum but may also be successfully used for restoring alignment of impacted nasal bones. Both of these instruments will cause damage to the nasal mucosa.

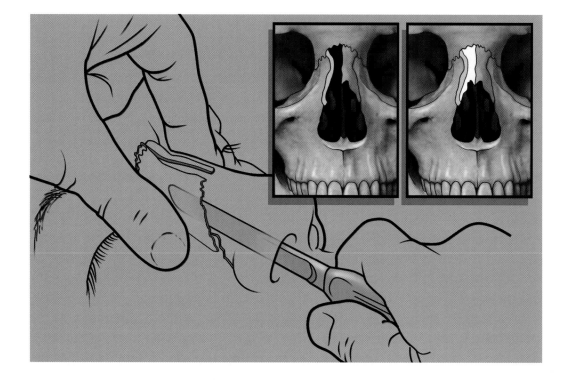

We prefer the use of the less traumatic Boise elevator; placing the elevator intranasally and the surgeon's thumb externally over the nasal bones permits detection of subtle osseous movements.[2]

To minimize nasal mucosal trauma, the Boise elevator should be used for reduction of nasal bone fractures.

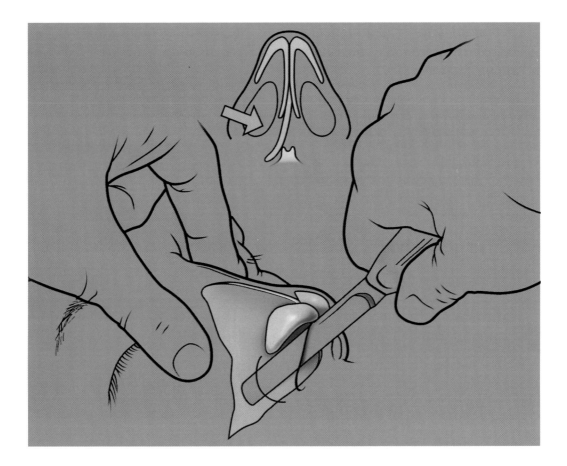

Reduction of the fractured nasal septum begins with relocating the displaced base into the vomerine groove. This may be accomplished with either the Asch forceps or blunt Boise elevator. If reduction of the septum is accomplished with a simple technique, it should be reexamined endoscopically or with a nasal speculum and headlight to ensure alignment of posterior elements. Nasal bone reduction should also be reassessed since shifting may occur during septal manipulation.[10] Comminuted nasal bones may be reduced and dorsal-posterior intranasal packing with Oxycel used to prevent collapse following reduction.

Acute septal reconstruction is considered for a patient with a nonreducible anterior or posterior-inferior septum, especially those with type IV fractures. This may be associated with a slightly increased risk of loss of traumatized nasal mucosa during undermining with subsequent septal perforation. Nevertheless, given the extremely high rate of posttraumatic nasal deformity secondary to malaligned or occult septal injury, the surgeon should perform a total anatomic septal reduction and/or reconstruction if the injury is acute and the septum is irreducible and posteriorly displaced.

If a septal fracture is identified, it must be anatomically reduced to prevent long-term nasal deviations. If the septal fracture cannot be reduced adequately, then submucous resection of the fracture should be performed.

A hemitransfixion or Killian incision is made, and bilateral inferior mucoperichondrial flaps are developed. Complete visualization of the septum is obtained to define the extent of the injury.

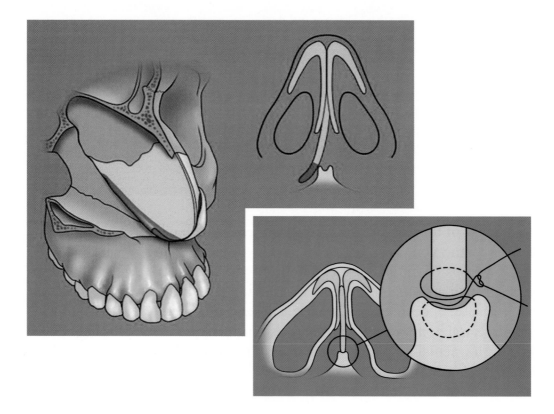

An inferior and posterior septal reconstruction to dislodge and align the septum and/or septal repositioning may be performed with anterior septal spine figure-of-eight sutures with a 5-0 PDS suture to keep the septum aligned and straight.

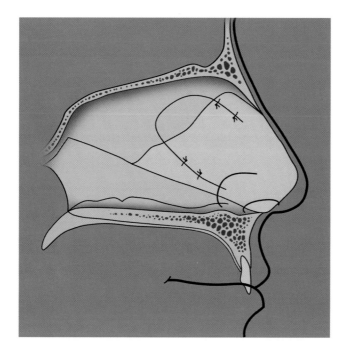

Reduced fractures of the septum are precisely reapproximated with through-and-through mucosal-septum-mucosal 4-0 chromic mattress sutures.

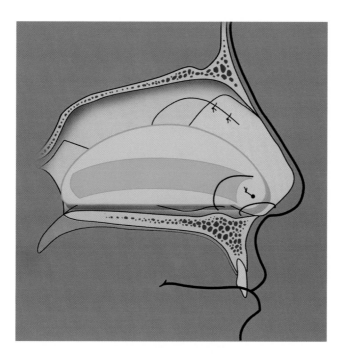

Doyle splints are recommended to further stabilize the caudal septum. Intranasal and external splints are used for 5 to 7 days, as are prophylactic antibiotics (cephalexin) and 3-day steroid dose pack (8 mg dexamethasone) to reduce postreduction nasal edema.

Clinical Algorithm

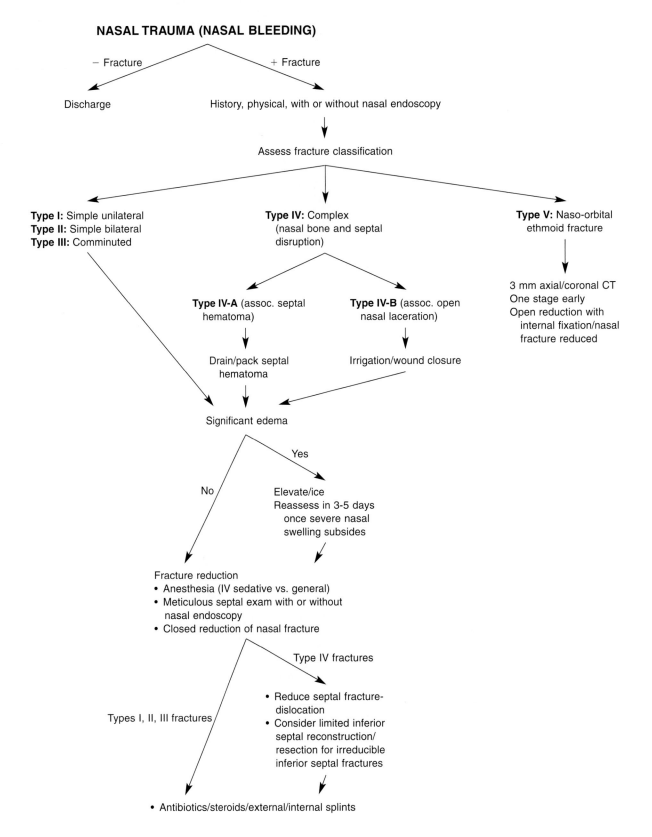

NASAL TRAUMA (NASAL BLEEDING)

− Fracture   + Fracture

Discharge   History, physical, with or without nasal endoscopy

Assess fracture classification

Type I: Simple unilateral
Type II: Simple bilateral
Type III: Comminuted

Type IV: Complex
(nasal bone and septal
disruption)

Type V: Naso-orbital
ethmoid fracture

Type IV-A (assoc. septal
hematoma)

Type IV-B (assoc. open
nasal laceration)

3 mm axial/coronal CT
One stage early
Open reduction with
internal fixation/nasal
fracture reduced

Drain/pack septal
hematoma

Irrigation/wound closure

Significant edema

Yes

No

Elevate/ice
Reassess in 3-5 days
once severe nasal
swelling subsides

Fracture reduction
• Anesthesia (IV sedative vs. general)
• Meticulous septal exam with or without
nasal endoscopy
• Closed reduction of nasal fracture

Type IV fractures

Types I, II, III fractures

• Reduce septal fracture-
dislocation
• Consider limited inferior
septal reconstruction/
resection for irreducible
inferior septal fractures

• Antibiotics/steroids/external/internal splints

We have formulated a clinical algorithm for acute nasal fracture management to minimize the incidence of posttraumatic deformity requiring revision septorhinoplasty. We caution, however, that an algorithm is merely a framework on which to base clinical decisions and does not supplant sound individualized clinical judgment.

The following points are emphasized:
1. The diagnosis of acute nasal fractures is based on a complete history and physical examination, including an intranasal examination, and not on radiographic studies.
2. In patients with significant posttraumatic swelling precluding immediate precise reduction, a clinical examination is performed, and local measures prescribed (i.e., ice, elevation) with follow-up in 3 to 5 days. Definitive treatment is be instituted 5 to 7 days after injury, depending on the edema of the nose. In isolated cases treatment can be delayed 10 to 12 days without significant problems with bone mobilization.
3. The septum is the key to nasal fracture management. All septal pathology, especially posteriorly, must be identified via the clinical examination and rigid nasal endoscopy. Significant septal fractures are directly visualized, and limited septal resection, reconstruction, and repositioning are considered.
4. This algorithm will yield improved long-term functional and aesthetic results; however, all patients should be initially counseled regarding the possibility of further nasal procedures.

Acute nasal fracture management has often been inadequate and associated with a high incidence of long-term nasal deformity. Primary factors contributing to poor long-term results include acute traumatic edema, unrecognized preexisting nasal deformity, and undetected posterior and inferiorly displaced septal fractures. Given these variables, we have devised a practice algorithm for acute nasal fracture management. This algorithm was developed and refined during the past 11 years in a series of 110 patients. However, we were not able to stratify these patients with regard to fracture type. The treatment failures were generally those patients with severe, difficult to reduce septal injuries, which emphasizes the importance of the septum. Further detailed data on the type of patients most prone to failure are presently being collected and will help further refine this algorithm.

Most reductions are performed 3 to 7 days after injury in the operating room with appropriate anesthesia. Irreducible septal injuries should be treated with limited inferior septal reconstruction in the acute phase to diminish second-degree nasal deformity. With this algorithm the need for extensive and difficult posttraumatic revision rhinoplasty should be significantly reduced.

■ KEY POINTS

■ Current management approaches to acute nasal fractures result in a high incidence of posttraumatic nasal deformity (14% to 50%).

■ Associated traumatic edema, preexisting nasal deformity, and occult septal injury account for most of the acute reduction failures.

■ Based on a detailed history and physical examination we have formulated a clinical algorithm for acute nasal fracture management.

■ We have had a 9% nasal revision rate in 110 patients treated in the past 11 years.

■ The low incidence of revision is attributed to complete nasal assessment (bony and septum), use of outpatient controlled general anesthesia, and primary septal reconstruction in patients with severe septal fracture-dislocations.

REFERENCES

1. Haug RH, Prather JJ. The closed reduction of nasal fractures: An evaluation of two techniques. J Oral Maxillofac Surg 49:1288, 1991.
2. Renner GJ. Management of nasal fractures. Otolaryngol Clin North Am 24:195, 1991.
3. Schultz RC, DeVillers VT. Nasal fractures. J Trauma 15:319, 1975.
4. Wang TD, Facer GW, Kern EB. Nasal fractures. In Gates GA, ed. Current Therapy in Otolaryngology–Head and Neck Surgery, vol 4, 1990, p 105.
5. Swearington JJ. Tolerances of human face to crash impact. Federal Aviation Agency, Oklahoma City, 1965.
6. Verwoerd CDA. Present day treatment of nasal fractures: Closed vs. open reduction. Facial Plast Surg 8:220, 1992.
7. Malianc JW. Rhinoplasty and restoration of facial contour: With specific reference to trauma. Philadelphia: FA Davis, 1947, p 29.
8. Kurihara K, Kim K. Open reduction and interfragment wire fixation of comminuted nasal fractures. Ann Plast Surg 24:179, 1990.
9. Murray JAM, Maran AGD. The treatment of nasal injuries by manipulation. J Laryngol Otol 94:1405, 1980.
10. Pollock RA. Nasal trauma: Pathomechanics and surgical management of acute injuries. Clin Plast Surg 19:133, 1992.
11. Crowther JA, O'Donoghue GM. The broken nose: Does familiarity breed neglect? Ann R Coll Surg Engl 69:261, 1987.
12. Waldron J, Mitchell DB, Ford G. Reduction of fractured nasal bones: Local versus general anesthesia. Clin Otolaryngol 14:357, 1989.
13. Cook JA, McRae DR, Irving RM, Davie LN. A randomized comparison of manipulation of the fractured nose under local and general anesthesia. Clin Otolaryngol 15:343, 1990.
14. Cook JA, Murrant NT, Evans KL, Lavelle RJ. Manipulation of the fractured nose under local anesthesia. Clin Otolaryngol 17:337, 1992.
15. Murray JA, Maran AGD, MacKenzie J, Raub G. Open v closed reduction of the fractured nose. Arch Otolaryngol 110:797, 1984.
16. Watson DJ, Parker RW, Slack WT, Griffiths MV. Local anesthesia versus general anesthesia in management of the fractured nose. Clin Otolaryngol 13:491, 1988.

17. Fry HJH. Interlocked stresses in human nasal septal cartilage. Br J Plast Surg 19:276, 1966.
18. Fry HJH. Nasal skeleton trauma and interlocked stress of nasal septal cartilage. Br J Plast Surg 20:146, 1967.
19. Mayell MF. Nasal fractures: Their occurrence, management and some late results. J R Coll Surg Edinb 18:31, 1973.
20. Wexler MR. Reconstructive surgery of the injured nose. Otolaryngol Clin North Am 8:549, 1975.
21. Gunter JP, Rohrich RJ. Management of deviated nose—importance of septal reconstruction. Clin Plast Surg 15:43, 1988.
22. Harrison DH. Nasal injuries: Their pathogenesis and treatment. Br J Plast Surg 32:57, 1979.
23. Adamson JE, Horton CE, Crawford HH, Tadeo RJ. Acute submucous resection. Plast Reconstr Surg 42:152, 1968.
24. Stranc MF, Robertson GA. Classification of injuries of nasal skeleton. Ann Plast Surg 2:468, 1979.
25. Humber PR, Horton CE. Trauma to the nose. In Starks RB, ed. Plastic Surgery of the Head and Neck. New York: Churchill Livingstone, 1989.
26. Logan M, O'Driscoll K, Masterson J. The utility of nasal bone radiographs in nasal trauma. Clin Radiol 49:192, 1994.
27. Dingman RO, Converse JM. The clinical management of facial injuries and fractures of the facial bones. In Converse JM, ed. Reconstructive Plastic Surgery, vol 2. Philadelphia: WB Saunders, 1977.

44

Management of the Deviated Nose*

Rod J. Rohrich, M.D. ▪ Jack P. Gunter, M.D.
Mark A. Deuber, M.D. ▪ William P. Adams, Jr., M.D.

*T*he deviated nose is one that varies from the straight vertical orientation of the face. Correction of this deformity presents a challenge because frequently a functional (airway obstruction) as well as an aesthetic problem must be addressed.[1-4] The anatomic basis of the deviation may be related to bony pyramid pathology, septal deformity, or a combination of the two.[5-7] The etiology may be congenital or acquired secondary to trauma or surgery. Severely injured noses represent a particularly difficult challenge for the surgeon involving both septal and asymmetric bony pathology.[8]

A major septal deformity is almost always a component of severely deviated noses.[9-12]

To consistently attain good aesthetic and functional results when correcting the deviated nose requires a thorough understanding of nasal anatomy[13] and physiology, accurate preoperative analysis and intraoperative diagnosis, an understanding of the physiology of cartilage and its healing,[14-16] and the skill to precisely execute the surgical steps required to alter and control the nasal septum. If both septal and bony deviations are present, they are corrected at the same setting. It is not necessary to stage the correction of the deviated nose.

*Abstracted in part from Rohrich RJ, Gunter JP, Deuber MA, Adams WP Jr. Management of the deviated nose. Plast Reconstr Surg (submitted for publication).

ANATOMY

A thorough understanding of normal nasal anatomy is prerequisite for the surgeon to achieve a good functional as well as aesthetic result.[17]

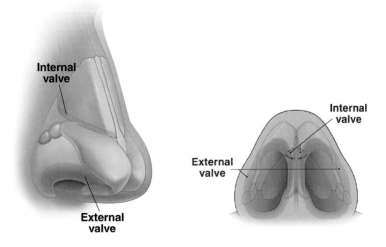

The nasal airway begins at the external nasal valve and comprises the lower lateral cartilages, the distal upper lateral cartilages, the head of the inferior turbinate, the caudal septum, and the remaining piriform aperture soft tissues. Just deep to this is the internal nasal valve, the narrowest portion of the normal nose. This is formed by the angle created between the caudal edge of the upper lateral cartilages and the dorsal septum. The nasal septum includes the quadrilateral cartilage, nasal spine, frontal spine, perpendicular plate of the ethmoid, vomer, and maxillary crest.

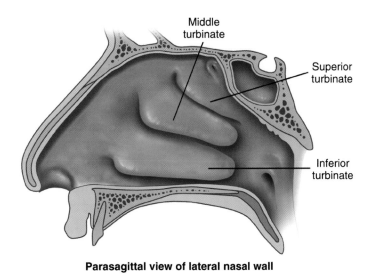

Parasagittal view of lateral nasal wall

Laterally, four turbinates are found (inferior, middle, superior, supreme) along with corresponding meatuses that drain the paranasal sinuses. The inferior turbinate is predominantly responsible for regulating airflow, whereas the middle turbinate serves to humidify the air.[18] Laterally, the nasal airway is also bounded by the upper lateral cartilages and the nasal bones. The nasal airway terminates at the choanae as the airflow passes into the nasopharynx.

PREOPERATIVE ASSESSMENT

Clinical analysis of the cause and anatomy of the nasal deviation is essential in planning corrective surgery. The deviated nose should be considered an osseocartilaginous unit in which all components potentially play a role. Critical components of the history include age, history of trauma, nasal airway complaints, and previous nasal surgery.

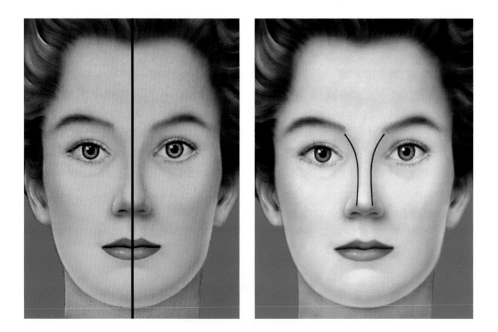

The external physical examination should include a detailed facial aesthetic analysis with emphasis on the deviation from the facial midline and the quality and shape of the dorsal aesthetic lines. The external examination concludes with an assessment of the shape and position of the nasal bones and the upper and lower lateral cartilaginous vaults. During the internal examination septal deviations and the bilateral status of the turbinates are assessed (see Chapter 5).

Critical components of the history include a history of nasal trauma, nasal airway complaints, allergies, and previous nasal surgery.

There are three basic types of nasal deviation, two of which have subtypes:
    Caudal septal deviation
        Straight septal tilt
        S-shaped septal tilt
    Concave deformity
        C-shaped dorsal deformity
        Reverse C-shaped deformity
    Concave/convex dorsal deformity

Caudal septal deviations cause significant airway compromise because they affect the anteroinferior part of the external nares. Two subtypes are commonly seen. The first and most common is a straight septal tilt off the vomer with no dorsal septal curvature, exhibiting a caudal septal deviation pushing the nasal tip off the midline, and without deviation of the nasal pyramid. The second subtype has a similar effect on the nasal tip but has an S-shaped curvature of the caudal septum that is more difficult to correct.

The second most common type is the concave deformity. The two subtypes are the C-shaped deformity with a left-sided concavity and the reverse C-shaped deformity with right-sided concavity. The least common type and most difficult to correct is the concave/convex deformity, also known as an S-shaped dorsal deformity with bony pyramid deviation.[19]

The goals of correction are both aesthetic and functional. The aesthetic goals include straightening the dorsum, defining the tip to enhance facial balance, and correcting bony asymmetries. Functionally, the goals are directed at improving the nasal airway, including straightening the septum, restoring the nasal valve integrity, and correcting any inferior turbinate hypertrophy.[8]

ETIOLOGY OF DEVIATION

Significant intrinsic and extrinsic forces produce nasal deviation.[20] These forces result in the septal distortion and deviation responsible for the functional and cosmetic deformity. The extrinsic forces are either secondary to scar contractures or congenitally asymmetric attachments of the osseocartilaginous skeleton, including attachments between the bony pyramid, the upper lateral cartilages, the lower lateral cartilages, and the septum. The intrinsic forces are those acquired or inherent septal cartilaginous abnormalities. In patients who have experienced nasal trauma these are predominantly represented by septal fractures of the caudal-inferior to the cephaloposterior septum, the horizontal septum, or the C-shaped central septal segment.[21,22]

Both intrinsic and extrinsic deforming forces are responsible for producing the aesthetic and functional deformity.

PRINCIPLES OF TREATMENT

Correction of the deviated nose is based on the six principles described be-low.[19,23] As with all rhinoplasty procedures, accurate preoperative planning and diagnosis are essential to successful outcomes.

Wide Exposure of Deviated Structures

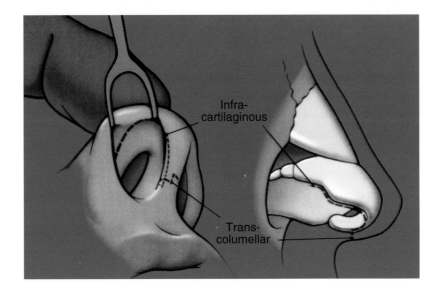

The open rhinoplasty approach is preferred for the management of the devi-ated nose, especially in patients with a high dorsal deviation. Any structure that is out of place must be freely mobilized of all attachments and replaced in its correct anatomic position. If the nasal bones are deviated, osteotomies must be performed; if the upper lateral cartilages are displaced, they should be freed from the septum and the lower lateral cartilages. Deviated portions of the septum must be widely mobilized to return them to the midline.

The exposure afforded by the open approach allows maximal accuracy in diagnosis and control in achieving optimal repair of the deviated nose.

Wide Release of Mucoperichondrial Attachments

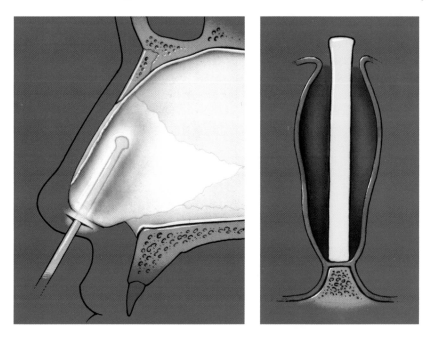

The mucoperichondrial attachments are conserved when possible to maintain the blood supply to the cartilage to minimize resorption. However, the mucoperichondrial attachments to a deviated portion of the septum must be widely released before the septum can be returned to the midline.

The mucoperichondrial attachments are widely released as an initial effort to return the septum to the midline.

After wide exposure the extrinsic deforming forces are sequentially released. The lower lateral cartilages are freed from the upper lateral cartilages at the scroll area with a cephalic trim.

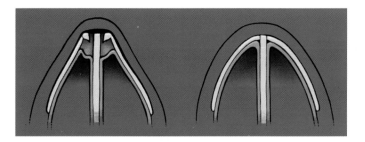

The upper lateral cartilages are divided and released from the septum. If the deformity is due to asymmetric upper lateral cartilages causing extrinsic twisting of the septum, this maneuver will actually result in straightening of the septum. Once this has been done, the septum can be visualized to accurately assess any intrinsic septal etiology of the deviation.

Straightening the Deviated Septum

Once the deviated septum has been widely mobilized and separated from the upper lateral cartilages, it must be straightened by addressing and correcting the intrinsic deforming forces. The goal is to straighten the septum while maximizing residual dorsal nasal support.

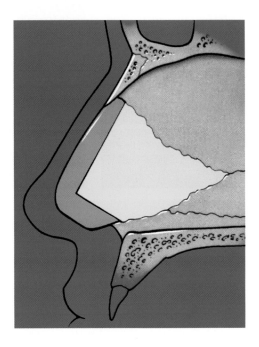

Initially the deviated portion should be resected, taking care to preserve at least an 8 to 10 mm dorsal and caudal L-strut. The resection may include septal cartilage, maxillary crest, vomer, and perpendicular plate of the ethmoid. The L-strut should remain attached to the perpendicular plate at the keystone area and the nasal spine–maxillary crest area.

At least an 8 to 10 mm dorsal and caudal L-strut must be preserved to prevent long-term nasal collapse.

If the caudal septum is deviated from the midline off the nasal spine, it must be anatomically reduced. This may be accomplished through the dorsal open approach with the release of the lower lateral cartilage attachments to the septum. The deviated portion of the caudal septum is then straightened.

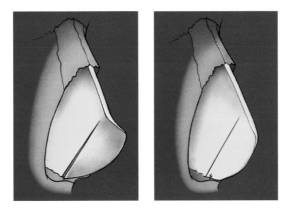

Straightening the septum may involve the development of a "swinging door" flap with vertical wedge sectioning of the septum at the point of caudal deviation if it is a type 1a deformity.

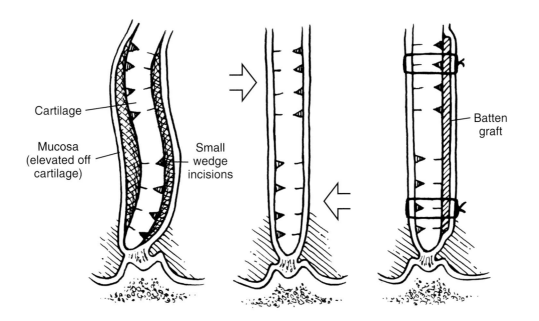

Not infrequently the deviated caudal septum (type 1b) requires the removal of small wedges of cartilage from the convex side with scoring only of the opposite side to destroy the cartilage memory and straighten the septum. It is then straightened and reduced to the midline with a 5-0 PDS suture secured to the periosteum of the nasal spine on the contralateral side of the original deviation (see Chapter 46). A batten septal graft is used to suture stabilize the now straightened caudal septum.

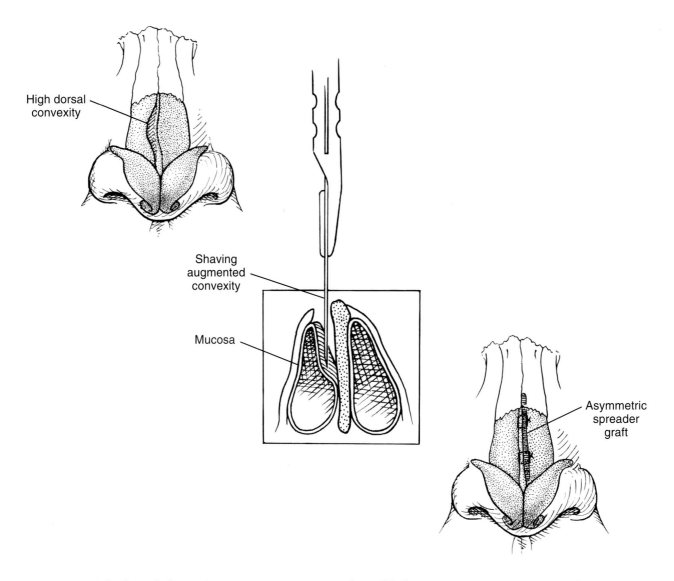

High dorsal deviations are now corrected. Mild deviations can sometimes be corrected by shaving the convexity from the upper lateral cartilage on the side of the deviation; the residual deformity is camouflaged with an asymmetric spreader graft. This combination will frequently be sufficient to correct minor C-shaped deformities of the dorsum (see Chapter 46). Cartilage scoring techniques may be necessary to help straighten the more severe high dorsal deviation.

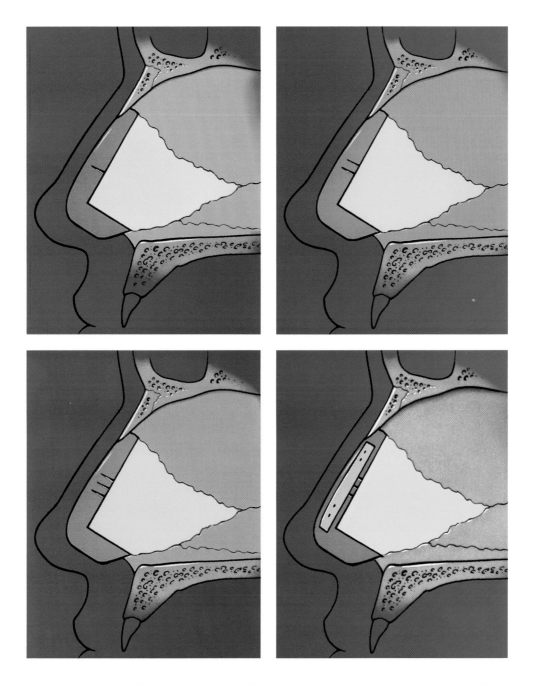

If a significant deformity persists despite these techniques, sequential inferior full-thickness cuts in the deviated portion of the dorsal septal cartilage are made up through 50% of the remaining dorsal L-strut. This will permit straightening of the deviated septum, but it will also weaken its support. Bilateral spreader grafts will be placed to maintain support and restore the dorsal aesthetic lines.

High dorsal deviations are straightened by making sequential inferior full-thickness cuts up through 50% of the deviated portion of the remaining L-strut.

After the septum has been straightened, the upper and lower lateral cartilages are reassessed for symmetry. Any remaining asymmetries should now be addressed by trimming the upper lateral cartilages and suture securing them to the septum before performing a lower lateral cephalic trim or any tip suture techniques.

Restoration of Septal Support

The height of the lower one half of the nasal dorsum, the midvault, is dependent on the support of the septum.

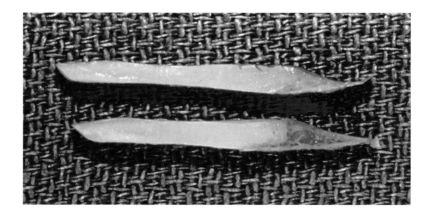

Long-term support is restored by buttressing the weakened dorsal septum with spreader grafts.[24-26] These grafts are ideally fashioned from the postero-inferior portion of the septal cartilage since it has the most consistent width and allows for harvesting the 30 to 35 mm length required. They are contoured to be 5 to 6 mm in height.

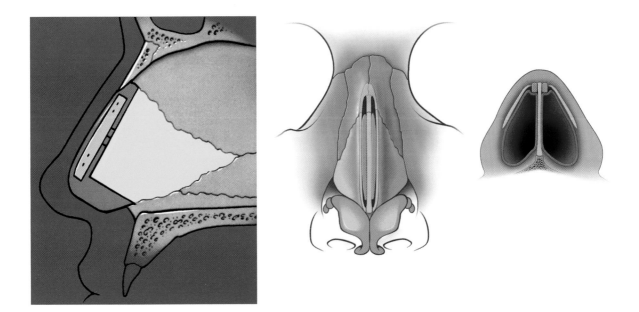

The spreader grafts are secured with two or three 5-0 PDS mattress sutures either unilaterally or bilaterally parallel to the dorsal septum according to the deformity being addressed.

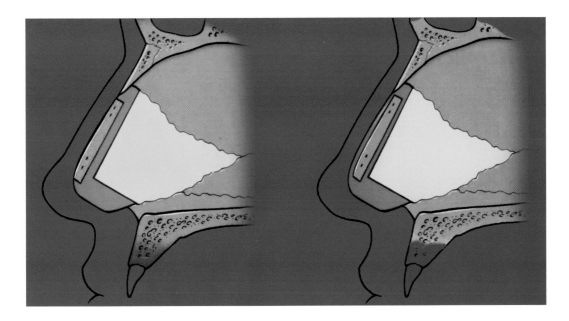

Asymmetric (unilateral) placement will allow for camouflaging of any residual deviation. Their position may be either visible at of above the dorsal septal plane or invisible below the septal plane, depending on whether widening of the midvault or elevation of the dorsum is desired.[27]

*The spreader grafts serve to maintain or restore the integrity
of the internal nasal valves, to restore the dorsal aesthetic lines,
and to strengthen and maintain long-term septal support.*

Submucosal Reduction of Hypertrophied Turbinates (if Present)

Septonasal deviations are a normal variant in human anatomy and do not typically lead to airway problems unless 50% to 60% of the anteroinferior airway is obliterated. This may lead to compensatory contralateral inferior turbinate hypertrophy. Even if airway obstruction is not present preoperatively, septal straightening may lead to narrowing of the anterior airway if inferior turbinate hypertrophy is present.

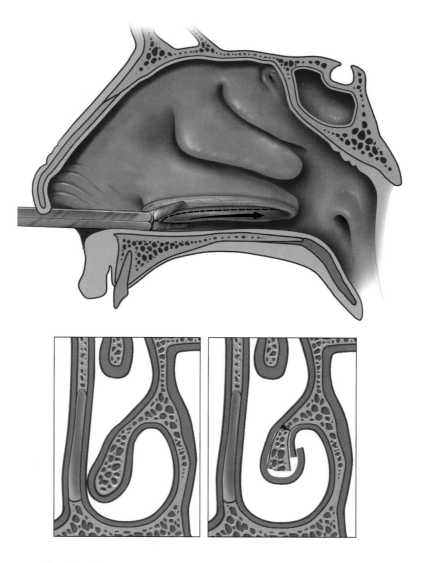

The hypertrophied inferior turbinates may subsequently interfere with septal repositioning and the postoperative airway. Submucosal reduction of the hypertrophied turbinate is performed to allow for an adequate postoperative airway (see Chapter 36) if needed after correction of the deviated septum.

Submucosal reduction of the anteroinferior turbinate with resection of the hypertrophied bone is critical to maintaining a straight septum and good nasal airway if inferior turbinate hypertrophy is present.

Precise Osteotomies

Accurately planned lateral and/or medial osteotomies will restore symmetry to the nasal pyramid. Prior to performing osteotomies the dorsal profile must be reassessed to determine if dorsal reduction of the bony pyramid is necessary. If a bony dorsal hump must be resected, the orientation of the nasal bones must be considered, especially if there is asymmetric bony deviation.

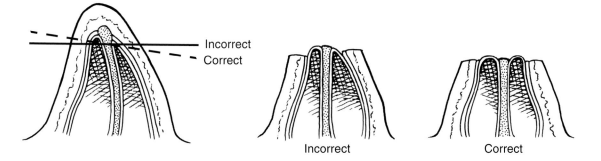

Less bone will need to be excised or rasped from the nasal bone on the deviated side that is more vertically oriented. This will prevent excessive reduction in nasal bone height of that side after the nasal bones are anatomically reduced (see Chapter 46).

In the setting of asymmetric nasal bones, rasping must be done obliquely, taking care to perform less reduction on the side of the more vertically oriented bone so that the nasal bones are symmetric after reduction with lateral osteotomies.

Lateral osteotomies alone will be sufficient only in the settings of bony pyramid deviation with symmetric nasal bones or a significant open roof. They are performed percutaneously with a 2 mm osteotome.

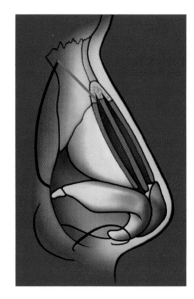

Deviation with any significant degree of bony asymmetries will require medial osteotomies as well.[20] These medial osteotomies are required to allow independent movement of the nasal bones. Adequate osteotomies must be performed to prevent greensticking, which may allow for re-deviation of the nasal pyramid in the postoperative period secondary to tissue memory (see Chapter 46). If planned, medial osteotomies should be performed prior to making the lateral osteotomies.

Medial osteotomies may be necessary in addition to lateral osteotomies in the setting of an asymmetric nasal pyramid.

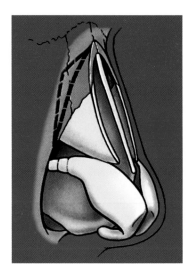

When nasal bone intrinsic convexity is present, double-level osteotomies will be necessary. Care should be taken not to excessively free up the periosteum of the nasal bones since comminution can result from multiple osteotomies and the periosteum can prevent the displacement of these comminuted fragments. Dorsal reduction and septal straightening should be addressed prior to the osteotomies while the nasal dorsum is still stable. Only minimal bony rasping and incremental cartilage incisions can be performed after the osteotomies.

OPERATIVE TECHNIQUE

The osseocartilaginous skeleton is exposed using the open rhinoplasty approach with a stair-step transcolumellar incision connected to bilateral vestibular infracartilaginous incisions. Once this has been accomplished, the lower lateral cartilages are separated from the upper lateral cartilages at the scroll area. A scroll-only cephalic trim is performed at this time. The nasal tip is now free from more proximal nasal deforming forces. The septal mucoperichondrial flaps are elevated using the Cottle elevator beginning at the anterior septal angle. The upper lateral cartilages are then separated and mobilized from the septum using a No. 15 blade.

Any nasal dorsal reduction surgery required is now performed followed by initial tip work. This sequence is critical in establishing the proper balance between the tip and the dorsum. If bony dorsal reduction is necessary, it is completed with the rasp. In the setting of asymmetric nasal bones, rasping must be performed obliquely, taking care to reduce the side of the more vertically oriented bone to a lesser degree so that the nasal bones are symmetric after lateral osteotomies.

Septal resection and cartilage graft harvesting are performed for a curved deviation, taking care to maintain at least an 8 to 10 mm L-strut dorsally and caudally. This resection may include septal cartilage, maxillary crest, vomer, and perpendicular plate of the ethmoid.

The septum is now addressed. If the caudal septum is deviated off the maxillary crest/vomer but does not have a curved deviation, it is anatomically reduced and secured in position with a figure-of-eight suture of 5-0 PDS to the periosteum of the contralateral nasal spine. If a significant intrinsic deviation is present, a "swinging door" flap technique is used by vertical sectioning of the septum at the point of deviation. Precise sequential scoring, morselization, or crosshatching must be performed for an extensive or S-shaped deformity.

Inferior full-thickness parallel cuts through 50% of the dorsal L-strut are made to correct the high dorsal deviation. Any remaining cartilaginous asymmetries are now addressed if present by trimming the upper lateral cartilages and/or performing lower lateral cephalic trims.

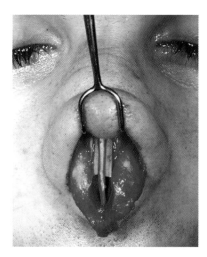

Spreader grafts are fashioned from the harvested septum and contoured to 5 to 6 mm in height and 30 to 32 mm in length. They are secured to the L-strut with at least two 5-0 PDS horizontal mattress sutures to restore support and internal nasal valve integrity. These are placed below the septal plane in an invisible position if midvault widening is not indicated or desired. Asymmetric spreader grafts may be used if necessary to camouflage any residual deformity to accurately restore the dorsal aesthetic lines.

The inferior turbinates are now assessed. If hypertrophy of the anteroinferior turbinate is present, we perform a limited submucous resection of the hypertrophied bone anteriorly followed by outfracturing of the posterior part of the turbinate.

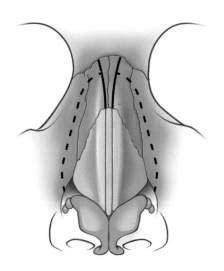

If there is a bony pyramid deviation present, then osteotomies are performed using the 2 mm external percutaneous osteotome. Generally lateral osteotomies are performed, but medial osteotomies will be necessary in the presence of asymmetric nasal bones that must be moved independently. For convex deformities of individual nasal bones mid-level (dual) osteotomies are performed as well. The periosteum is preserved as much as possible so that displacement of any fragments does not occur in the event of comminution.

Final tip refinement is then performed followed by skin redraping, meticulous closure, and standard internal and external splinting.

It is important to have a perfectly straight nose prior to completion of the rhinoplasty and closure.

CASE ANALYSES

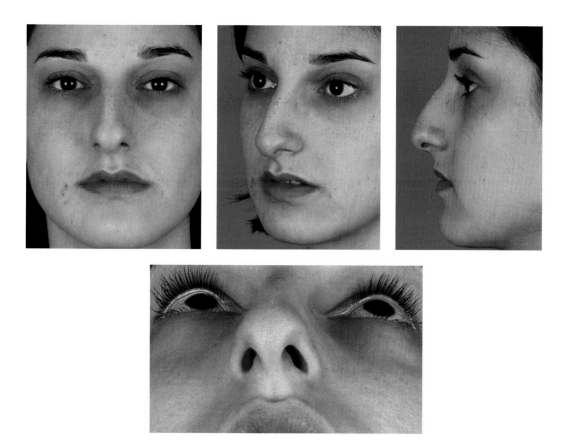

This 19-year-old primary rhinoplasty patient had a history of deviated nose and nasal airway obstruction. She had a high C-shaped dorsal spinal deviation and a bulbous tip with short nasal bones and thin skin. She requested functional and aesthetic improvement. The frontal view best demonstrates the short nasal bones with the C-shaped deformity, narrow midvault, and dorsal aesthetic lines that are disrupted in the keystone area. She also had a bulbous tip. The patient had thin skin showing bifidity as well as an excess in infratip projection with periapical hypoplasia. On the lateral view the patient exhibits a low radix with a prominent dorsal cartilaginous hump, short upper lip, a slight excess tip projection, and normal nasal length. The nasolabial angle was 105 degrees. The oblique view confirmed the caudal septal and nasal tip deviation to the right.

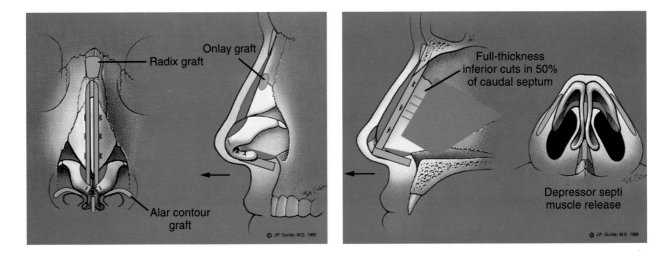

The operative goals included:
- Correction of dorsal deviation
- Redefinition and widening of dorsal aesthetic lines
- Redirection of dorsal hump and straightening of nose
- Refinement of nasal tip
- Correction of nasal airway obstruction
- Release and transposition of depressor septi muscle to lengthen upper lip

The surgical plan called for:
- Open rhinoplasty
- Component dorsal hump reduction
- Septal reconstruction and septal graft harvest
- Inferior full-thickness cuts in 50% of the L-strut
- Bilateral spreader grafts to widen the dorsum after separation of the upper lateral cartilage from the septum
- Radix augmentation of 5 mm with morselized cartilage graft
- Reconstruction of tip with a columellar strut secured with intercrural sutures
- Interdomal and transdomal sutures as well as infratip cap graft to correct bifidity
- Left dorsal onlay graft to correct irregularity of left osseocartilaginous vault
- Depressor septi muscle release and transposition
- Caudal bone resection of 3 mm secured with 5-0 PDS sutures to nasal periosteum
- No nasal osteotomies
- Bilateral alar contour grafts to correct alar weakness

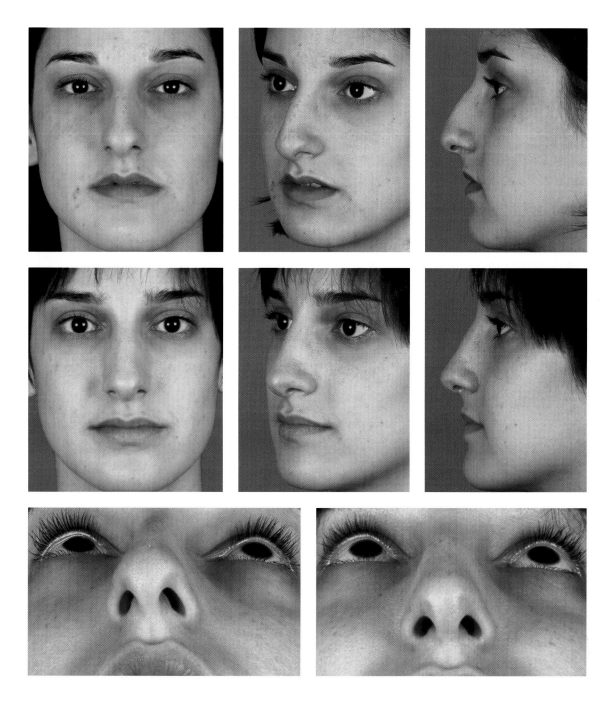

The patient is shown 2 years postoperatively. Note the straight nasal dorsum with balanced dorsal aesthetic lines. The bulbous tip is corrected and infratip lobular projection improved. The lateral view reveals a normal radix with normal length and projection and improved nasal infratip lobular area. The nasolabial angle is now 95 degrees and the dorsum straight. The oblique view demonstrates correction of the high midvault dorsal deviation and bulbous tip. The basal view shows the improved columella to tip relationship and symmetry of the external nares.

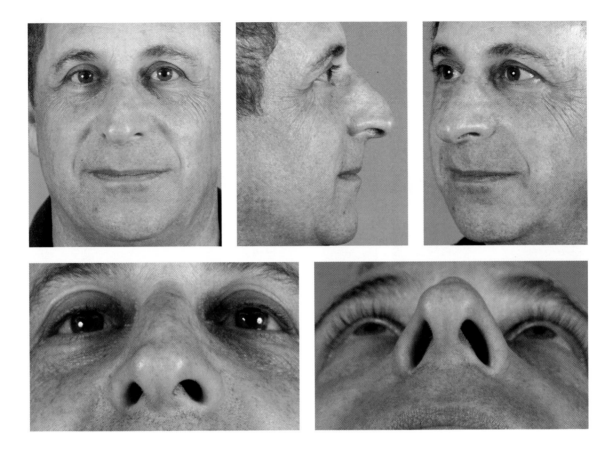

This 55-year-old man complained of his large nose, excessive nasal length and tip projection, and dorsal hump with a significant reverse C-shaped deformity. He had Fitzpatrick type II thin skin, reverse C-shaped dorsal deviation, long nose, and bulbous tip. The lateral view best demonstrated the long nose with excess dorsal convexity, excess tip projection, and high radix with a significant reversed C-shaped deformity. The nasolabial angle measured 95 degrees. The oblique view revealed the dorsal convexity and excess nasal length and deviation. The basal view showed the dorsal convexity deviating the nose to the right, bulbous tip, and alar collapse bilaterally (more on the right than the left) with deviation of the nose caudally into the left nostril.

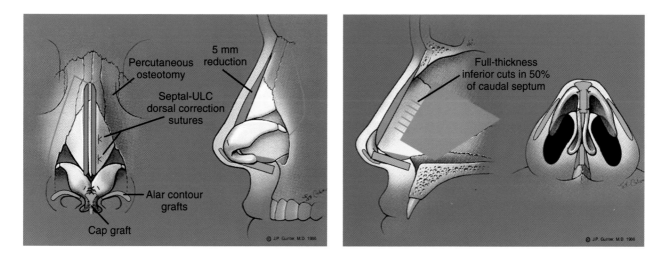

The operative goals included:
- Reduction of nasal length and tip projection
- Reduction of dorsal hump
- Refinement of nasal tip
- Correction of dorsally deviated dorsum
- Narrowing of bony nasal base
- Prevention of alar collapse

The surgical plan called for:
- Open rhinoplasty
- Exposure of dorsal framework and reduction of dorsal hump
- Septal harvest and septal reconstruction
- Inferior full-thickness cuts through 50% of the septum caudal to the deviated part of the septum and proceeding distally
- Suturing of septum with 5-0 PDS horizontal mattress sutures to upper lateral cartilage to maintain dorsal correction
- Securing columellar strut graft with intercrural sutures
- Placement of interdomal and transdomal sutures to refine nasal tip
- Placement of bilateral alar contour grafts to correct alar notching
- Reduction of caudal septum 3 mm and suturing with 5-0 PDS to anterior nasal spine to straighten caudal septum
- Bilateral external nasal bone osteotomies to narrow nasal base (low to low)

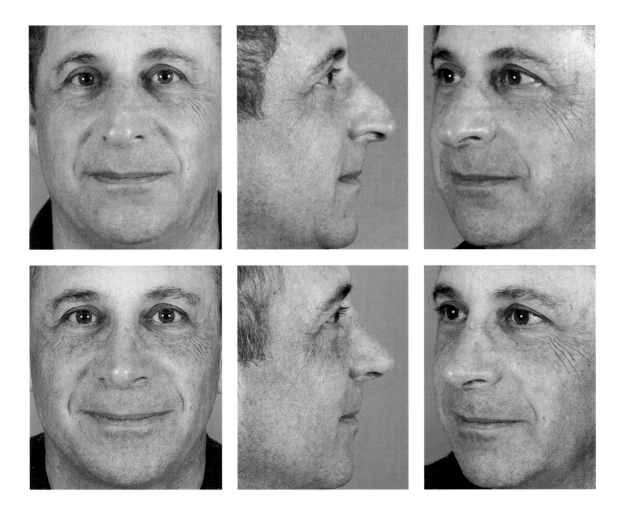

The patient is shown 9 months postoperatively with a straight nose and improved nasofacial balance. The nasal length as well as tip projection is normal. Note the straight dorsum and improved dorsal aesthetic lines on the lateral and oblique views.

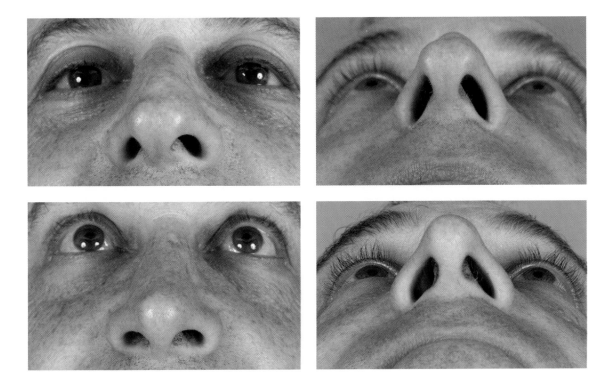

The basal view reveals correction of alar notching. However, slight fullness of the left caudal septum persists; palpation shows this to result from soft tissue at the feet of the crura that has retained memory from the long-standing septal deviation.

■ KEY POINTS

■ Severely dorsally deviated noses almost always have a major septal deformity as a component. Straightening the septum is the key to achieving good functional and aesthetic results.

■ Nasal deviations can be classified into three basic types: The straight septal tilt off the vomer, the C-shaped and reverse C-shaped deformities (usually without bony pyramid deviation), and the S-shaped deformity involving a deviated bony pyramid.

■ The open rhinoplasty approach is preferred for correction of the deviated nose. All deviated structures should be widely mobilized to allow for replacement in a correct anatomic position.

■ Mucoperichondrial attachments should be maintained when possible; however, they must be widely released from the deviated parts of the septum and osseocartilaginous skeleton. Intrinsic and extrinsic deforming forces must be completely released to achieve adequate correction.

■ The septum is then straightened; this may involve resection of the deviated portion, scoring and/or morselization, and anatomic reduction to the midline with a 5-0 PDS suture to the contralateral periosteum of the nasal spine.

■ Parallel full-thickness cuts through 50% of the dorsal L-strut should be made for a high dorsal septal deviation to allow the septum to be straightened, but this will result in long-term loss of support.

■ To restore septal support, spreader grafts 5 to 6 mm in height and 30 to 32 mm in length should be secured to the dorsal septum with at least two 5-0 PDS sutures. These will also maintain the integrity of the internal nasal valves and if placed asymmetrically will camouflage any residual septal deviation. Dorsal aesthetic lines will be restored to normal.

■ Contralateral inferior turbinate hypertrophy follows severe septal deviation. This must be addressed with submucous resection of the hypertrophied bone and outfracturing of the inferior turbinate to allow adequate room for septal repositioning and to maintain patency of the airway postoperatively.

■ If bony pyramid deviation is present, precisely planned osteotomies should be performed using the external percutaneous osteotome. These may include lateral osteotomies, medial osteotomies if bony asymmetry requiring independent nasal bone movement is present, or double-level osteotomies if intrinsic nasal bone deviation is present. When the nasal pyramid is asymmetric, dorsal reduction must be done obliquely to prevent excess bone removal from the more vertically oriented side, which would become evident after anatomic repositioning of the nasal bones.

REFERENCES

1. Brian DF. The management of the deviated nose. J Laryngol Otol 95:471, 1981.
2. Dingman RO, Natvig P. The deviated nose. Clin Plast Surg 4:145, 1977.
3. Johnson CM, Anderson JR. The deviated nose—its correction. Laryngoscope 87:1680, 1977.
4. Planos J. The twisted nose. Clin Plast Surg 4:55, 1977.
5. Bernstein L. Submucous operations on the nasal septum. Otolaryngol Clin North Am 6:675, 1973.
6. Edwards N. Septoplasty: Rational surgery of the nasal septum. J Laryngol Otol 89:875, 1975.
7. McKinney P, Shively R. Straightening the twisted nose. Plast Reconstr Surg 64:176, 1979.
8. Rohrich RJ, Adams WP Jr. Late salvage of nasal injuries. Operative Tech Plast Surg 5:342, 1998.
9. Dingman RO. Correction of nasal deformities due to defects of the septum. Plast Reconstr Surg 18:291, 1956.
10. Gorney M. Septum in rhinoplasty. In Millard DR, ed. Symposium on Corrective Rhinoplasty, vol 13. St Louis: CV Mosby, 1976, p 180.
11. Killian G. The submucous window resection of the nasal septum. Ann Otol Rhinol Laryngol 14:363, 1905.

12. Spector M. Partial resection of the interior turbinates. Ear Nose Throat J 61:28, 1982.

13. Converse JM. Corrective surgery of nasal deviations. Arch Otolaryngol 52:671, 1950.

14. Fry H. Interlocked stresses in human nasal septal cartilage. Br J Plast Surg 19:276, 1966.

15. Fry H. Nasal skeletal trauma and the interlocked stresses of the nasal septal cartilage. Br J Plast Surg 20:146, 1967.

16. Gibson T, Davis B. The distortion of autogenous cartilage grafts: Its cause and prevention. Br J Plast Surg 10:257, 1958.

17. Teichgraeber JF. Management of the nasal airway. Dallas Rhinoplasty Symp 12:225, 1997.

18. Courtiss EH, Gargan TJ, Courtiss GB. Nasal physiology. Ann Plast Surg 13:214, 1984.

19. Rohrich RJ. Discussion of Guyuron B, Uzzo CD, Scull H. A practical classification of septonasal deviation and an effective guide to septal surgery. Plast Reconstr Surg 104:2210, 1999.

20. Byrd HS, Salomon J, Flood J. Correction of the crooked nose. Plast Reconstr Surg 102:2148, 1998.

21. Verwoerd CDA. Present day treatment of nasal fractures: Closed versus open reduction. Facial Plast Surg 8:220, 1992.

22. Murray JA, Maran AGD, MacKenzie J, et al. Open versus closed reduction of the fractured nose. Arch Otolaryngol 110:797, 1984.

23. Gunter JP, Rohrich RJ. Management of the deviated nose. Clin Plast Surg 15:43, 1988.

24. Sheen JH, Sheen AP. Aesthetic Rhinoplasty, 2nd ed. St Louis: Quality Medical Publishing, 1998 (reprint of 1987 ed.).

25. Sheen JH. Spreader grafts: A method of reconstructing the roof of the middle nasal vault following rhinoplasty. Plast Reconstr Surg 73:230, 1984.

26. Rohrich RJ, Sheen J. Secondary rhinoplasty. In Grotting JC, ed. Reoperative Aesthetic and Reconstructive Plastic Surgery. St Louis: Quality Medical Publishing, 1995.

27. Rohrich RJ, Hollier LH. Use of spreader grafts in the external approach to rhinoplasty. Clin Plast Surg 23:255, 1996.

45

The Crooked Nose:
An Algorithm for Repair

H. Steve Byrd, M.D. ▪ James D. Burt, M.B.B.S., F.R.A.C.S.

*C*orrection of the crooked nose necessitating repair of a deviated dorsal or caudal septum remains one of the most challenging problems in rhinoplasty. Accomplished surgeons tend to be divided as to the best surgical approach. An anatomic reconstruction provides optimal contour and nasal dimensions at the risk of weakening the supporting bony and cartilaginous skeleton, creating the potential for collapse.[1-4] Alternatively, camouflage techniques preserve maximal structural support but may require aesthetic compromise in patients with overly prominent dorsums and dorsal aesthetic lines that are wide, divergent, or asymmetric.[5,6] (Both groups are characterized by aggravating recurrences and revision rates.)

Anatomic reconstruction of the crooked nose provides optimal contour and nasal dimension at the risk of weakening the osseocartilaginous support.

We will describe a sequence of repair that provides structural realignment with release of deforming forces while preserving or reconstructing the key skeletal support.

RELEASE OF DEFORMING FORCES

Forces causing cartilaginous septal deviation may be extrinsic or intrinsic to the septal cartilage. Extrinsic forces include those secondary to deviation of the nasal pyramid, forces acting through the attachments of the upper lateral cartilages, and forces from deviation or injury to the vomer, perpendicular plate of the ethmoid, or maxillary crest.

Deforming forces responsible for cartilaginous septal deviation may be either intrinsic or extrinsic.

Release of these extrinsic forces may allow correction of the cartilaginous septal deformity; failure to achieve complete release contributes to recurrence. Intrinsic deforming forces may be secondary to the growth and development of the septal cartilage or due to injury to the cartilage itself. Intrinsic deviating forces must be overcome by weakening the cartilage or by overpowering the deforming forces with sutures or grafts.

Exposure

An open rhinoplasty with a dorsal approach to the septum is preferred for both dorsal and caudal septal deviations. This is achieved through an infracartilaginous incision connected to a transcolumellar step incision, which allows complete degloving of the tip and midvault with dissection over the perichondrium. If deviation of the nasal pyramid is present, dissection is extended in a subperiosteal plane over the bony dorsum.

Lower Lateral Cartilages

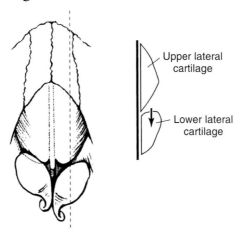

Deforming forces in the cartilaginous midvault frequently extend into the tip, producing asymmetry, buckling, and deviation of the lower lateral cartilages. Detachment of the lower lateral cartilages from the upper scroll by the addition of an intercartilaginous incision or through direct release sparing the mucosal incision frees the tip from these deforming forces. Furthermore, this maneuver allows caudal and downward retraction of the lower lateral cartilages, improving visualization of the dorsal and caudal septum.

Release of the lower lateral cartilages from the upper scroll frees the tip from deforming forces.

Septal Degloving

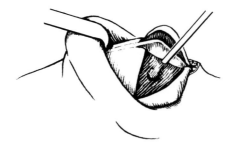

Dorsal submucoperichondrial degloving of both sides of the septum is undertaken. This is begun at the anterior septal angle using scalpel dissection with the lower lateral cartilages retracted caudally and down. The caudal 1 cm of the septum is routinely dissected with a No. 15 blade down to its attachments with the nasal spine. As the dissection proceeds cephalad along the caudal septum, the perichondrium is less densely adherent and can be elevated with a Cottle elevator over the remainder of the septum, perpendicular plate, and cephalad portion of the vomer. The final step in septal degloving involves dissection in the subperiosteal plane over the vomerine-maxillary crest. The transition from the subperichondrial septal plane to the subperiosteal plane is best achieved by initiating the subperiosteal plane from the spine cephalad, thereby elevating the mucoperiosteum away from the point of breakthrough and avoiding a mucosal tear or buttonhole.

Detachment of the Upper Lateral Cartilages From the Septum

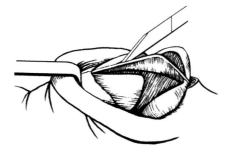

The first extrinsic force on the septal cartilage to be released is the attachment of the upper lateral cartilages to the dorsal septum. This release is achieved by sharply extending the subperichondrial dissection of the dorsal septum across the upper lateral cartilages flush with the septal sidewall. This submucosal release preserves the integrity of the lining while freeing the dorsal septum from any deforming forces resulting from previous injury or deformity of the nasal sidewall.

Nasal Bones

The next extrinsic force on the septal cartilage to be released is that produced by deviation of the bony pyramid. In some patients the bony and cartilaginous skeletons are actually shifted in opposite directions. In these patients correction of the bony deviation may actually worsen the septal deformity.

The deformity of the bony pyramid can generally be separated into one of three categories: a symmetric pyramid that is deviated from the aesthetic midline, a deviated pyramid with a prominent dorsum, and a deviated pyramid with asymmetry of the nasal bones.

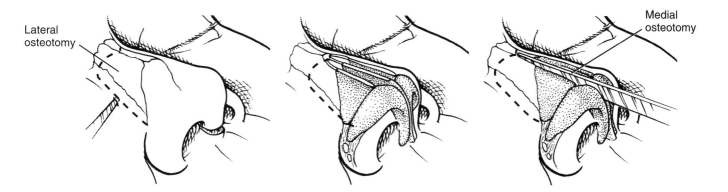

In the first category a shift of a symmetric pyramid to midline is achieved through lateral percutaneous osteotomies and greenstick fracture of the perpendicular plate of the ethmoid, preserving the roof of the bony dorsum. In the second category resection of the prominent bony dorsum is followed by lateral percutaneous osteotomies. The open roof of the dorsum allows independent and differential movement of the nasal bones. In the third category medial osteotomies followed by lateral percutaneous osteotomies are performed. The medial osteotomies are necessary to break the continuity of the bony dorsum, thereby allowing independent and differential movement of the nasal bones without reducing dorsal height. Lateral percutaneous osteotomies are required for each category. These osteotomies must be carefully executed with a sharp 2 mm osteotome, avoiding branches of the angular artery and vein so that bleeding and swelling are minimized.[7] The medial periosteum and mucosal lining should be preserved.

Lateral percutaneous osteotomies are required for all categories of osseous deformity.

SEPTAL REPAIR

After release of all extrinsic forces and the deviated septum, including repositioning of the bony nasal pyramid, the intrinsic forces on the dorsal and caudal septum are repaired in a graduated approach.

Septal Resection

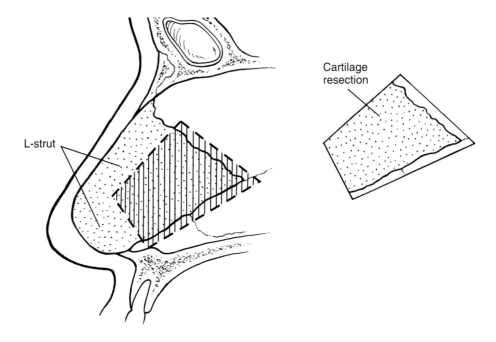

Significant intrinsic and extrinsic deforming forces in the dorsal and caudal septum are eliminated by midseptal resection that includes the attached perpendicular plate of the ethmoid and vomer. This large segment of cartilage and bone should be resected in continuity while preserving an 8 to 10 mm dorsal and caudal L-strut of septal cartilage. The resected bone and cartilage are preserved for later use as grafts when reconstruction is begun.

Midseptal resection is used to overcome significant intrinsic and extrinsic deforming forces.

Caudal Septal Repositioning

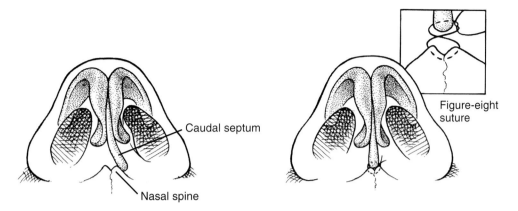

If the caudal base of the L-strut is not positioned in the aesthetic midline, it should be sharply detached from the maxillary crest and nasal spine and suture affixed to the midline. It should be emphasized that congenital deformity and injury may contribute to an off midline position of the spine and maxilla, thereby producing malposition and deviation through the attached base of the caudal septum. Once the base of the caudal septum is fully detached and mobilized, it can be readily held in the midline by suture fixation to the periosteal and soft tissue attachments of the maxilla.

Correction of the Septal L-Strut

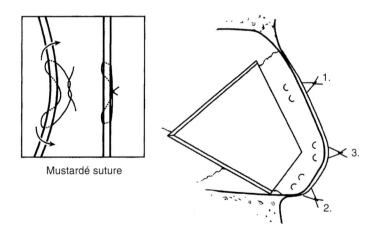

Following release of the upper lateral cartilage correction of the proximal bony deviation, resection of the midseptal deformity, and repositioning of the base of the caudal septum, the dorsal and caudal L-strut may have minimal residual deformity or deviation. When the L-strut is straight, scoring, morselization, or partial transection is unnecessary, and the surgeon should proceed with grafts or repair.

When curvature or deviation remains in the L-strut, the residual intrinsic deforming forces should be countered by permanent horizontal control sutures. These control sutures are placed in a Mustardé configuration.[8] The axis of the suture is exactly perpendicular to the concave surface of the cartilage, and the knot is placed on the convex side. As the suture is tightened, it effectively shortens the cord length of the convex surface, thereby straightening the cartilage. If the cartilage is resistant to bending, light scoring of the concave surface may be necessary. Scoring should be limited to a degree that allows the suture to produce straightening but that minimizes structural weakening. The curvature of the dorsal and caudal L-strut should each be controlled with independent sutures, and frequently a third obliquely oriented suture is required to reorient the anterior septal angle.

Should deformity of the septal L-strut persist, permanent horizontal control sutures are used to achieve straightening.

TIP AND MIDVAULT RECONSTRUCTION
Structural Repair

Once all intrinsic and extrinsic deforming forces have been released and the residual septal L-strut has been repositioned in the midline and straightened with sutures, the tip and midvault must be reconstructed to preserve the structural integrity and functional outcome. Septal support grafts and accurate suture reconstruction of the released cartilages are the keys to this phase of the algorithm.

Septal Extension Grafts

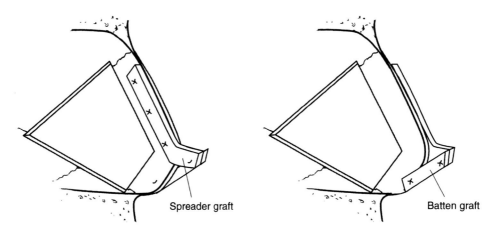

Spreader graft   Batten graft

Grafts from the resected portion of the midseptum and perpendicular plate of the ethmoid are added to increase the strength of the L-strut and to provide tip support. They are secured either flush with the dorsal septum as a spreader graft[5] or recessed below the caudal septal edge as a batten graft. These septal extension grafts are secured to the septal L-strut with multiple mattress sutures and extend as a coupled pair into the tip lobule complex. Any inherent curvature of these grafts is neutralized by its partner as they are sandwiched to embrace the septal L-strut. By using the opposing forces of the two grafts, scoring and morselization are generally not needed to maximize the strength of the grafts.

When the septal extension graft is placed in the spreader graft position flush with the dorsal septum between the upper lateral cartilage and septum, it serves to widen the cartilaginous midvault.[5] In the presence of dorsal septal deviation the spreader graft is usually required on the concave side of the deformity since the upper lateral cartilage on the concave side will bow in toward the deviation and will need to be laterally displaced to correct the concavity. When midvault outward bowing is present on the convex side of the dorsum, the extension graft should be placed as a batten graft below the junction of the septum and the upper lateral cartilage. Batten grafts may also be placed in an oblique position across the anterior septum at the junction of the dorsal and caudal L-strut to strengthen and straighten the septal angle.

In addition to supporting the septum, we prefer the septal extension graft for controlling tip position and definition.[9] By securing the position of the tip to an extension of a fixed facial structure, control of tip projection and rotation is maintained without the use of a columellar strut. The graft extends into the tip lobule complex with its inferior extent at the cephalic border of the junction of the medial and middle crura (columellar-lobular angle). From this point it extends up between the domes to create the desired columellar-lobular angle and degree of tip projection. From its domal extent it drops back to the anterior septal angle, securing the desired level of differential between the anterior septum and the tip. In noses with thin skin the desired differential is approximately 6 mm, whereas in noses with thick skin it should be increased to 10 mm. The angle incorporated into the extension graft at the domes dramatically affects the dorsum-tip relationship. Measured from a plane vertical to the face, an angle of 45 degrees or less will produce a supratip break, whereas an angle greater than 60 degrees will result in a straight dorsum.

Anterior septal extension grafts extend into the tip lobule complex with its inferior extent at the cephalic border of the junction of the medial and middle crura (columellar-lobular angle).

Repair of the Upper Lateral Cartilages

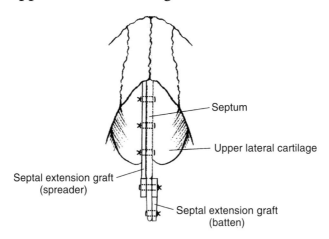

Repair of the Lower Lateral Cartilages

Viewed from above the dorsal septum and extension grafts should be in the exact aesthetic midline. Slight variations can be corrected as the upper lateral cartilages are secured to the dorsum through the use of clocking sutures. These corrections are accomplished by using the attachments of the upper lateral cartilages to nasal bones to pull the septum back to midline with permanent sutures. On the concave side of the deformity the upper lateral cartilage is sutured to the extended spreader graft, whereas on the convex side it is sutured directly to the dorsal septum to eliminate the outward bowing.

Repair of the Lower Lateral Cartilages

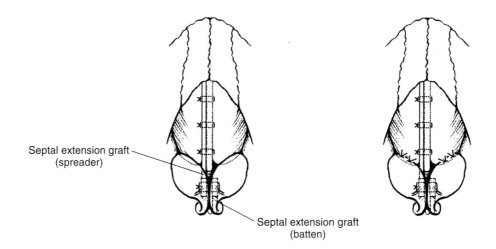

The symmetry of the lateral crus and domes is evaluated while viewing from above. The interdomal ligament is sutured to the domal segment of the extension graft, thereby securing tip projection and rotation. Points along the cephalic border of the lateral crus are held to the anterior septal angle at the point where the extension graft joins the septum. These points are adjusted until ideal symmetry between the sides is achieved, and they are sutured to the septum and extension graft at these points. A second suture attaches the midportion of the cephalic border of the lateral crus back to the upper lateral cartilage scroll. The cephalic border of the lateral crus between the domes and point of fixation to the anterior septum is trimmed to conform to the profile contour of the extension graft. Minimal trimming is required, and any residual convexity or depression in the lateral crus is corrected by a combination of lateral crural spanning sutures or alar spreader grafts.[7,10]

Soft Tissue Repair

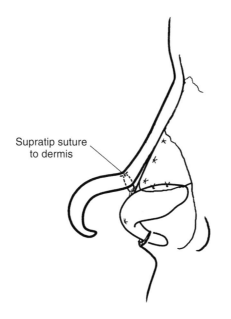

Aside from closure of mucosal and skin incisions, it is useful to suture the soft tissue ligament at the junction of the dorsum and tip lobule complex (supratip ligament) to the anterior septal angle. This subcutaneous closure helps reduce dead space in the supratip and improves the predictability of definition between the dorsum and tip. Closure of the septal mucosa with through-and-through mattress sutures completes the repair. A small mucosal perforation on one side of the septum will allow blood to drain from the space if there is a tendency for it to accumulate. Splints or packs are generally not used.

CASE ANALYSIS

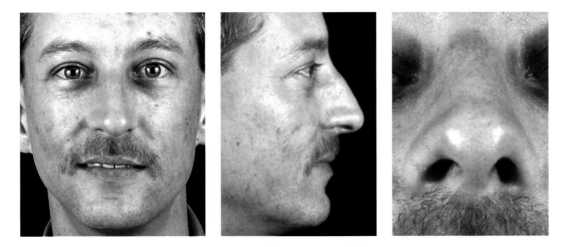

This 33-year-old man with a crooked nose as a result of an old nasal fracture had a C-shaped deformity of the septum to the right with complete airway obstruction on the right side. The dorsal aesthetic lines were indistinct due to the nasal deviation and a tip that was off midline.

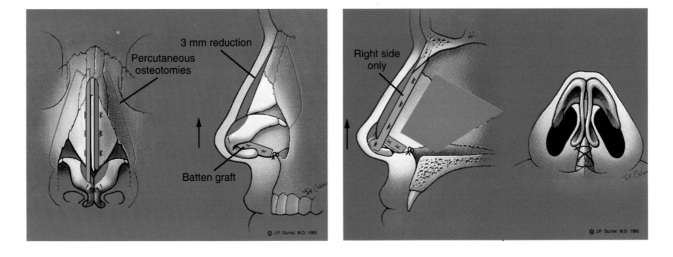

An open primary rhinoplasty was performed to release the extrinsic and intrinsic forces. Treatment included a small cephalic trim, septal degloving and release of the upper lateral cartilages from the septum, 3 mm osseocartilaginous reduction, septal resection, percutaneous lateral osteotomies, repositioning of the caudal septal L-strut with a nasal spine suture, and placement of a right-sided septal extension graft in the spreader position and a left-sided batten graft to control tip projection and stabilize the L-strut. A horizontal control suture was used on the caudal septum to straighten this as well as suture techniques on the tip.

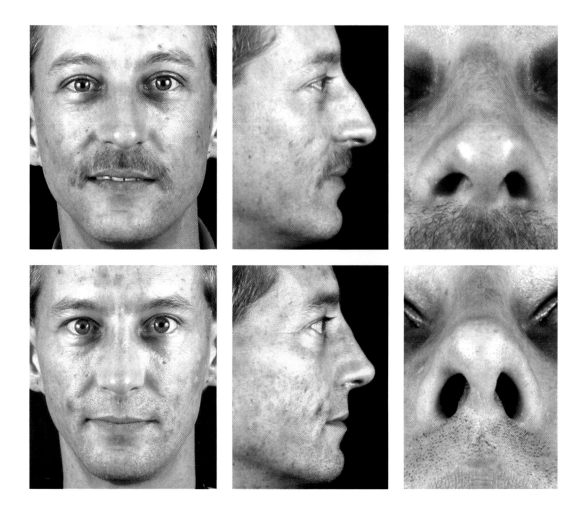

The result is seen 1 year after correction of the crooked nose deformity. The patient's airway has remained patent.

■ KEY POINTS

■ An anatomic reconstruction of the nose is generally preferred when deviation involves the dorsal and caudal septum. Camouflage techniques are reserved for sidewall depressions when the airway is normal and there is no compensatory outward bowing on the opposite side.

■ The algorithm we propose removes all extrinsic forces on the residual septal L-strut, preserves maximal intrinsic integrity by minimizing scoring and employing control sutures, increases the strength and structure of the L-strut while improving midvault (internal valve) physiology through the use of extended spreader and batten grafts, frees the tip from deforming forces carried through the septum, and provides control of tip projection, rotation, and shape through extension grafts off the septum.

■ Questions have been raised as to the physiologic validity of extended spreader grafts placed along the dorsal septum that would possibly blunt or obliterate the internal valve angle. In our experience the normal 10- to 15-degree internal valve angle is of diagnostic significance since it allows the surgeon to identify an overly narrow midvault when the angle is reduced. However, when the angle is blunted or reduced from the use of a spreader graft, any loss of airway space from this change is more than compensated for by the lateral displacement of the cartilaginous sidewall. Airway function has universally improved.

REFERENCES

1. Johnson CM, Anders JR. The deviated nose: Its correction. Laryngoscope 87:1680, 1977.
2. Rees TD. Surgical correction of the severely deviated nose by extramucosal excision of the osseocartilaginous septum and replacement as a free graft. Plast Reconstr Surg 78:320, 1986.
3. Jugo SB. Total septal reconstruction through a decortication approach in children. Arch Otolaryngol Head Neck Surg 113:173, 1987.
4. Gunter JP, Rohrich RJ. Management of the deviated nose. The importance of septal reconstruction. Clin Plast Surg 15:43, 1988.
5. Sheen JH, Sheen AP. Aesthetic Rhinoplasty, 2nd ed. St. Louis: Quality Medical Publishing, 1998 (reprint of 1987 ed.).
6. Constantian MB. An algorithm for correcting the asymmetrical nose. Plast Reconstr Surg 83:801, 1989.
7. Tebbetts JB. Open rhinoplasty: More than an incisional approach. Rethinking the logic, sequence, and techniques of rhinoplasty. Dallas Rhinoplasty Symp, p 67, 1993.
8. Mustardé JC. The treatment of prominent ears by buried mattress sutures: A ten-year survey. Plast Reconstr Surg 39:382, 1967.
9. Byrd HS, Andochick S, Copit S, Walton KG. Septal extension grafts: A method of controlling tip projection, rotation, and shape. Plast Reconstr Surg 100:999, 1997.
10. Gunter JP, Rohrich RJ. Correction of the pinched nasal tip with alar spreader grafts. Plast Reconstr Surg 90:821, 1992.
11. Byrd HS, Salomon J, Flood J. Correction of the crooked nose. Plast Reconstr Surg 102:2148, 1998.

The illustrations on pp. 817 to 818 and 821 (bottom) to 825 are reprinted from Byrd HS, Salomon J, Flood J. Correction of the crooked nose. Plast Reconstr Surg 102:2148, 1998.

46

Innovative Surgical Management of the Crooked Nose

Dean M. Toriumi, M.D. ▪ Deborah Watson, M.D.

$\mathcal{S}$uccessful management of the crooked nose deformity requires accurate preoperative diagnosis, knowledge of the structural anatomy of the nose, and awareness of any long-term consequences of different surgical techniques. Deviated segments of the nose are usually shifted back to the midline by manipulating cartilage, performing osteotomies, or realigning other structural attachments. However, nasal structures cannot be altered in a way that will compromise major nasal support structures. Absolute correction of the deviated nose is difficult because of the complexity of the structural defect and the highly visible, well-defined subunits of the nasal dorsum. For example, the nasal structure may be aligned in the midline, but the nose may appear crooked because of a residual concavity or convexity along one of the borders of the dorsal nasal subunit. Natural lighting from above will pass tangentially over such contour defects and cast shadows that can accentuate dorsal irregularities and create the illusion of a crooked nose.

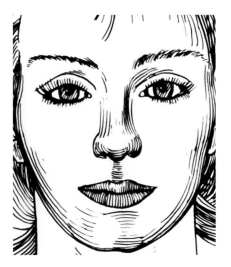

Ideally, a contour line created in part by shadows extends from the brow and dorsal nasal subunit to the tip-defining point. Any break or deviation of the dorsal nasal contour line may give the nose a crooked or irregular appearance. Absolute correction of the crooked nose deformity will require the surgeon to become familiar with conventional methods (septoplasty, osteotomies, tissue excision, grafting, etc.) as well as to be able to improvise when encountering variant nasal anatomy.

We will describe a graduated approach to the crooked nose, highlighting novel techniques that feature more aggressive tissue modification without loss of nasal support or compromise of nasal function.

Any break or deviation of the dorsal nasal contour line may give the nose a crooked or irregular appearance.

SUPPORT MECHANISMS OF THE NOSE

The major support mechanisms of the lower third of the nose include (1) the lower lateral cartilages, (2) the fibrous attachment between the cephalic margin of the lateral crura and the caudal margin of the upper lateral cartilage, (3) the soft tissue attachment between the cephalic margin of the medial crura and the caudal margin of the nasal septum, and (4) the interdomal ligament attaching the domes to the anterior septal angle.[1] Two of these major support mechanisms of the nose (attachment of the medial crura to the caudal septum and the interdomal ligament) are dependent on the structural integrity of the caudal region of the nasal septum. If the caudal septum is compromised to the point where it cannot provide support to the lower third of the nose, there may be a significant loss of tip support and projection.

Manipulation of the cartilaginous nasal septum must be performed in a manner that preserves a continuous cartilaginous strut between the bony septum at the osseocartilaginous junction (rhinion) and the posterior septal angle at the nasal spine.

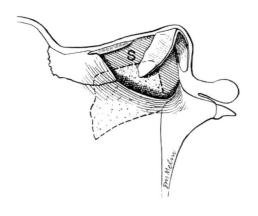

An L-shaped strut of septal cartilage composed of an anterior (dorsal) and caudal segment will act to support the lower lateral cartilages at the interdomal ligament and at its connection to the medial crura. The width of the strut should be at least 1.5 cm and composed of rigid straight cartilage. If the cartilage of the L-shaped septal strut is crooked or unstable, support of the lower third of the nose may become compromised. The significance of the support provided by the caudal septum can be demonstrated by performing a full transfixion incision and observing the resultant decrease in nasal tip projection.

Therefore the integrity of the L-shaped septal strut and all of its support attachments must be strengthened or reconstituted if these attachments are weakened or divided.

An L-shaped strut of septal cartilage composed of an anterior (dorsal) and caudal segment will support the lower lateral cartilages at the interdomal ligament and at its connection to the medial crura.

The nose can be divided into thirds, with the upper third supported primarily by bone and the lower two thirds supported primarily by cartilage. The difference in tissue composition between the upper third and lower two thirds of the nose necessitates different methods of treatment. Modification of the contour of the upper third of the nose requires primarily bony work using osteotomies and rasps, whereas modification of the lower two thirds of the nose entails primarily cartilage and soft tissue manipulation. Correction of deformities of the cartilaginous lower two thirds of the nose is most difficult because of the inherent memory of cartilaginous tissues and their tendency to persist in a deviated state.

Modification of the contour of the upper third of the nose requires primarily bony work using osteotomies and rasps, whereas modification of the lower two thirds of the nose entails primarily cartilage and soft tissue manipulation.

UPPER THIRD OF THE NOSE

Before shifting the bony nasal vault back to the midline the dorsal profile must be assessed to determine if reduction of a dorsal hump will be required. If a dorsal hump is to be resected, the orientation of the bony vault must be taken into account in the actual hump removal. In the severely deviated bony vault less bone may need to be excised from the nasal bone on the side of deviation that more closely approximates a vertical orientation. This maneuver will prevent excessive reduction in height of the vertically oriented nasal bone.

Less bone may need to be excised from the nasal bone on the side of deviation that more closely approximates a vertical orientation.

If the deviated segment is limited to the upper third of the nose, bilateral medial and lateral osteotomies will usually permit the bony vault to be shifted back to the midline. Not infrequently, however, inadequate osteotomies may result in a greenstick fracture, and the bony nasal vault may deviate during the postoperative period because of the memory of the tissues. In some cases double lateral osteotomies can be performed to ensure complete mobilization of the bony vault and decrease the likelihood of postoperative deformity. Execution of double lateral osteotomies may actually result in comminution of the nasal bones and not two distinct cuts in the bone. Therefore special care must be taken not to free up the periosteum from the nasal bones because comminuted segments of bone may become displaced.

> *Inadequate osteotomies may result in a greenstick fracture, causing the bony nasal vault to deviate during the postoperative period.*

LOWER TWO THIRDS OF THE NOSE

In most crooked noses the lower two thirds of the nose is at least partially involved in the deformity. In these cases the upper lateral cartilages may need to be freed from the anterior (dorsal) border of the nasal septum to allow these cartilaginous structures to reorient themselves in the midline. If the lower two thirds of the nose is not reoriented after osteotomies, the nose may shift back toward the preoperative orientation and heal in a crooked position because of the memory of the deviated cartilaginous structures.[2]

> *Failure to reorient the lower two thirds of the nose after osteotomies may result in the nose shifting back toward the preoperative position.*

NASAL VALVE

The nasal valve is a triangular-shaped opening defined by the caudal margin of the upper lateral cartilage, the nasal septum, and the floor of the piriform aperture.[3] Inferomedial collapse of the caudal margin of the upper lateral cartilage can result in significant compromise of the cross-sectional area of the nasal valve with subsequent nasal obstruction. In some cases the inferior turbinate influences the cross-sectional area of the nasal valve, and its positioning must be taken into account when performing functional nasal surgery.

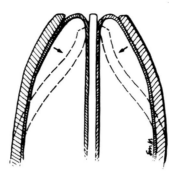

When the upper lateral cartilages are divided from the nasal septum, there is a significant risk of inferior and medial collapse of the upper lateral cartilages with subsequent compromise of the nasal valve.[4] Other maneuvers that can increase the degree of inferomedial collapse of the upper lateral cartilages include cephalic trim of the lateral crura, cutting the mucosa that connects the septum and upper lateral cartilages, and infracture of the nasal bones.

Dividing the upper lateral cartilages from the nasal septum may contribute to inferior and medial collapse of the upper lateral cartilages with subsequent compromise of the nasal valve.

OPERATIVE TECHNIQUE

To prevent valve collapse, several special surgical maneuvers can be implemented to help preserve the normal position of the upper lateral cartilages. During the septoplasty segment of the operation a hemitransfixion incision can be used to access the septum.

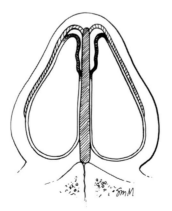

Bilateral subperichondrial flaps can be elevated all the way up to the point where the nasal septum meets the upper lateral cartilage at the apex of the nasal vault.[4]

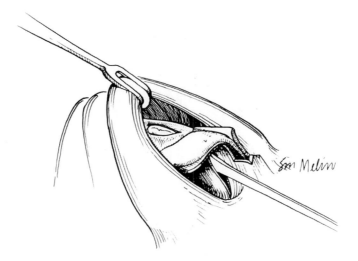

A Freer elevator can then be advanced to the apex of the nasal vault and used to divide the upper lateral cartilage from the nasal septum without violating the intranasal mucosa. Preservation of the intranasal mucosa will help prevent collapse of the upper lateral cartilages because the mucosa will support the cartilages and minimize inferomedial displacement. The open approach provides direct visualization of this dissection and allows the surgeon to manipulate the nasal septum from above (open approach) and below (hemitransfixion incision). After soft tissue is dissected off the nasal dorsum, the Freer elevator can be inserted into the hemitransfixion incision, which can then be directly visualized as the instrument is used to divide the upper lateral cartilage from the nasal septum.

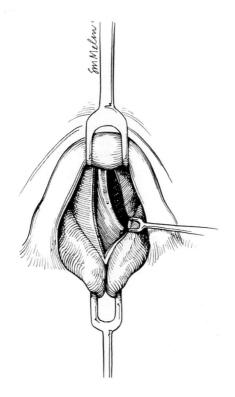

Once the nasal septum is released from the upper lateral cartilages, the actual degree of deviation of the anterior (dorsal) segment of the L-shaped septal strut can be determined. A deviated L-shaped septal strut can be visualized from above (open approach) after attachments to the upper lateral cartilages have been released. In this case the primary component of the deviation is in the region of the anterior septal angle. If only a minor cartilaginous deviation exists, the nose may shift to the midline with little difficulty after medial and lateral osteotomies are completed. At this point the upper lateral cartilages are sutured to the septum near the anterior septal angle to prevent collapse of the upper lateral cartilages.

The upper lateral cartilages are sutured to the septum near the anterior septal angle to prevent their collapse.

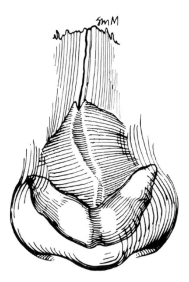

In some cases a significant residual deviation of the anterior (dorsal) border of the nasal septum will be noted. These deviations may involve the entire cartilaginous septum or could represent an isolated deformity of the caudal segment of the L-shaped septal strut. Patients with a C-shaped deformity have a dorsal concavity on one side of the nose and a convexity on the opposite side. If the caudal septum is in the midline, camouflaging techniques can be used to correct mild to moderate C-shaped deformities of the L-shaped septal strut so that the dorsal nasal subunit appears straight. With the septum exposed from above by the open approach the anterior (dorsal) border of the nasal septum can be shaved in a tangential plane on the convex side to allow the upper lateral cartilage to move medially. This conservative cartilage shave is performed to reduce the prominence of the convex component of the septal deformity without compromising the integrity of the L-shaped septal strut or nasal valve.

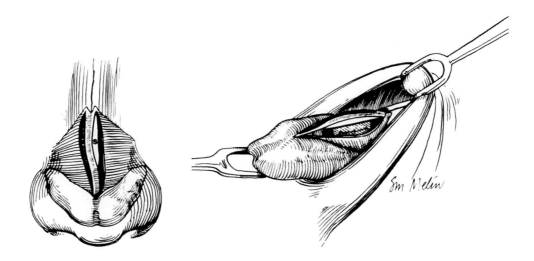

To help efface the concave component of the septal deformity, a unilateral planoconvex spreader graft can be inserted between the anterior (dorsal) border of the nasal septum and the upper lateral cartilage.[5] The graft is inserted above the intact intranasal mucosa to prevent contamination or exposure of the graft. This spreader graft will act to efface the concavity of the C-shaped deformity and also help preserve the cross-sectional area of the nasal valve. The graft is carefully carved from septal cartilage to a size that will fill the concave component of the C-shaped deformity. It should be made slightly larger than the defect to account for changes in the ipsilateral upper lateral cartilage. The graft can be sutured into position with a 5-0 PDS mattress suture that incorporates the nasal septum and graft. The needle can be straightened before suturing to allow more precise suture placement. Once the graft is in position, both upper lateral cartilages are sutured to the septum near the caudal end of the spreader graft. At this point the skin can be redraped and the deformity examined and palpated. If a residual concavity exists, a separate onlay cartilage graft can be placed lateral to the upper lateral cartilage to completely efface the defect. This method of camouflaging the C-shaped deformity does not correct the underlying anterior (dorsal) septal deviation. If the patient suffers from nasal airway obstruction secondary to the septal deviation, more aggressive maneuvers may be necessary to straighten the cartilaginous dorsum and open the airway. Spreader grafts on both sides of the septum are more effective than a unilateral spreader graft and are used to create a straight dorsal septum and maintain airway patency.

A separate onlay cartilage graft can be placed lateral to the upper lateral cartilage to completely efface the residual defect.

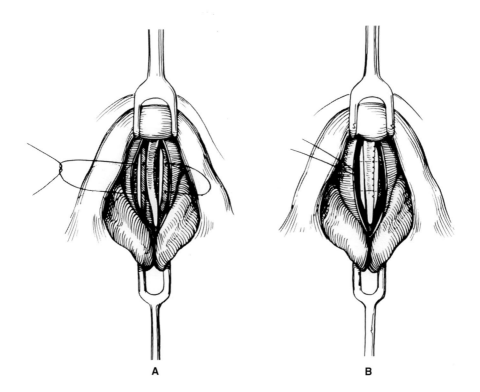

A   B

With larger C-shaped deformities bilateral spreader grafts or ethmoid bone stenting grafts can be used to straighten the deformed anterior (dorsal) segment of the L-shaped septal strut *(A)*. If appropriate cartilage is not available, thin ethmoid bone can be harvested from the nasal septum and carefully cut into rectangular grafts measuring 5 to 12 mm in length and 3 to 5 mm in width. A fine rasp can be used to file down any irregularities of the bone grafts, which must be relatively thin and flat before placement. Large Keith needles can be used to hand drill two holes into each bone graft. The holes must be just large enough to allow introduction of a straightened needle on the 5-0 PDS suture that will be used to fix the graft into position. If available, a low-speed hand-held drill can be used to drill the holes into the bone grafts. The holes should be separated by at least 3 mm and must be positioned so that the holes in each graft are opposite corresponding holes in the contralateral graft *(B)*. Working with this thin bone is difficult because it may fracture while being manipulated. In the future stiff, moldable resorbable polymer sheets or plates may be used instead of ethmoid bone to stent the crooked cartilage into a straight orientation.

Bilateral spreader grafts or ethmoid bone stenting grafts can be used to straighten the deformed dorsal septum.

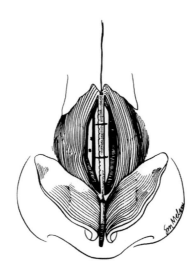

Before the spreader grafts or ethmoid bone stenting grafts are sutured into position, the deviated cartilage must be lightly crosshatched in a vertical direction on the concave side of the C-shaped deformity to help release the memory of the cartilage. The spreader grafts or bone grafts are sutured on opposite sides to sandwich the deviated cartilage and stent it into a straight orientation. A thicker graft can be placed on the concave side of the deformity to accommodate anatomic changes in the upper lateral cartilage.[6] A single 5-0 PDS mattress suture is used to fix the bone grafts into position with about 1 mm of septal cartilage above the edge of the grafts. This rim of cartilage along the anterior (dorsal) border will provide camouflage so that the grafts will not be visible or palpable along the dorsum of the nose. Once in position the deviation of the cartilage should be corrected without loss of support provided by the L-shaped septal strut. If available, a thin cartilage graft can be used as an onlay graft over the reconstructed nasal dorsum to ensure the stenting grafts are camouflaged.

After all of the grafts are in position the most anterocaudal corner of the upper lateral cartilage should be sutured to the region of the nasal septum near the anterior septal angle. This suture should be used whenever the upper lateral cartilages are divided from the septum and will help prevent inferomedial collapse of the upper lateral cartilages.

The caudal margin of the septal cartilage provides support for the lower third of the nose via attachments to the domes (interdomal ligament) and medial crura. If the caudal septum is severely deviated, there may be significant loss of nasal tip support with loss of tip projection. Major loss of caudal septal support can also result in an overly short, overrotated nose or a retracted columella. Therefore caudal septal deviations must be corrected for support purposes as well as for correction of airway obstruction. Relatively minor caudal septal deviations can be corrected by using cartilage manipulation and suturing techniques. Severe caudal septal deviations may require replacement of the deformed segment of the nasal septum with a straight piece of cartilage. Replacement of the deformed caudal segment of the nasal septum is an effective method for correcting the overly short, overrotated nose or retracted columella.

If the caudal septum is severely deviated, there may be significant loss of nasal tip support with loss of tip projection.

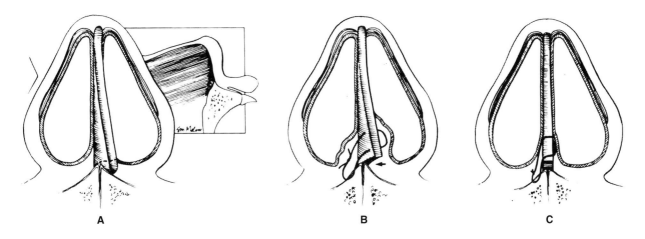

A **B** **C**

When the posterior septal angle is subluxated off the maxillary crest–nasal spine, the caudal septum can be fixed in the midline by trimming and suturing the posterior septal angle to the nasal spine region *(A)*. This technique is most effective when the anterior septal angle is in relatively good position and provides adequate tip support but the posterior septal angle is being forced off midline from compression on the nasal spine. Through a hemitransfixion incision a small triangle of cartilage at the posterior septal angle can be excised to allow the caudal septum to swing back to the midline *(B)*. The concave side of the deviation can be lightly crosshatched to release the memory of the cartilage. Finally, the deviated caudal septum is sutured to periosteum on the opposite side of the nasal spine to fix the septum in the midline *(C)*. When placing this suture care should be taken to avoid pulling down the posterior septal angle since this could result in a decrease in nasal tip projection.

If the posterior septal angle is subluxated off the maxillary crest–nasal spine, the caudal septum can be fixed in the midline by trimming and suturing the posterior septal angle to the nasal spine region.

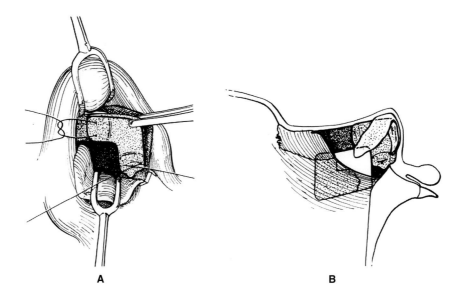

A   B

When the caudal septum, anterior septal angle, or a significant portion of the L-shaped septal strut is severely deviated or fractured, the deformed segment of nasal septum can be replaced.[7] If necessary, a major segment of the L-shaped septal strut can be replaced with an L-shaped piece of cartilage taken from another area (posteroinferior) of the nasal septum. Straight autologous septal cartilage harvested from the posteroinferior septum is the preferred grafting material for the L-shaped graft because it will not resorb or warp. The replacement L-shaped strut must be sutured to a stable cartilage remnant at the osseocartilaginous junction (rhinion) and nasal spine *(A)*. If no cartilage remnant exists in the region of the nasal spine, the L-shaped septal strut graft can be sutured to the periosteum in the region of the nasal spine. In the overrotated nose or retracted columella deformity the caudal length of the L-shaped strut can be increased to lengthen the nose or reorient the columella. The caudal extension of the graft can be sutured between the medial crura to act as a columellar strut and provide a stable structure to support the medial crura and domes *(B)*. If a caudal extension graft is used, anterior and caudal positioning is critical to set appropriate nasal length and projection. The mucosal incisions are closed after approximating the mucoperichondrial flaps and fixing the L-shaped septal strut between the flaps with a running catgut mattress suture. Finally, stiff intranasal septal splints (Reuter bivalve splint, Xomed-Treace, Jacksonville, Fla.) should be sutured on both sides of the septum to compress the flaps and support the L-shaped septal strut graft for at least 5 days. These patients should be kept on antibiotics for 7 to 10 days after surgery. Replacement of severely deformed L-shaped struts can provide a stable reconstruction with excellent dorsal nasal contour and long-term stability. However, if an appropriate cartilage replacement graft cannot be harvested from another region of the septum, this technique cannot be used.

The septal strut graft can be sutured between the medial crura to act as a columellar strut and provide a stable structure to support the medial crura and domes.

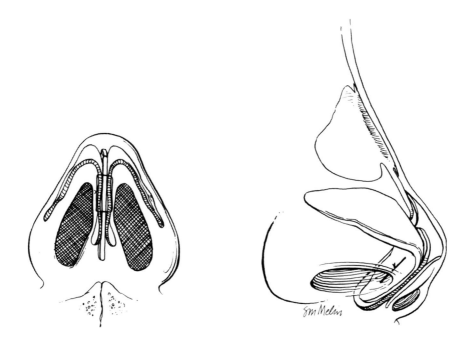

Noses that exhibit deviations of the caudal portion of the nasal septum and anterior septal angle frequently demonstrate a loss in nasal tip support and projection. After the L-shaped septal strut is corrected or reconstructed, a sutured-in-place columellar strut can be placed in a well-defined pocket between the medial crura.[4,8] These struts will act to increase tip support and create a stable medial crural–columellar strut complex that can then be fixed to a straight caudal septum via a precisely placed septocolumellar suture.[4,9]

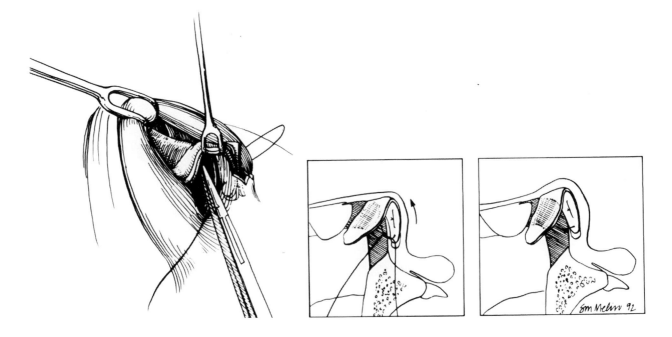

A temporary 5-0 Prolene suture is placed high on the caudal septum and low on the medial crural–columellar strut complex to preserve tip projection and stabilize the nasal tip. When a transfixion incision is used, this suture will support the tip while new fibrous attachments develop between the caudal septum and medial crural–columellar strut complex. The septocolumellar suture must be used in combination with a sutured-in-place columellar strut and only provides temporary support. These sutures can be left in place for up to 3 weeks or until the suture proves to be bothersome to the patient. In cases where maximal tip support is needed a 5-0 Prolene buried septocolumellar suture from low on the columellar strut (sutured between the medial crura) to high on the caudal septum can be left in place under the mucosa to provide long-term support. Properly placed buried septocolumellar sutures (low on the columellar strut to high on the caudal septum) can be used to increase nasal tip projection.[9]

A sutured-in-place columellar strut placed in a well-defined pocket between the medial crura will increase tip support and create a stable medial crural–columellar strut complex.

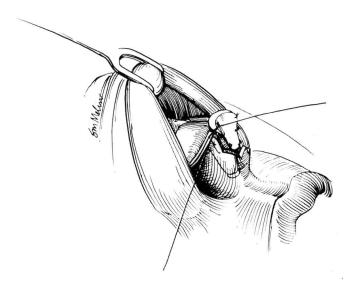

Sutured-in-place shield-shaped tip grafts can be used to provide increased tip projection, support, and a bidomal tip configuration.[4] Abnormal nasal development may have resulted in asymmetric lower lateral cartilages in some crooked noses. In such cases dome division with cartilage resection may be necessary to attain domal symmetry. When the domes are divided, however, the cartilages should be reconstituted with a suture to maintain an intact lower lateral cartilage structure.[4] The sutured-in-place shield-shaped tip graft can be fixed to the caudal margin of the medial crura to stabilize the lower lateral cartilages and help hide tip asymmetries. For maximal tip support a shield-shaped tip graft can be sutured to the caudal margin of the medial crural–columellar strut complex that is fixed to the caudal margin of a stable L-shaped septal strut via a septocolumellar suture. This structure concept of preservation or reconstitution of support mechanisms using specialized suture and grafting techniques can provide desirable contour changes without weakening the nasal structure.[4] Application of the structure concept in the management of the crooked nose can yield excellent results that will not deteriorate with the passage of time.

When the domes are divided, the cartilages should be reconstituted with sutures to maintain an intact lower lateral cartilage structure.

POSTOPERATIVE CARE

Patients undergoing major cartilage grafting are maintained on oral antibiotics for the first week after surgery. Any nasal packing is removed within 24 hours after surgery, and intranasal septal splints are kept in place for 5 days. Patients are asked to refrain from blowing their noses for at least 2 weeks to prevent any intranasal contamination of the grafts. If the open approach was used, sutures are removed from the transcolumellar incision after 5 days, and anti-tension taping is continued for at least 2 weeks.

The external nasal cast is removed relatively early (postoperative day 5) to allow careful examination of the nasal contour and initiation of nasal exercises to ensure a straight dorsal nasal contour. At 5 days the nasal bones are not completely healed, and a slight shift in the bony nasal vault may be corrected by applying repeated pressure to the malpositioned nasal bone. The possibility of such an exercise is discussed before surgery so patients are not confused about the necessity of such management.

CONCLUSION

Management of the crooked nose is difficult because of the complexity of the structural abnormalities resulting in the deformity and the conspicuous nature of the dorsal nasal contour line of the nose. Effective management requires aggressive yet thoughtful application of techniques that stress the importance of proper diagnosis, good exposure, preservation and reconstitution of major support structures, and application of the structure concept. The successful surgeon is able to correct the crooked nose deformity without compromising nasal support or nasal function.

■ KEY POINTS

- ■ A continuous cartilaginous strut between the osseocartilaginous junction and the nasal spine must be preserved. An L-shaped strut of septal cartilage composed of a dorsal and caudal segment is sufficient to maintain support of the lower nasal third.

- ■ Complete medial and lateral osteotomies are usually required to shift the bony vault back to the midline. Occasionally double lateral osteotomies are required to ensure complete mobilization of the nasal bones.

- ■ The integrity of the nasal valve can be compromised if the upper lateral cartilages are divided from the nasal septum. If this maneuver is used to correct a middle vault deviation, the upper lateral cartilages should be sutured back to the septum to prevent collapse of the upper lateral cartilages.

- Bilateral splinting spreader grafts to straighten a dorsal septal deformity not only treat the deformity, but also will correct airway obstruction.

- The caudal septum provides support for the lower third of the nose; therefore any deviations must be corrected by cartilage manipulation, cartilage replacement, and/or suturing techniques. Once corrected the caudal septum should be fixed in the midline by securing it to the periosteum of the nasal spine.

- Anterior and caudal positioning of a caudal extension graft is critical to attain appropriate nasal length and projection.

- Columellar struts will increase tip support and create a stable medial crural–columellar strut complex, particularly when they are secured to a straight caudal septum with a septocolumellar suture.

- Shield-shaped tip grafts increase tip projection, provide tip support, and produce a bidomal tip contour. These grafts can be sutured to the caudal margin of the medial crura to stabilize the lower lateral cartilages and hide tip asymmetries.

REFERENCES

1. Jancke JB, Wright WK. Studies on the support of the nasal tip. Arch Otolaryngol 93:458, 1971.
2. Anderson JR. Straightening the crooked nose. Trans Am Acad Ophthalmol Otolaryngol 76:938, 1972.
3. Sheen JH. Spreader graft: A method of reconstructing the roof of the middle nasal vault following rhinoplasty. Plast Reconstr Surg 73:230, 1984.
4. Johnson CM, Toriumi DM. Open Structure Rhinoplasty. Philadelphia: WB Saunders, 1990.
5. Sheen JH, Sheen AP. Aesthetic Rhinoplasty, 2nd ed. St. Louis: Quality Medical Publishing, 1998 (reprint of 1987 ed.).
6. Toriumi DM, Johnson CM. The crooked nose. Operative Tech Otolaryngol Head Neck Surg 1: 252, 1990.
7. Briant TDR, Middleton WG. The management of severe nasal septal deformities. J Otolaryngol 14:120, 1985.
8. Anderson JR. The dynamics of rhinoplasty. In Proceedings of the Ninth International Congress of Otolaryngology. Excerpta Medica International Congress Series, No. 206. Amsterdam: Excerpta Medica, 1969, p 708.
9. Berman WE. Surgery of the nasal tip. Otolaryngol Clin North Am 8:563, 1975.

PART EIGHT

Special Considerations and Advances

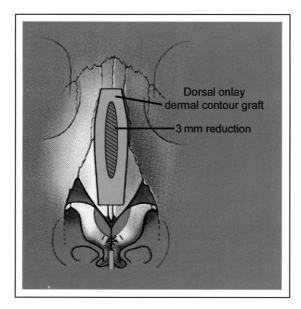

Dorsal onlay
dermal contour graft

3 mm reduction

Importance of the Depressor Nasi Septi Muscle: An Anatomic Study and Clinical Application

Rod J. Rohrich, M.D. • William P. Adams, Jr., M.D.
Bang Huynh, M.D. • Arshad R. Muzaffar, M.D.

*T*he plunging nasal tip remains a difficult problem in rhinoplasty and is accentuated by an active depressor septi muscle, diagnosed by a drooping nasal tip and shortened upper lip during animation (smiling).[1-12]

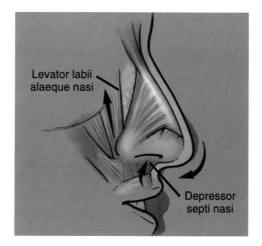

The depressor septi is a small, paired muscle located on either side of the nasal septum, originating from the medial crural footplates. Previous techniques have generally addressed this problem by resecting the depressor septi.[5-8]

Although the anatomy and function of the depressor septi have been described,[1-4] anatomic variations have not been previously studied. The purpose of this study was to delineate the anatomic variations of the depressor septi muscle in fresh cadaver dissections and correlate our findings with our clinical experience to develop an applied clinical rhinoplasty algorithm.

The routine preoperative rhinoplasty examination should include an assessment of the depressor septi muscle. In our series we identified 32 patients preoperatively who demonstrated dynamic shortening of the upper lip and inferior displacement of the nasal tip. Dissection and transposition of the depressor septi muscles were performed as an adjunct to rhinoplasty in this subgroup. Our anatomic study and operative techniques, including clinical examples, are presented below.

The plunging nasal tip remains a difficult problem in rhinoplasty and is accentuated by an active depressor septi muscle, diagnosed by a drooping nasal tip and shortened upper lip during animation (smiling). Preoperative diagnosis, intraoperative division, and transposition of the depressor septi muscle can enhance the lip-tip relationship in rhinoplasty.

ANATOMIC STUDY

The depressor septi muscles were dissected in 55 fresh cadavers. The muscles were exposed by an external incision along the nasal base. The skin was removed, revealing the plane of the orbicularis oris and depressor septi muscles. Dissection was continued cephalad toward the nasal septum to allow visualization of the anterior nasal spine, the medial crural footplate, the medial crus of the lower lateral cartilage, and the septal cartilage. Anatomic variations of the depressor septi muscles were recorded.

CLINICAL STUDY AND OPERATIVE TECHNIQUE

During the preoperative rhinoplasty examination patients were asked to smile so that any dynamic component of the depressor septi muscle on the nasal tip and upper lip could be assessed. Patients with an active depressor septi muscle as evidenced by drooping of the nasal tip and shortening of the upper lip on smiling were candidates for transoral depressor septi muscle transposition during rhinoplasty.

Our operative technique for transposition of the depressor septi includes the following steps:

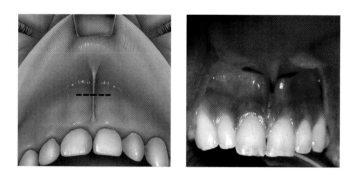

An 8 to 10 mm horizontal incision in the upper labial sulcus is centered on the frenulum.

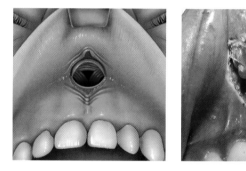
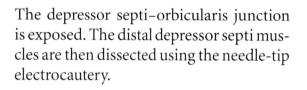

The depressor septi–orbicularis junction is exposed. The distal depressor septi muscles are then dissected using the needle-tip electrocautery.

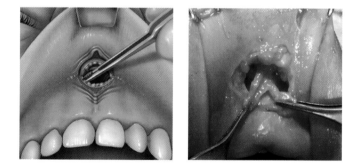

The depressor septi muscles are released near their origin with the orbicularis (type I) or periosteum (type II).

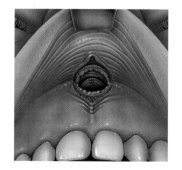

The depressor septi muscles are transposed and their cut ends sutured together with 4-0 chromic catgut sutures.

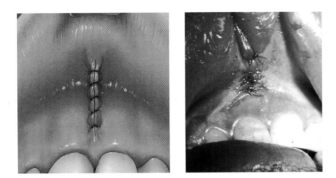

The horizontal intraoral incision is closed vertically, thereby lengthening the upper lip.

The long-term aesthetic results of this procedure were evaluated after 1 year.

ANATOMIC FINDINGS

TYPE I	TYPE II	TYPE III
Orbicularis oris	Periosteum	Diminutive
(N = 34, 62%)	(N = 12, 22%)	(N = 9, 16%)

Three types of depressor septi muscles were identified. Type I depressor septi muscles (62%) are visible and identifiable and can be traced to full interdigitation with the orbicularis oris from their origin at the medial crural footplate. Type II muscles (22%) are visible and identifiable but, unlike the first group, insert into periosteum and demonstrate little or no interdigitation with the orbicularis oris. The third group, type III (16%), includes instances when no or only a rudimentary depressor septi muscle is visible.

CLINICAL FINDINGS

All patients with an active depressor nasi septi muscle on preoperative examination demonstrated an identifiable depressor nasi septi muscle on exploration. In all cases the drooping nasal tip and short upper lip were improved following dissection and transposition of the depressor septi muscle. No evidence of relapse was evident at up to 2-year follow-up.

CASE ANALYSIS

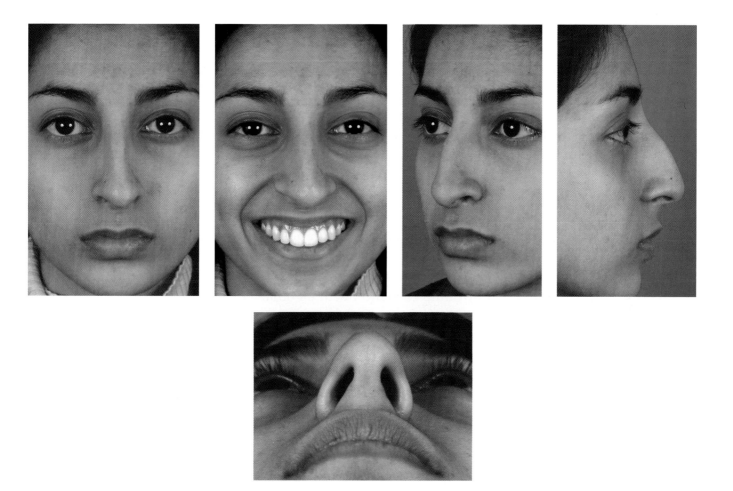

This primary rhinoplasty patient requested aesthetic correction of her nose. Specifically, she was concerned with the dorsal hump, inadequate tip projection, short upper lip, and narrow midvault area with a high dorsal deviation. The frontal view showed that she had Fitzpatrick type III skin with adequate facial proportions. She had thin skin and narrow dorsal aesthetic lines with a C-shaped dorsal deviation of the nasal tip to the left. Asymmetric alar flaring (right more than the left) and an asymmetric bulbous tip were noted. The frontal and animated frontal views demonstrated an active depressor septi muscle that shortened the upper lip and depressed the nasal tip. On the lateral view a high radix with a 5 mm dorsal hump and excess tip projection and length with a short upper lip were seen. She had a nasolabial angle of 90 degrees. The oblique view and overhead view confirmed dorsal midvault narrowing and deviation. The basal view revealed that she had alar notching bilaterally with periapical hypoplasia and a wide columellar base.

The operative goals included:
- Dorsal hump reduction
- Straightening of the dorsally deviated nose
- Widening and straightening of the dorsal aesthetic lines
- Decreasing tip projection and refining of the nasal tip
- Releasing and transposing of the depressor septi muscle to improve the tip to upper lip relationship

The surgical plan consisted of:
- An open approach via a stair-step transcolumellar incision
- Exposure of the nasal dorsum and separation of the upper lateral cartilage from the septum
- Incremental cartilaginous hump reduction of 5 mm using angled septal scissors and bony hump reduction with a Foman rasp
- Septal reconstruction and septal graft harvest
- Placement of bilateral spreader graft using three 5-0 PDS horizontal mattress sutures to straighten and strengthen the nasal dorsum as well as widen the dorsal aesthetic lines
- Cephalic trim that preserved 6 mm of the lower lateral cartilage
- Columellar strut secured with an intercrural suture of 5-0 PDS
- Placement of interdomal and transdomal sutures for tip refinement using 5-0 PDS
- Placement of bilateral alar contour grafts to correct alar notching
- No nasal osteotomies
- Release and transposition of depressor septi muscle via an upper lip transfrenulum incision

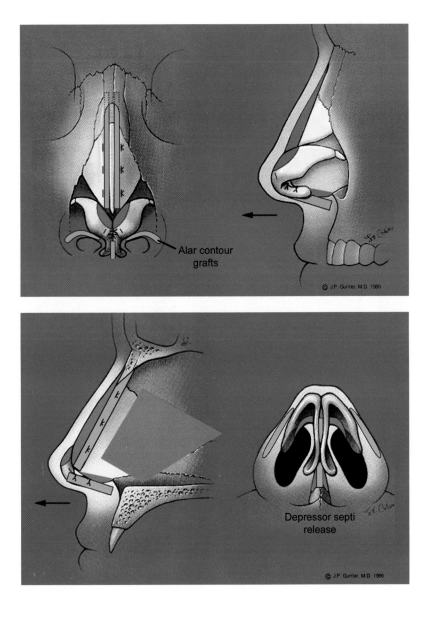

Alar contour grafts

Depressor septi release

© J.P. Gunter, M.D. 1986

© J.P. Gunter, M.D. 1986

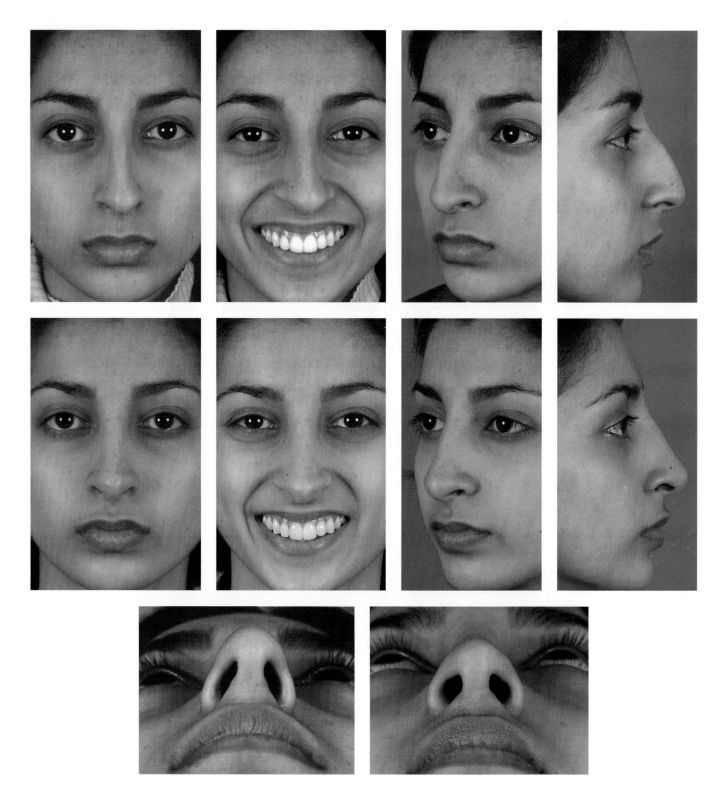

The patient is shown 2 years postoperatively with a straight dorsum and wider dorsal aesthetic lines. Note the improved tip refinement. The lateral view reveals a straight dorsum and refinement and a nasolabial angle of 95 degrees. The oblique and overhead views show a straight nose with good dorsal aesthetic lines. The basal view shows correction of the alar notching and a narrower columella and a straightened nasal tip.

> *In patients with an active depressor septi muscle preoperatively a depressor septi muscle was identified 100% of the time. Depressor septi release enhanced the rhinoplasty result.*

DISCUSSION

The importance of the depressor septi muscle in rhinoplasty has been recognized for some time. In 1976 Wright[9] reported that an "overactive" depressor septi muscle contributes to drooping of the nasal tip and that this phenomenon could be diagnosed by the "smile test" (i.e., the nasal tip drops slightly when the patient smiles).

In 1983 Ham et al.[10] reported that the depressor septi was responsible for "tension at the tip and on the dorsum of the nose" and recommended transection of the depressor septi to remedy this problem.

Cachay-Velasquez[6] in 1992 described the "rhino-gingivolabial syndrome of the smile." He emphasized the importance of facial animation in revealing aesthetic imperfections that may otherwise go unnoticed when the face is in repose. Specifically, the rhino-gingivolabial syndrome includes drooping of the nasal tip, elevation and shortening of the upper lip, and increased maxillary gingival show. The author attributed this syndrome to "hypertrophy" of the depressor septi muscles. His method for correction of this condition involved excision of the depressor septi muscles as well as partial excision of the orbicularis and nasalis muscles through a transfixion incision. After many years of clinical experience with this technique he reported no cases of nasal airway obstruction, contrary to Converse's admonition to preserve the function of this muscle.[11]

Lawson and Reino[7] described a related method termed reduction columelloplasty involving en bloc removal of soft tissue, including the depressor septi muscle, through a full-thickness diamond-shaped excision between the feet of the medial crura that allows direct visualization and suture plication of the splayed medial crura. As in the technique of Cachay-Velasquez, this method results in decreased interalar distance as well as enhanced tip projection and an augmented nasolabial angle.

Mahe and Camblin[2] have noted that transection of the depressor septi muscle may fail to produce lasting results because of reattachment of the muscle. Attempts have been made to prevent this occurrence by placing cartilage at the site of the transection.

De Souza Pinto et al.[12] have recently reported their "dynamic rhinoplasty" technique. The authors use a Z-plasty incision based on the frenulum and combine release of the medial fasciculi of the depressor septi with either horizontal or vertical plication of the intermediate fasciculi, depending on whether the patient has a short or a long upper lip, respectively. They describe a somewhat complicated classification system that delineates six different groups of patients with drooped or upright nasal tips, short or long upper lips, and the two "special cases" of the black nose and the mouth breather. However, aside from the manipulation of the lateral fasciculi described for the black nose, the only significant difference in the treatment of the depressor septi in the other groups seems to be the direction of plication in short or long upper lips as described above.

We attempted to further delineate the anatomic basis for modification of the depressor septi muscle by examining its anatomic variations. Having defined three different types of depressor septi muscles, we have developed an applied algorithm for treatment of the drooping tip/short upper lip complex in rhinoplasty.

Routine preoperative examination of the rhinoplasty patient should easily identify those patients who demonstrate a drooping nasal tip and shortened upper lip on animation, particularly on smiling. In such patients (types I and II) dissection and transposition of the distal depressor septi muscles and suturing together of the cut ends (which prevents the "reattachment" described by Mahe and Camblin) reliably and effectively correct this dynamic facial deformity. Dissection and transposition rather than excision of tissue provide fullness to the central upper lip. Follow-up of up to 2 years shows well-maintained aesthetic results without signs of relapse.

Transoral depressor septi muscle transposition enhances the tip-lip relationship, provides relative upper lip lengthening, gives relative fullness to the upper lip, and maintains tip rotation/projection on animation.

In patients with dynamic drooping of the nasal tip and shortening of the upper lip (i.e., type I and II depressor septi muscles) the transoral depressor septi muscle transposition procedure should be employed to attain the optimal aesthetic rhinoplasty result.

■ KEY POINTS

■ The depressor septi muscle can accentuate a drooping nasal tip and short upper lip on animation.

■ Dissection and transposition of the depressor septi muscle during rhinoplasty can improve the tip–upper lip relationship in appropriately selected patients.

■ Three variations of the depressor septi muscle were delineated: type I, inserted fully into the orbicularis oris (62%); type II, inserted into periosteum and incompletely into the orbicularis oris (22%); and type III, no or rudimentary depressor septi muscle (16%).

■ In our study 32 patients were identified preoperatively with an active depressor septi muscle diagnosed by a drooping nasal tip and shortened upper lip on animation. This subgroup underwent dissection and transposition of the depressor septi during rhinoplasty with correction of the deformity in 100% of cases.

■ Transoral depressor septi muscle transposition is a valuable adjunct to rhinoplasty in patients with a type I or II muscle variant and may be identified on the preoperative evaluation with the smile test.

■ In appropriately selected patients transoral depressor septi muscle transposition improves the tip-lip relationship and enhances the aesthetic result in rhinoplasty.

REFERENCES

1. Figallo E. The nasal tip: A new dynamic structure. Plast Reconstr Surg 95:1178, 1995.
2. Mahe E, Camblin J. Le muscle depresseur de la pointe. Ann Chir Plast 19:257, 1974.
3. Mahe E, Camblin J. La résection du muscle depresseur de la pointe dans les rhinoplasties esthétiques. Ann Oto-Laryngol 92:381, 1975.
4. De Souza Pinto EB, Da Rocha RP, Filho WQ, Neto ES, Zacharias KG, Amancipo EA, de Camargo AB. Anatomy of the median part of the septum depressor muscle in aesthetic surgery. Aesthetic Plast Surg 22:111, 1998.
5. Cachay-Velasquez H, Laguinge R. Aesthetic treatment of the columella. Ann Plast Surg 22: 370, 1989.
6. Cachay-Velasquez H. Rhinoplasty and facial expression. Ann Plast Surg 28:427, 1992.
7. Lawson W, Reino A. Reduction columelloplasty: A new method in the management of the nasal base. Arch Otolaryngol Head Neck Surg 121:1086, 1995.
8. Cetinkale O, Tulunay S, Cokneseli B. Augmentation of the columella-labial angle to prevent the "smiling deformity" in rhinoplasty. Aesthetic Plast Surg 22:106, 1998.
9. Wright WK. Symposium: The supra-tip in rhinoplasty: A dilemma. II: Influence of surrounding structure and prevention. Laryngoscope 86:50, 1976.
10. Ham KS, Chung SC, Lee SH. Complications of Oriental augmentation rhinoplasty. Ann Acad Med Singapore 12:460, 1983.
11. Converse JM, ed. Plastic and Reconstructive Surgery. Philadelphia: WB Saunders, 1964, p 702.
12. De Souza Pinto EB, Muniz ADC, Erazo PJ, Abdalla PCSP. Dynamic rhinoplasty: Treatment of the tip muscles. Perspect Plast Surg 12:21, 1999.

48

The Supratip Break

H. Steve Byrd, M.D. • James D. Burt, M.B.B.S., F.R.A.C.S.
William P. Adams, Jr., M.D.

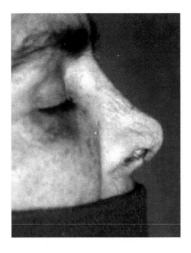

The supratip break is the point cephalad to the nasal tip where the contour lines of the nasal dorsum rise toward the tip-defining points. It thereby characterizes a nose in which tip projection slightly exceeds the profile line of the dorsum. It is frequently a desired aesthetic characteristic of the Caucasian nose, but its control during rhinoplasty can be most challenging.

The supratip break is the point cephalad to the nasal tip where the contour lines of the nasal dorsum rise toward the tip-defining points.

ANATOMY

The supratip break is a consequence of the difference in projection between the domes of the lower lateral cartilages and the plane of the dorsal septum. Measurements obtained at the time of open rhinoplasty and in fresh cadaver specimens suggest that the supratip break becomes evident in thin-skinned noses when the difference is between 6 to 7 mm (i.e., the dome projecting points project 6 to 7 mm above the plane of the anterior dorsal septum). In thick-skinned noses a differential of approximately 10 mm is required for the supratip break to be seen.

Tip projection is the single most critical variable to be controlled in creating the supratip break. In thin-skinned noses the supratip break becomes evident when the difference in projection between the dorsal septum and the dome projecting points is 6 to 7 mm (10 mm in thick skin).

The other important anatomic finding characterizing the presence of the supratip break has to do with the angle formed between a perpendicular line through the domes and the cephalic border of the lower lateral cartilages.

In addition to the vertical difference in projection, the angle formed by the perpendicular plane between the dome projecting points and the cephalic margins of the lower lateral cartilages is important.

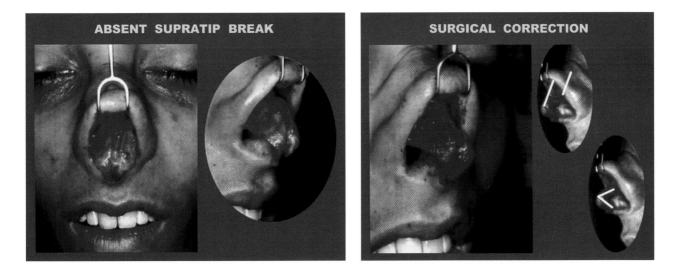

If the angle is open (45 degrees or more), the dorsal profile line flows smoothly onto the nasal tip without a definitive angle. When the cephalic alae form an angle less than 45 degrees and when the differential is present, the subtle break between the dorsal profile line and the nasal tip will occur. As the thickness of the nasal skin increases, the differential between the dorsal septum and the domes must increase and similarly the angle should also increase. In thick-skinned noses a differential of 10 mm with an angle of 30 degrees is needed for a supratip break.

With these anatomic findings relevant to the supratip break defined the surgical goals can now be formulated to accomplish this aesthetic entity. The number one variable that must be controlled at the time of rhinoplasty to create a supratip break is tip projection. This control almost always involves the use of a columellar strut to secure tip projection. My preference is an anterior septal extension graft that not only locks the domes and lower lateral cartilages to the desired plane of projection but also allows the medial, intermediate, and domal segments to be configured and shaped in a manner that is preferred. Furthermore, the anterior septal extension graft serves as a useful jig to cause the cephalic border of the lower lateral cartilages to form the angle previously described with the perpendicular line through the domes.

Either a columellar strut or anterior septal extension graft may be appropriate to achieve and maintain tip support, depending on the stability of the caudal border of the septum.

The surgical choice between a columellar strut and an anterior septal extension graft should be made on the basis of the stability of the caudal border of the septum. If the caudal septum is stable, the anterior septal extension graft is the preferred modality. However, if the caudal septum is weak or unstable, then a columellar strut must be used to support the tip. Once tip support is secured, the cartilaginous and bony dorsum can then be reduced to satisfy the remainder of the differential between the dorsal profile line and the tip.

Patients with weak lower lateral cartilages characterized by retracted alar margins, drooping tip, absent supratip break, prominent dorsum, and acute columellar-lip angle provide the greatest challenge in creating an aesthetic break between the dorsum and the tip. In these patients most of the characteristics are from a failure of the lower lateral cartilages to provide adequate tip support. Accordingly, a very well-planned structural adjustment for tip support must be achieved if the desired aesthetics are to be accomplished. This may involve supporting grafts resting on the anterior maxillae.

CASE ANALYSES

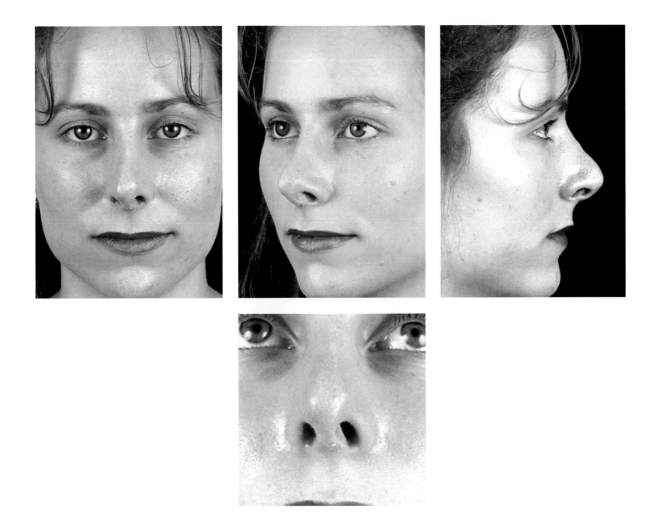

This 30-year-old woman had a nasal deformity with a remote history of nasal trauma but no previous surgery. Her primary complaint was that her nose was too large and full in the tip area. Analysis showed she had thin skin with washed-out dorsal aesthetic lines. Her nasal bridge was deviated slightly to the left and her tip to the right due to a septal deflection. She had a supratip deformity as well as an overprojecting tip.

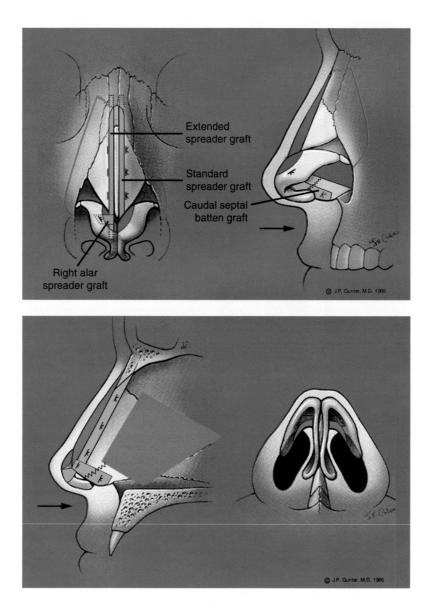

A right-sided extended spreader graft and left-sided batten graft were used to aid in straightening the nose as well as give her the optimal relationship with approximately 7 mm between the caudal septum and the tip-defining points in her thin skin to produce the supratip break.

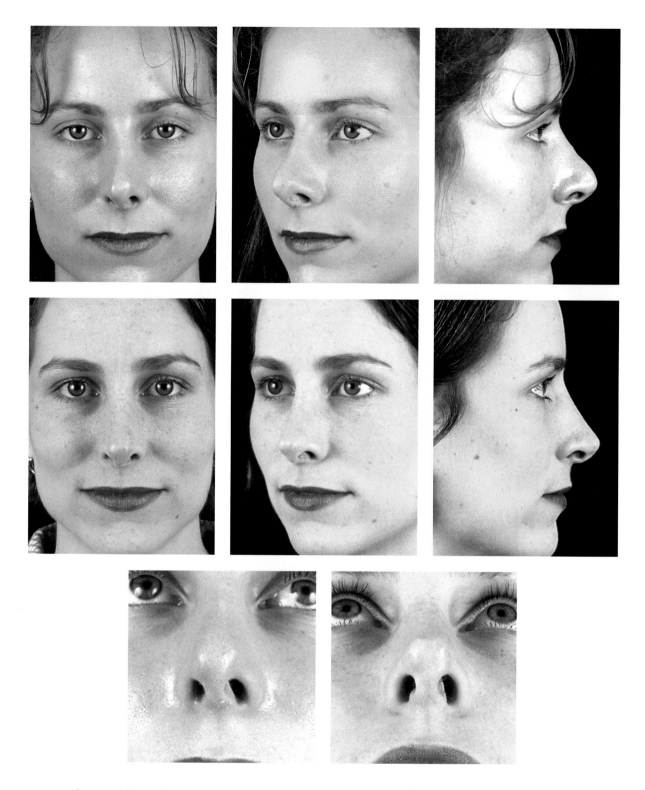

The results at 2 years demonstrate a more harmonious nose that is midline and a more refined dorsum with the desired subtle supratip break.

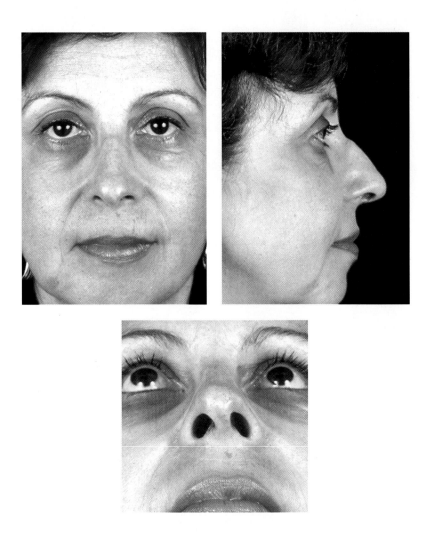

This 45-year-old woman complained of a dorsal hump and drooping tip. Analysis showed she had an underprojected nose with a large osseocartilaginous dorsal hump and slightly bulbous tip.

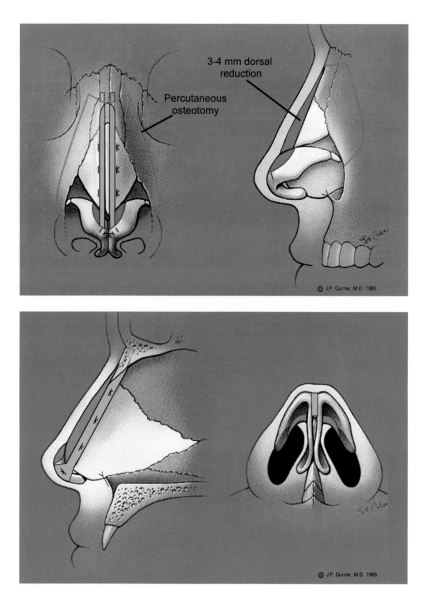

This was addressed with an osseocartilaginous dorsal hump reduction of approximately 5 mm, percutaneous osteotomies, and extended spreader and batten septal extension grafts to control her tip projection as well as produce a supratip break.

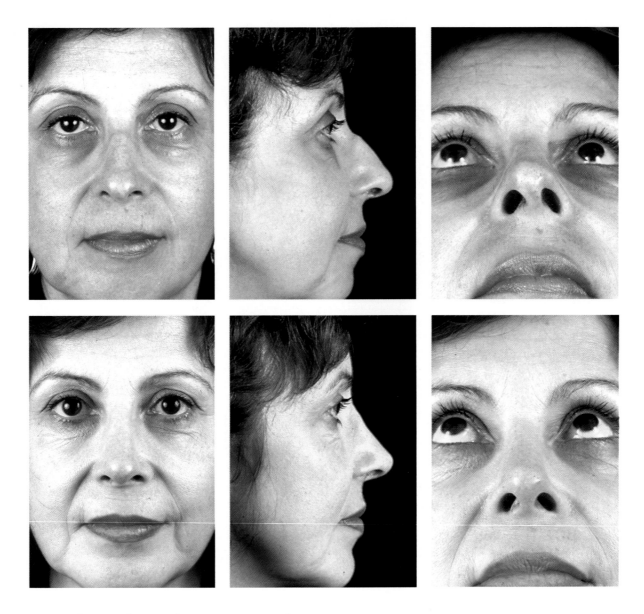

The results are shown at 14 months.

■ KEY POINTS

■ To produce a supratip break, the surgeon must consider the skin thickness, leaving a tip-defining point to caudal septal differential of 6 to 7 mm in thin-skinned patients and 10 mm in thick-skinned patients.

■ Supratip break may also be facilitated by geometry of an extended septal extension graft in the spreader position to produce the desired differential.

REFERENCES

1. Byrd HS, Barton FE Jr. Acquired deformities of the nose. In McCarthy JG, ed. Plastic Surgery, vol 3. Philadelphia: WB Saunders, 1990, pp 1924-2008.
2. Byrd HS, Hobar PC. Rhinoplasty: A practical guide for surgical planning. Plast Reconstr Surg 91:642, 1993.
3. Byrd HS, Andochick S, Copit S, Walton G. Septal extension grafts: A method of controlling tip projection, rotation, and shape. Plast Reconstr Surg 100:999, 1997.
4. Byrd HS, Salomon J, Flood J. Correction of the crooked nose. Plast Reconstr Surg 102:2146, 1998.

49

Role of AlloDerm in the Correction of Nasal Contour Deformities

Rod J. Rohrich, M.D. • Brian J. Reagan, M.D. • Joseph M. Gryskiewicz, M.D.

*N*asal augmentation with an emphasis on obtaining a natural, nonoperative appearance has become the focus of rhinoplasty today. As we have come to understand that nasal skin cannot be expected to contract in a consistent fashion, nasal augmentation has become an increasingly accepted rhinoplasty technique. Graft material is often needed to obtain desired outcomes. Autologous material, either septal or ear cartilage, is always preferred. However, when a patient has an inadequate source of autologous material, allograft material can obtain the desired results.

Current techniques for nasal augmentation using autologous material have certain inherent drawbacks. Cartilage grafts may cause unsightly irregularities over time. Secondary rhinoplasty patients often have a significantly depleted source of cartilage. Harvesting of autologous rib adds to the complexity and morbidity of the procedure. As a result, much interest has focused on the development of alternative soft tissue substitutes. Ideal characteristics of a soft tissue substitute include the following:
1. Biocompatible
2. Easily obtainable
3. Inexpensive
4. Nonimmunogenic
5. Nonresorbable
6. Easily stored

An alternative approach to the correction of nasal contour deformities using AlloDerm as onlay grafts will be described.

BACKGROUND

AlloDerm is freeze-dried acellular allogeneic dermis. Originally designed as a skin substitute for burn reconstruction, its use as a soft tissue filler has expanded impressively as surgeons came to recognize its clinical utility. Following harvest from a cadaver the epidermis and cellular components are removed via chemical leaching to leave an intact network of collagen and extracellular proteins. The graft is then freeze-dried to allow easy storage and shipment.[1]

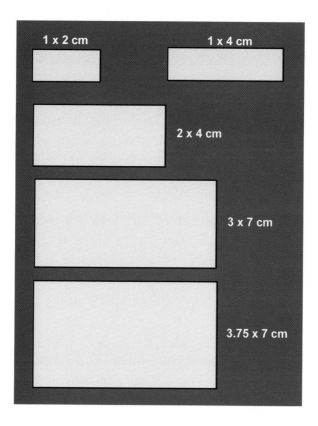

AlloDerm is available in many sizes. The thickness of the AlloDerm grafts depends on the specific size ordered and ranges from 0.3 to 1 mm. Generally, we use the 3 × 7 cm size sheet, which is 1 mm thick and is adequate for any type of contour correction, especially involving the nasal dorsum. AlloDerm is shipped at ambient room temperature. On receipt it should be stored under refrigeration at 2° to 8° C (36° to 46° F). The refrigerated shelf life of AlloDerm is 2 years.

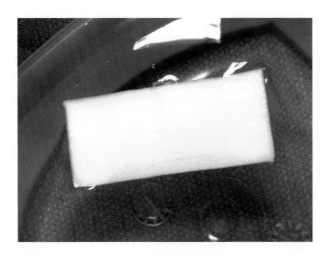

Prior to application the grafts are rehydrated with two washes in sterile saline or lactated Ringer's solution. This step takes a minimum of 10 minutes and is described in each packet insert. Samples of the donor skin are tested to rule out contamination by bacteria and fungi. No case of disease transmission has ever been reported.

AlloDerm grafts have been used extensively for both reconstructive and cosmetic purposes.[2-6] Laboratory investigations show that AlloDerm does not incite an inflammatory response or an allergic reaction.[2,7] Rather it provides a matrix for ingrowth and subsequent replacement by the host tissue. The rate at which AlloDerm is replaced may be dependent on the characteristics of the wound bed.

AlloDerm possesses many qualities of an ideal soft tissue graft. It is biocompatible and nonimmunogenic. There is an adequate supply, and shelf life is sufficient to allow storage and easy access. A 3 × 7 cm sheet, which is generally adequate for any nasal augmentation, is affordable at $500. The rehydrated sheet is pliable and easy to use. Partial resorption has been reported with AlloDerm grafts, but overall survival has generally been described to be excellent.[3,8,9]

INDICATIONS

AlloDerm is useful in primary and secondary rhinoplasty for dorsal augmentation, correction of dorsal irregularities, tip grafting, or camouflage over autologous grafts. Patients undergoing ethnic rhinoplasties (African-American, Asian) requiring significant dorsal elevation and patients with depleted sources of autologous cartilage undergoing secondary rhinoplasties are particularly amenable to the use of AlloDerm grafts.

AlloDerm is used in primary and secondary rhinoplasties for dorsal augmentation, correction of dorsal irregularities, tip grafting, or camouflage over autologous grafts.

OPERATIVE TECHNIQUE

The open rhinoplasty approach is preferred except in tertiary procedures when the patient's skin shows signs of vascular compromise. Open rhinoplasty allows for superior intraoperative diagnosis and facilitates the placement and suture stabilization of the graft. However, the use of a closed approach has also been described.[9]

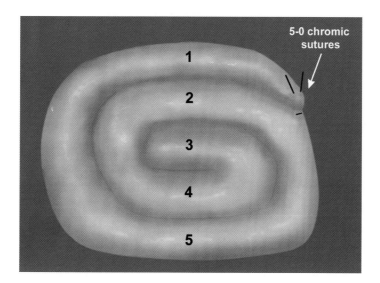

After proper preoperative diagnosis of the deformity and adequate exposure of the nasal skeleton, the AlloDerm grafts are rolled and trimmed to the desired shape. Multiple layers may be delivered for dorsal augmentation. This is accomplished by first folding the graft on itself. This creates a graft approximately 3 × 1 cm with the depth determined by the number of layers used.

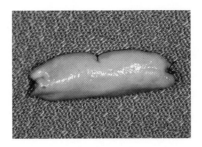

Once the appropriate thickness has been determined, the graft is tapered and sutured to itself at key points along the length and ends using 5-0 chromic catgut.

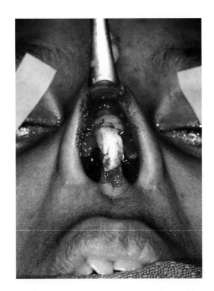

The graft is then delivered to the dorsum where stay sutures of 5-0 chromic are used to secure its position. A 5-0 rapidly absorbing chromic suture can also be placed through the skin and tied to stabilize the graft. This stitch usually pulls off when the splint is removed on the seventh postoperative day. Onlay camouflage tip grafts are simply trimmed to the desired shape. They can be placed directly over the alar cartilages or on top of cartilage grafts to yield a smoother contour. Again, 5-0 chromic stay sutures to underlying support structures are used to secure the grafts. Tip onlay grafts can be stacked in multiple layers if needed.

Multiple layers may be used for dorsal augmentation. Onlay camouflage tip grafts trimmed to the desired shape can be placed directly over the alar cartilages or on top of cartilage grafts for a smoother contour.

CASE ANALYSES

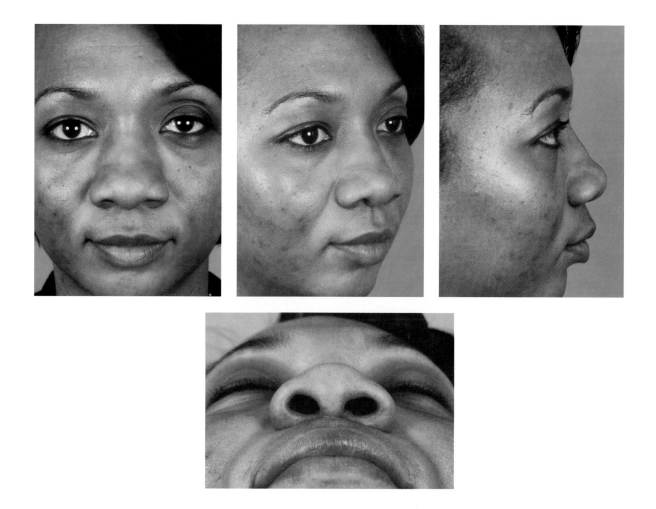

This 45-year-old woman desired more dorsal and tip projection. In addition, she requested that her wide alar base be corrected. She wanted to avoid a rib or ear cartilage donor scar. She had thick skin, a wide nasal vault with excessive alar flaring, and an ill-defined bulbous tip. The lateral view showed a low radix, maxillary protrusion, alar flaring, and decreased nasal tip projection.

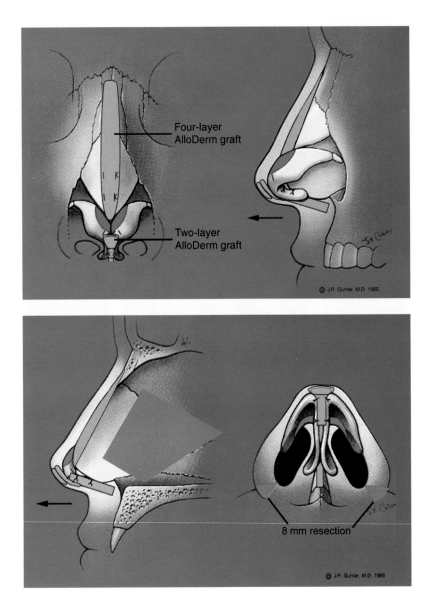

The operative plan included:
- Open rhinoplasty approach
- Septal cartilage harvest
- Dorsal preparation with 2 mm of dorsal rasping
- AlloDerm graft (four layer) to dorsum with suture fixation to upper lateral cartilage using 5-0 plain catgut
- Cephalic trim
- Columellar strut fixed with intracrural suture
- Tip definition with interdomal and transdomal sutures as well as a Sheen infratip lobule graft covered with a two-layered AlloDerm graft
- Type 1 alar base resection (8 mm)

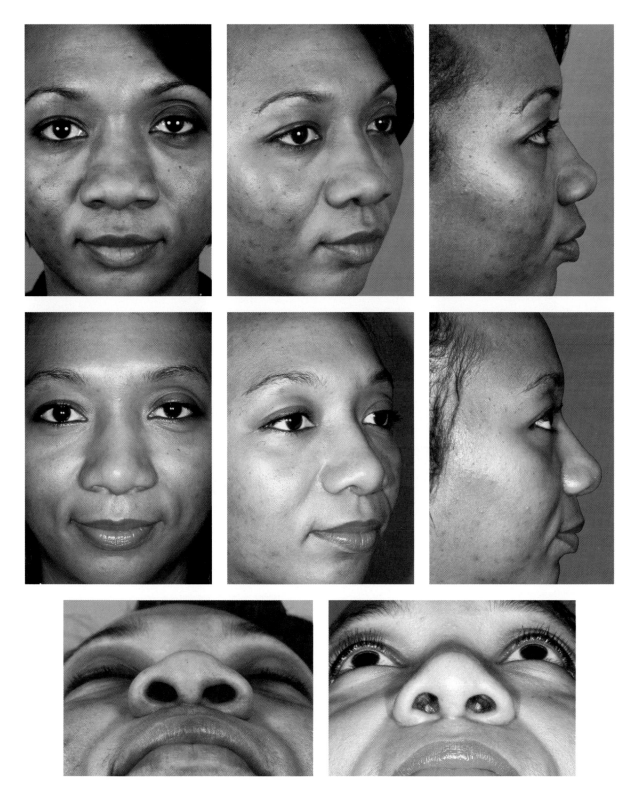

The increased dorsal height, increased nasal tip projection, and improved definition are shown 15 months postoperatively.

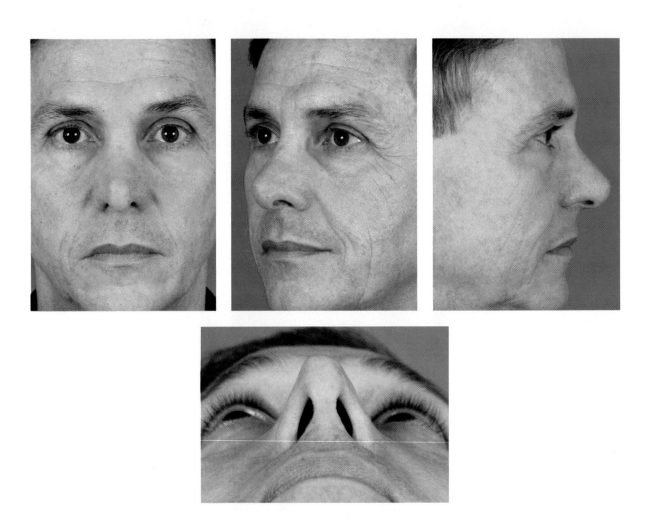

This 50-year-old man, who had undergone two nasal procedures elsewhere, complained of nasal airway obstruction, a saddlenose deformity, and a feminine nasal tip. The frontal view demonstrated good facial proportions, moderately thin skin, a dorsum that was widened and flat with no dorsal aesthetic lines, and alar pinching. On the lateral view a low radix, adequate tip projection, and a 90-degree nasolabial angle were evident.

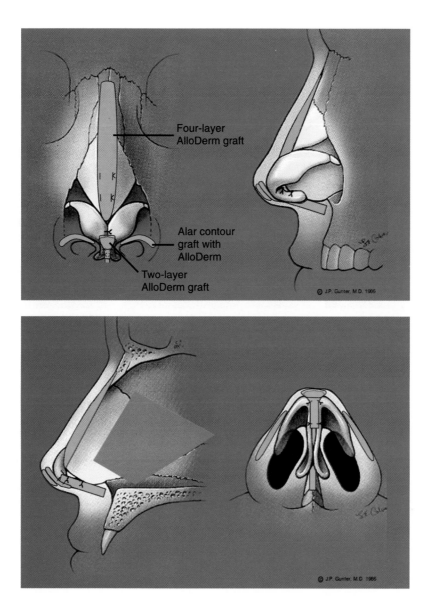

The operative plan included:
- Open rhinoplasty
- Septal reconstruction with inferior turbinate resection (bilateral, submucosal)
- Dorsal preparation with subperiosteal bony dorsum undermining
- Dorsal augmentation with a four-layer AlloDerm graft
- Columellar strut secured with 5-0 PDS suture
- Intercrural and intradomal sutures and an onlay infratip (Sheen) cartilage graft covered with an AlloDerm tip graft secured with a 5-0 plain catgut
- Lateral alar contour grafts with AlloDerm to correct alar pinching
- No osteotomies

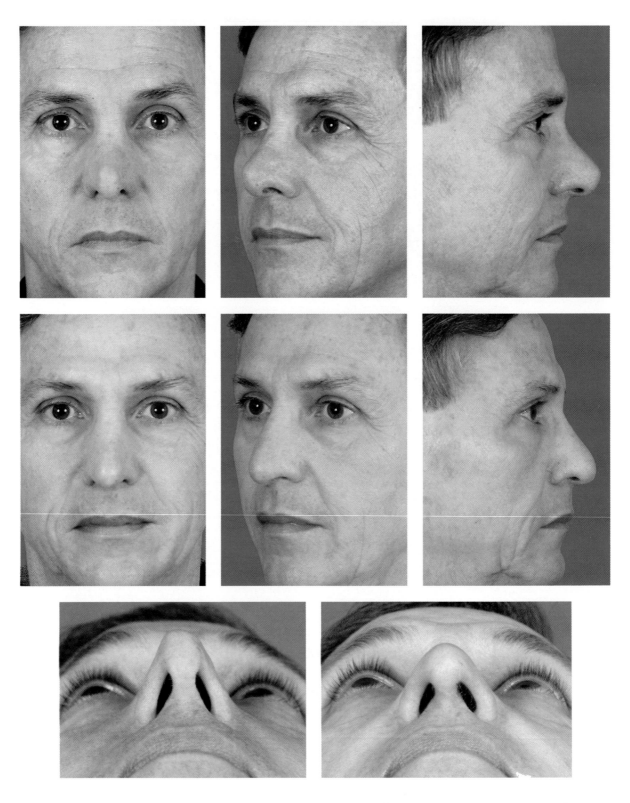

At 18 months dorsal nasal augmentation with AlloDerm is well maintained. The AlloDerm grafts have a natural feel. The saddlenose deformity and alar pinching have been corrected.

CONCLUSION

Dorsal augmentation in a primary rhinoplasty for an ethnic nose or an over-resected nose in secondary procedure are two examples of the usefulness of AlloDerm. In addition, tip grafts can be helpful to camouflage tip irregularities or can be placed over cartilage grafts to provide a smoother contour, especially in the thin-skin patient.

The open rhinoplasty approach lends itself well to the use of AlloDerm. It facilitates accurate intraoperative diagnosis of the deformity and allows easy delivery and suture stabilization of the graft. AlloDerm should not be used alone for support of the nasal tip. Two-year follow-up shows good long-term results with the use of this material.

■ KEY POINTS

■ AlloDerm is useful for primary and secondary dorsal augmentation, tip grafting, and camouflage over autologous grafts.

■ AlloDerm may be applied in multiple layers.

■ This graft material should not be used alone for tip support.

■ Long-term results over 2 years show good results with minimal resorption.

■ Resorption is more common over the bony dorsum and in the thin-skin patient.

REFERENCES

1. Livesy S, Herndon D, Hollyoak M, et al. Transplanted acellular allograft dermal matrix. Transplantation 60:1, 1995.
2. Wainwright D, Madden M, Luterman A, et al. Clinical evaluation of an acellular allograft dermal matrix in full-thickness burns. J Burn Care Rehab 17:124, 1996.
3. Jones F, Schwartz B, Silverstein P. Use of a nonimmunogenic acellular dermal allograft for soft tissue augmentation. Aesthetic Surg Q 16:196, 1996.
4. Kridel R, Foda H, Lunde K. Septal perforation repair with acellular human dermal graft. Arch Otolaryngol Head Neck Surg 124:73, 1998.
5. Tobin H, Karas N. Lip augmentation using an AlloDerm graft. Oral Maxillofac Surg 56:722, 1998.
6. Schwartz B. The use of a permanent dermal allograft for lip augmentation. Presented at the Sixty-fifth Annual Scientific Meeting of the American Society of Plastic and Reconstructive Surgeons, Dallas, 1996.
7. Reagan B, Madden M, Huo J, et al. Analysis of cellular and decellular allogeneic dermal grafts for the treatment of full-thickness wounds in a porcine model. J Trauma 43:458, 1997.
8. Gryskiewicz J, Rohrich RJ, Reagan B, Schwartz BM. The use of AlloDerm for the correction of nasal contour deformities. Plast Reconstr Surg 107:561, 2001.
9. Rohrich RJ, Reagan B, Adams W, et al. Early results of vermilion lip augmentation using acellular allogeneic dermis: An adjunct in facial rejuvenation. Plast Reconstr Surg 105:409, 2000.

50

Managing the Alar Base

Robert M. Oneal, M.D.

*A*lar base surgery can be used to correct a number of deformities of nostril size and asymmetry as well as a constellation of alar base and sidewall abnormalities. Determining the specific location and extent of resections is dependent on accurate preoperative diagnosis.

ANATOMY AND PREOPERATIVE ASSESSMENT

Three variations, as originally described by Sheen,[1] are seen in deformities of the relationship between nostril size and alar size and shape:
1. Appropriate-size nostrils with excess alar lobule or alar flare
2. Large nostrils but less excessive than the alar lobule excess
3. Nostrils and alar lobules equally enlarged

However, given the multiple variations seen clinically, assessment of the specific alar deformity is important in addition to noting the size of the nostril. These subdivisions of alar abnormalities include increased intra-alar width, increased length of the sidewall or alar flaring, high alar attachment, and intrinsic thickness or hanging of the alar sidewall. The frontal view is best for assessing whether the flare of the alar base is lateral to a line dropped from the medial canthus. However, the basal view is essential to assess the relative alar sidewall length and shape and the exact configuration of the nostril sill and the nostril size. The basal view as well as the oblique view is useful for assessing the alar attachment relative to the columella.

The alar base must be assessed from the frontal, basal, and oblique views.

PRINCIPLES OF TREATMENT

The following treatment approaches, alone or in combination, in most cases correct the many variations of deformities described above. Not infrequently different techniques or a combination of them will be needed on the two sides to correct asymmetries.

Reduction of Alar Flaring With or Without Reduction of the Circumference of the External Nares by Nostril Sill Excision

Alar flaring is the most common indication for alar base modification and requires careful preoperative assessment for correction.[1] The configuration of the alar base that extends beyond a vertical line dropped from the medial canthus must be noted.

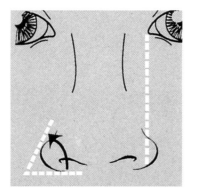

Also the angle of the vertical plane of the alar lobule and the horizontal plane of the nasal base must be documented. This angle should be less than 90 degrees, indicating that the vertical plane of the alar lobule diverges laterally as it meets the horizontal plane of the nasal base.

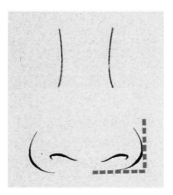

If the alar plane is perpendicular to the nasal plane, alar resection should be approached with caution or avoided.

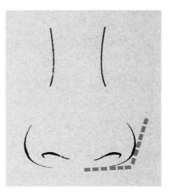

Resection may produce an obtuse angle of the alar base and an unattractive appearance.

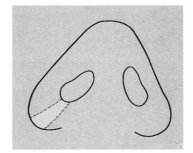

If the nostril circumference is also too large, then the nostril floor excision can extend into the vestibule, which will reduce the nostril circumference.

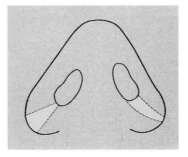

Any diminution of the nostril circumference can be avoided by limiting the excision to the nostril sill (right side). In rare instances the nostril can be made smaller with minimal reduction of alar positioning (left side).

Reduction of the Length of the Alar Sidewall or Reduction of a Large Alar Lobule by Alar Base Excision

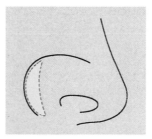

An excessively long sidewall or a disproportionately long nostril with or without some bowing of the alar base is an indication for reduction. A significant set back of the tip that would lead to alar sidewall redundancy may also be compensated for by alar base excision. Depending on individual circumstances, it may occasionally be necessary to combine techniques of alar base plus nostril floor excision.[2,3] In general, it is important to measure the width of the alar base resection carefully with the caliper and then tattoo the exact location of points on opposite sides of the excision in the nostril rim with methylene blue. I have found the most effective closure is to use one or two buried 5-0 or 6-0 clear PDS sutures in the dermis and carefully approximate the skin with 6-0 fast-absorbing gut.

Repositioning the Alar Base to the Nostril Sill

When there is a high-arching nostril with a more superior attachment of the alar base, repositioning of the alar base downward by selective nostril floor excision will help to produce some favorable straightening of the alar margin.

Sculpturing the Alar Sidewall or the Alar Base Itself

Alar sculpturing may be indicated if there is a need to raise a thick hanging alar sidewall relative to a normal columella, change the contour of the free alar margin, or thin a thick alar rim. Although sculpting can be very effective, such patients should be selected carefully. Occasionally a patient may have narrow nostrils associated with thick sidewalls and a widened columella. The particular techniques useful in such cases are well described by Millard.[4] Thinning of the sidewalls, removing the soft tissue from the columella, and suturing the feet of the medial crus close together may produce a more physiologic nostril opening. When the patient has long alar sidewalls and a hidden columella, anteriorly based chondrocutaneous flaps, as described by Millard,[5] can rotate the excessive lateral wall tissue into the columella and produce a more harmonious balance between the alar sidewalls and the columella on the lateral projection.

COMPLICATIONS

Complications after modification of the alar base include visible scars, notching of the nostril sill, asymmetry, and excessive narrowing of the nostrils. The scars are usually well hidden, and in carefully selected cases these techniques can produce satisfactory results. However, the patient should be forewarned about the residual scar. An external incision may be objectionable to some patients. My experience is that this scar is usually not too prominent in darker skinned individuals, and more often than not the advantages far outweigh the disadvantages.

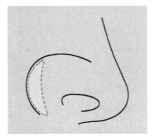

Other concerns can be minimized by attention to a few important technical details. By placing the inferior incision for alar base excision just above the alar facial groove a more natural configuration and a better scar can be obtained than by carrying the excision right in the groove. The nostril floor should only be excised and carried into the vestibular skin area if the nostril itself needs to be narrowed. It is possible to excise the alar base or to modify the nostril flow without excising any vestibular skin, depending on the needs of the individual patient. It is generally best to take a conservative approach, particularly when reducing nostril circumference, since it is relatively simple to go back and excise a little bit more, but it is very difficult to enlarge a stenotic nostril.

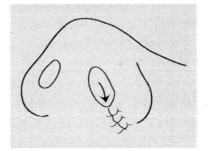

Sheen[1] has pointed out the potential for an unnatural appearance as well as potential notching from a straight-line scar in the nostril sill.

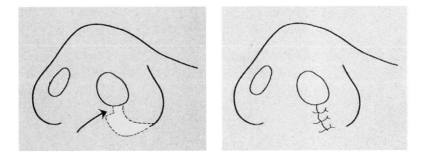

The medial flap described by Sheen effectively avoids these problems and helps maintain a more natural configuration of this area.

To avoid the straight-line closure, he creates a medial buttress that changes the direction of the scar and helps evert the skin edge. The combination helps avoid notching. The surgeon can also bevel the lateral side to get more eversion of the closure area. It should also be mentioned that the alar lobule can be a donor site for a composite graft. Indications might be correction of asymmetries that are sometimes seen with a cleft lip or nose or repositioning of a unilateral high alar rim with a lateral vestibular release and insertion of the alar base composite graft.

A medial flap can be used to prevent notching of the nostril sill.

Undercorrection is a problem. Guyuron[6] has pointed out the amount of alar narrowing achieved using the increased width is not a ratio of 1:1. It may have to be as much as 1.5 or 2:1 to get enough permanent correction. In severe cases where there seems to be lateral tension the alar cinch procedure, as described by Regnault and Daniel,[2] using deepithelialized flaps sutured to the anterior nasal spine helped to prevent relapse. The worst complication in my opinion is overcorrection and nostril stenosis. Obviously this is to be avoided by carefully assessing the need to remove any vestibular skin, which in many cases is not necessary, and to replace the tissue if too much seems to have been removed. Long-term correction can be accomplished with a composite graft, perhaps from the opposite alar base, or the flap described by Constantian[7] brought in from the adjacent cheek.

CASE ANALYSES

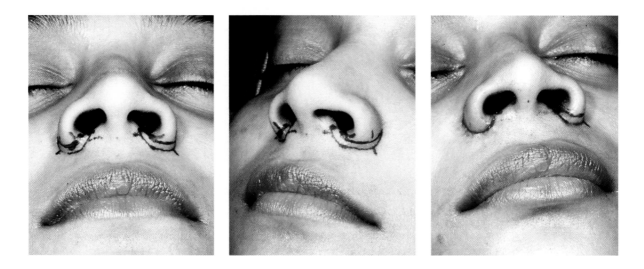

This patient had alar flaring, increased interalar width, and an enlarged nostril circumference. The markings have been made for combined alar base and nostril sill excision. The oblique view shows the extent of alar base resection planned. The basal view shows the patient after excision and closure of the right side.

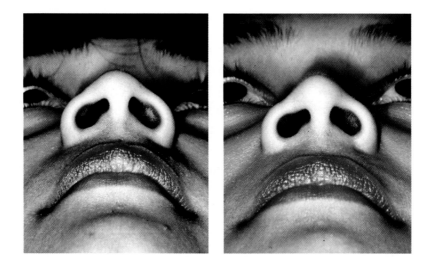

The reduction in interalar distance and decrease in nostril circumference are seen at 1 year.

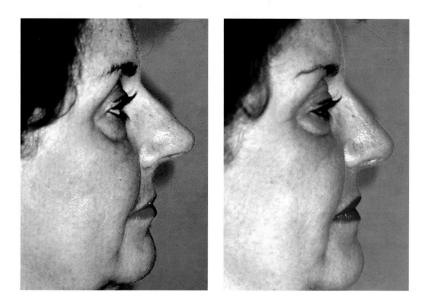

This patient had increased tip projection and increased nostril size.

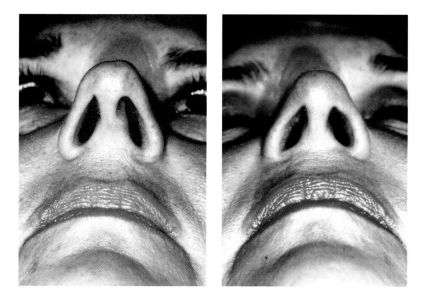

The reduction of tip projection, shortened alar sidewalls, and decrease in nostril size are seen at 1 year.

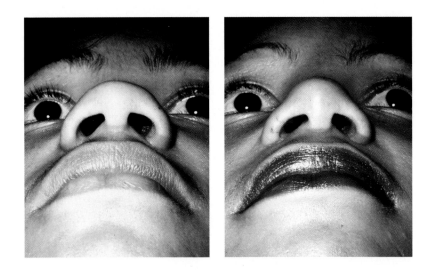

This patient had alar flaring and normal nostril size. Note the reduction in alar flaring without nostril size reduction 1 year postoperatively.

■ KEY POINTS

■ Three variations in the alar base are seen: appropriate-size nostrils with excess alar lobule or alar flare, large nostrils but less excessive than the alar lobule excess, and nostrils and alar lobules equally enlarged.

■ A medial flap helps prevent notching of the nostril sill.

■ Placing the inferior incision for alar base excision just above the facial groove produces a more acceptable scar.

REFERENCES

1. Sheen JH, Sheen AP. Aesthetic Rhinoplasty, 2nd ed. St. Louis: Quality Medical Publishing, 1998, pp 252-282 (reprint of 1987 ed.).
2. Regnault P, Daniel RK, eds. Aesthetic Plastic Surgery. Boston: Little, Brown, 1993, p 145.
3. Tardy ME, Younger MK, Cheng E. The overprojecting tip. Facial Plast Surg 4:327, 1987.
4. Millard DR. Alar margin sculpturing. Plast Reconstr Surg 40:337, 1967.
5. Millard DR. Versatility of chondromucosal flap in the nasal vestibule. Plast Reconstr Surg 50: 580, 1972.
6. Guyuron B. Precision rhinoplasty. Part II: Prediction. Plast Reconstr Surg 81:500, 1988.
7. Constantian M. An alar base flap to correct nostril and vestibular stenosis and alar base malposition in rhinoplasty. Plast Reconstr Surg 101:1666, 1988.

51

Alar Resection and Grafting*

Jack H. Sheen, M.D.

*T*he goal of alar resection today is to ensure relatively symmetric, non-surgical-appearing nostrils that are in harmony with the overall facial characteristics. The diversity of alar configurations requires a flexible approach that can be adapted to individual variations. This may require narrowing the nostril, reducing a large alar lobule, or repositioning an alar rim. Whatever the goal, it must be achieved with aesthetic efficiency, that is, with maximal improvement at minimal cost. Too often the alar base is narrowed at the expense of natural-appearing nostrils. Because problems resulting from alar surgery are for the most part permanent and disfiguring, careful planning is requisite.

The most frequent problems resulting from alar resection are nostril–alar lobule disproportion and visible scarring or distortion of the nostril, commonly seen as notching of the sill. In my view a naturally flaring alar base is far preferable to these deformities.

*Modified from Sheen JH, Sheen AP. Aesthetic Rhinoplasty, 2nd ed. St. Louis: Quality Medical Publishing, 1998 (reprint of 1987 ed.).

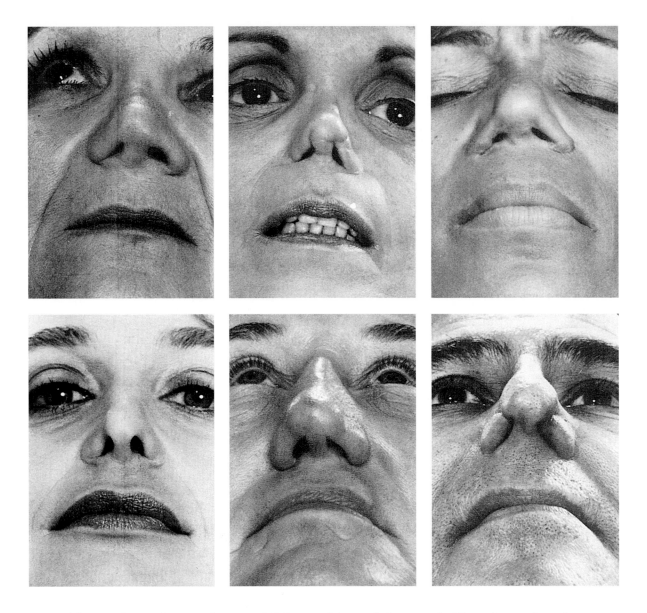

The patients shown above exhibit notching of the nasal sill and varying degrees of nostril-alar disproportion and asymmetry after alar resection. Adopting a two-surface concept and using a technical maneuver that I call the medial flap can help prevent a potentially disastrous result and create symmetric, well-contoured nostrils.

PATIENT EVALUATION

Patients requiring alar resection may have a variety of alar base configurations. For example, they may have thick alar lobules with small nostrils or wide flaring nostrils with thin alar lobules. The nasal sill may be long or shortened by encroachment of the medial crus. Obviously no single resection technique will adequately correct all the combinations of problems. Before alar resection is undertaken it is important to identify which components of the alar base should be altered and to tailor the operation accordingly. Reduction of the width of the alar base should not be performed at the expense of nostril size or alar contour.

When evaluating the alar base it is helpful to think in terms of two surfaces: the cutaneous or lobular surface and the vestibular surface. Considered independently, each contributes to a varying degree to the width and contour of the alar base. Therefore each surface can be managed independently with different types and amounts of resection. Tissue resection from the vestibular side decreases the size of the nostril. Tissue resection from the cutaneous side modifies the alar lobule and may indirectly affect the contour (not the size) of the nostril. Thus the questions to be addressed are do both the nostril and the alar lobule need to be reduced and, if so, in what proportion?

The cutaneous or lobular surface and the vestibular surface contribute to a varying degree to the width and contour of the alar base.

Standard wedge resections designed to narrow the alar base may do so at the expense of nostril size. Thus the solution may be worse than the problem. However, if the cutaneous and vestibular aspects of the nares are considered separately, narrowing can be well controlled in terms of nostril size and nostril-lobular proportion.

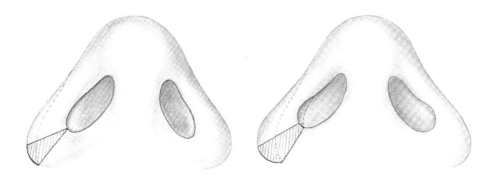

Patients requiring alar resection can be categorized into types I and II. Type I patients have appropriately sized nostrils but excessive alar lobules. Only the lobules should be reduced without excising the vestibular skin. Type II patients have large nostrils and excessive alar lobules. Correction involves resection of lobular as well as vestibular skin.

OPERATIVE TECHNIQUE
Type I: Cutaneous Resection

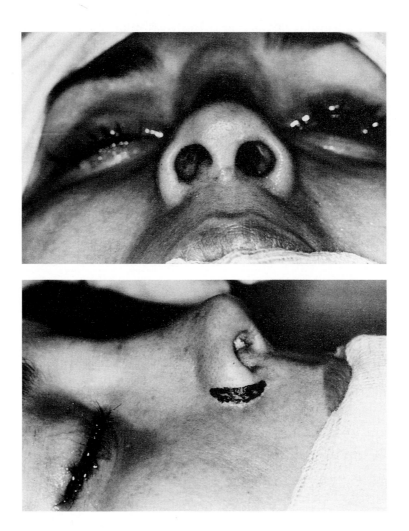

This patient has nostrils of normal size and a wide alar base. Excising only the alar lobule will reduce the width of the base and preserve the size of the nostrils while improving their contour. The markings extend along the entire border of the alar lobule and measure approximately 3 mm.

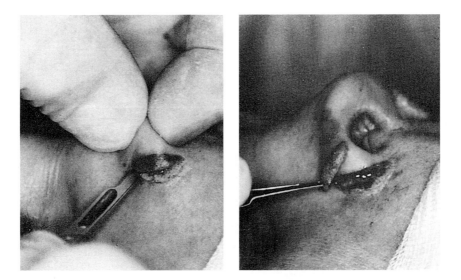

The tissues are held with the surgeon's forefinger and thumb to avoid forceps marks. A carefully controlled cut is made just 1 mm on the nasal side of the alar-facial junction, creating a very small cuff. With a No. 15 blade the incision is beveled so that the deepest edge will extend to, but not through the vestibular side. The resected alar wedge measures approximately 3 × 13 mm. The vestibular skin remains intact.

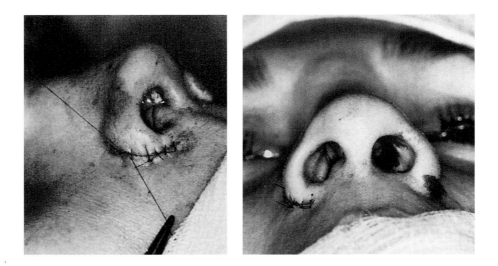

The incision is closed with 6-0 nylon sutures. A comparative view of the resected and unresected sides demonstrates the cutaneous resection has reduced the alar lobule and created a nostril with a more elliptical contour.

Type II: Vestibular and Cutaneous Resection With Preservation of the Medial Flap

Most patients requiring reduction of the nasal base also require some reduction in the size of the nostril.

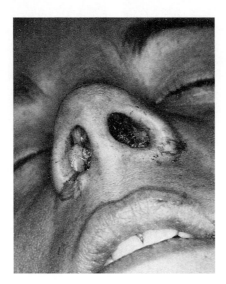

This patient has nostrils that flare slightly and moderately large alar lobules that are rotated laterally. More lobular skin than vestibular skin must be resected to rotate the lobule medially.

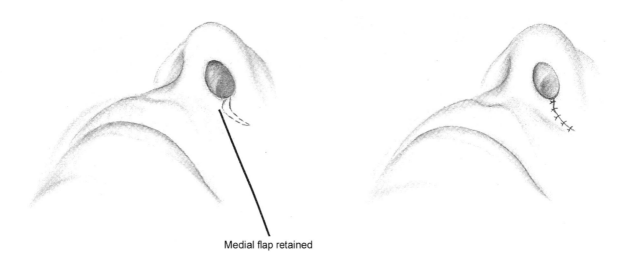

Medial flap retained

The use of a medial flap produces a natural-appearing nasal sill when vestibular skin is resected.

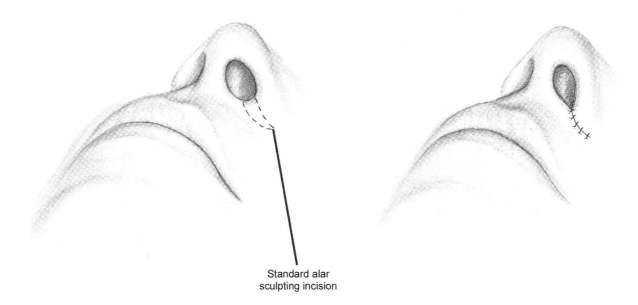

Standard alar
sculpting incision

If the tissues are resected, an unnatural, surgical notching of the nasal sill will
result.

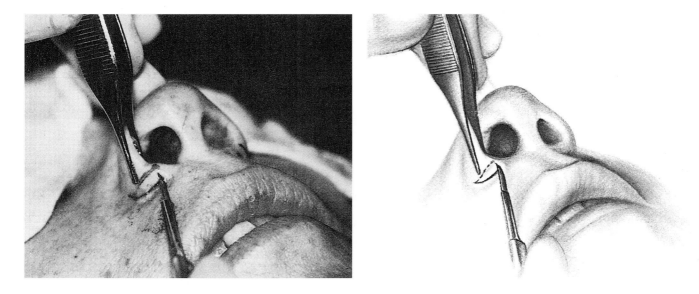

After the planned excision has been marked, an incision is made with a No. 11
blade extending medially along the alar base and stopping short of the last 2
to 3 mm.

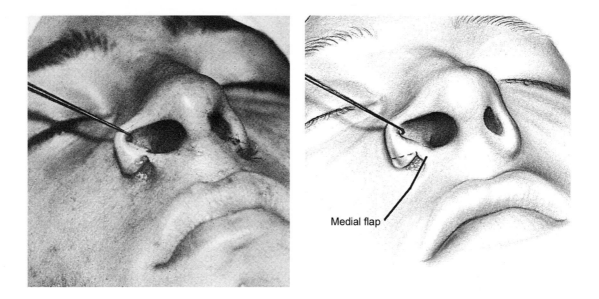

The surgical distortion of the nasal sill can be prevented by preserving a small triangle of skin at the medial edge of the incision (the medial flap) using a back cut. Except for a small segment of the nasal sill, the inferior cut has been made. The nostril is pulled laterally to demonstrate the medial flap. The medial flap is used in all cases of vestibular resection to ensure a smooth nasal sill.

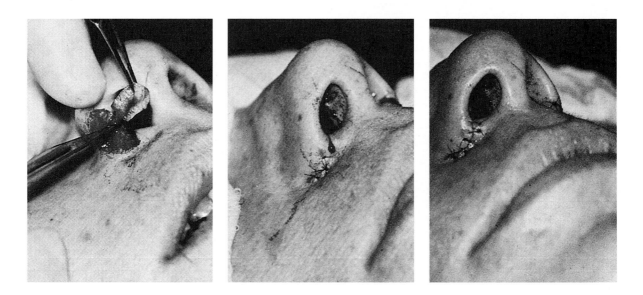

The superior cut is made, excising the wedge of tissue. The retained medial flap can be seen. This patient's nasal sill maintains its natural continuity because of preservation of the medial flap. The flap is shown before and after suture placement.

CASE ANALYSES
Large Alar Lobule, Flaring Nostril

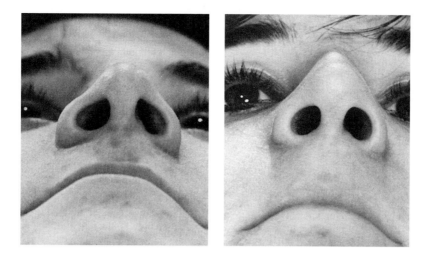

In this case the need for reduction is greater on the cutaneous surface of the ala. Because the nostrils flare but are not excessively large, only minimal vestibular resection is necessary to recontour the nostrils. A type II alar resection was performed, resecting approximately 3 mm from the cutaneous surface and 1 mm from the vestibule. Note the smooth continuity of the nostril perimeter following the medial flap technique.

Broad Alar Base, Relatively Small Nostrils

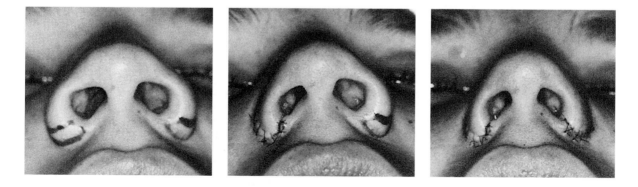

The alae are marked before resection. The ratio of cutaneous to vestibular resection is 2:1. The sides are compared intraoperatively. At the completion of the operation the contour of the nostrils is improved and the alar base is sufficiently narrowed without compromising nostril size.

Long Nasal Sill

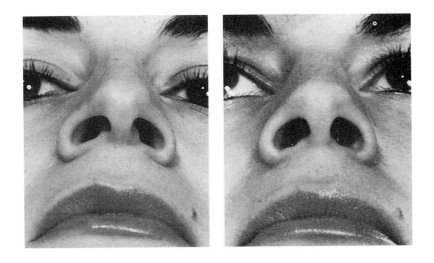

The alar incision encroaches on the nasal sill, allowing more resection medially and less laterally. Symmetry and alar notching are of particular concern because of the thinness of these alar lobules. Preservation of a medial flap ensures the smooth contour of the nasal sill.

Disproportionately Thick Alar Lobule

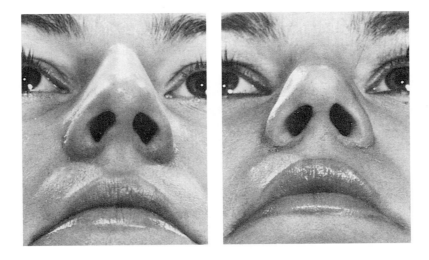

This patient has thick alar lobules and nostrils of appropriate size. The vestibule was incised for repositioning only. The ratio of cutaneous to vestibular resection was 3:1. The proportion of alar lobule to nostril is now correct.

Thin Alar Lobules

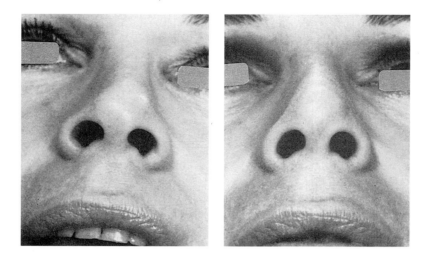

Like the last patient, this patient's nostrils are naturally notched. The medial flap was placed just lateral to the notch to ensure continuity. The cutaneous and vestibular surfaces are parallel. Equal amounts of tissue were resected from each side.

Normal Nasal Sill, Very Thin Alar Lobules

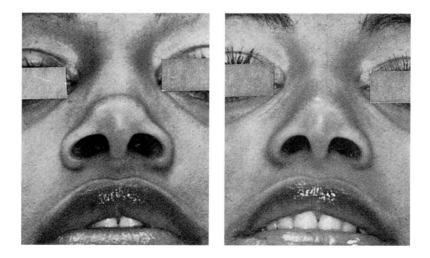

This patient has exceptionally thin alar lobules. The nostril curves around and enters the nasal sill without the usual lobular thickening. Such patients present special problems because the margin for error is small. The surgeon must resect tissues conservatively. The continuity of the nasal sill on the basal view is good postoperatively, although there is a slight notch on the patient's left nostril at the point of resection. The medial flaps have been preserved.

Disproportionately Long Nostril

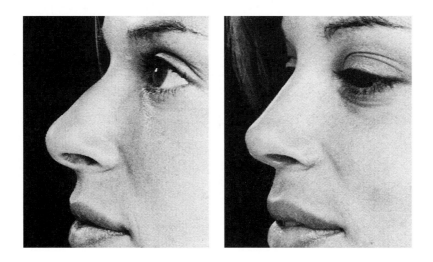

This patient's nostrils are too long for the tip lobule. The nostril-tip proportion has been improved by the resection of 1.5 mm of vestibular skin and 2 mm of lobular skin. She is a type II patient.

Long, Arching Nostril

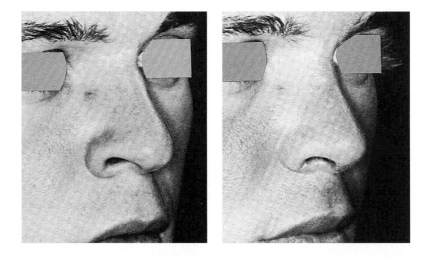

Nostrils that arch up and insert below the columella give the definite impression of a snarl. This unpleasant aspect of this patient's nasal base was corrected by effectively decreasing the length of the nostril. Nostril shortening was accomplished by resection of 2 mm of the vestibule and 3 mm of the lobule.

ALAR LOBULE GRAFTING

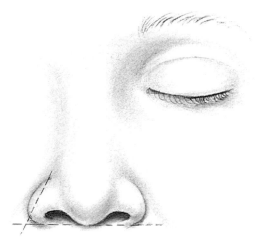

An important consideration in planning alar resection is the position of the vertical plane of the alar lobule relative to the horizontal plane of the nasal base. Ideally, the lobular plane should not be perpendicular to the basal plane but should slightly diverge laterally. Extreme lateral divergence is evident in flaring nostrils that need to be moved medially.

The position of the vertical plane of the alar lobule relative to the horizontal plane of the nasal base is a key consideration.

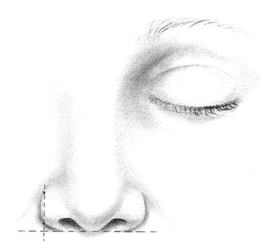

If the alar plane is perpendicular to the basal plane, alar resection should not be done.

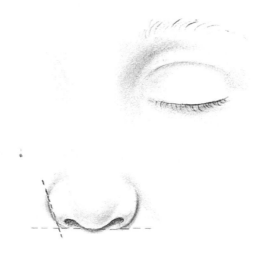

Wedge resections would cause a disproportionately narrow nasal base, resulting in a bowling pin appearance.

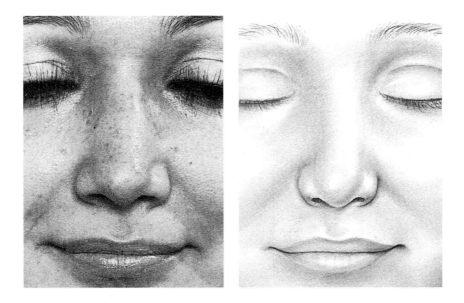

The nasal base that appears broad may have alar and basal planes that are perpendicular. Although it may appear that alar resections would be beneficial, they probably would not. The drawing illustrates the likely aesthetic result if alar resections were done.

The Alar Lobule as a Composite Graft

As a variation on robbing Peter to pay Paul, tissue can be taken from the alar lobule as a composite graft and used to (1) expand the nostril or (2) reposition an alar rim. In either case some lobular tissue is taken where it is excessive, or at least can be spared, to correct an area of tissue deficit at the nostril sill or in the vestibular wall.

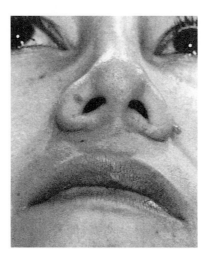

This patient demonstrates nostril-lobular disproportion resulting from alar resection. The nasal base remains wide, whereas the nostrils are unacceptably small. She is an ideal candidate for nostril expansion using part of the alar lobule as a free graft.

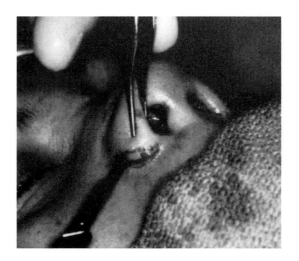

An appropriately sized graft is marked. With a No. 15 blade an angled cut is made so that the medial end of the incision is just lateral to the vestibule.

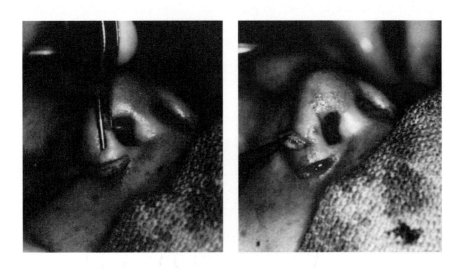

The superior incision completes the resection. An elliptical graft measuring about 3 × 11 mm is removed.

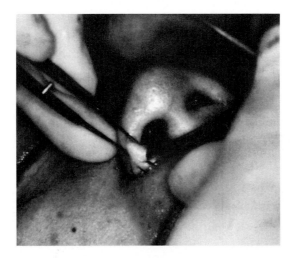

Following wound closure with 6-0 nylon suture a second incision is made nearby, going from the vestibular side and angled to avoid contact with the first incision.

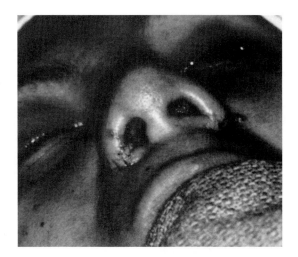

The composite graft is inset and secured at the ends with 5-0 catgut. The entire perimeter of the graft is carefully sutured with 7-0 chromic suture. The expansion of the nostril is immediately apparent.

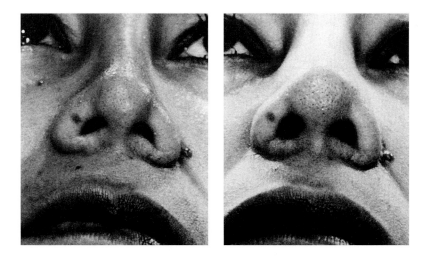

The patient is shown 2 years after surgery. The improvement in nostril size is striking. The alar lobules appear thinner and less bulky. That such small grafts should have such a dramatic effect is surprising. (Likewise, the small amount of tissue resection that can cause deformity is surprising.)

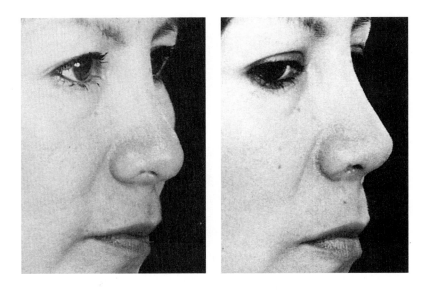

The effect of nostril expansion is less apparent on the oblique view. Also, no visible scarring or deformity of the alar lobule is evident.

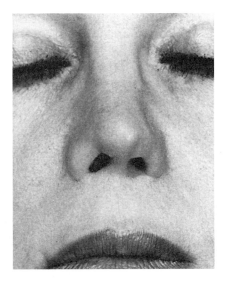

This nostril asymmetry resulted from multiple operations. A composite graft from the ear, placed in the vestibular wall, was planned to lower the right alar rim. A composite graft from the right alar lobule was planned to expand the left nostril. Even though the right nostril seems small, remember that only a small graft is needed to improve the contralateral side.

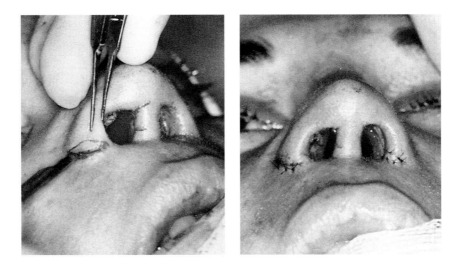

A type I alar resection (cutaneous) is done. The maximum width of the ellipse is 3 mm. Following routine closure the left nasal sill is split at a point that allows maximal nostril expansion (usually at the site of the old incision). The graft is inset and carefully sutured around its perimeter with interrupted 7-0 chromic suture.

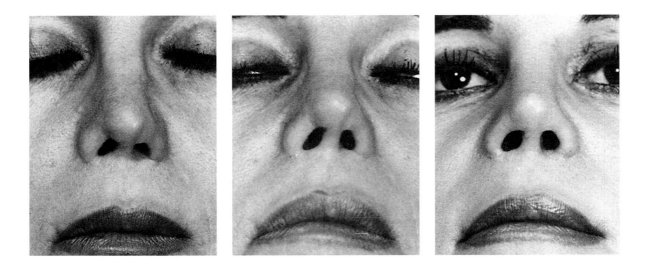

The preoperative asymmetry is most apparent on the frontal view because of the asymmetry in position of the alar rims. On the basal view the left nostril can be seen to be somewhat smaller than the right. The left nostril has been successfully expanded by the contralateral lobular composite graft. The contour improvement in the right nostril is the result of the composite ear graft placed in the vestibule.

Lowering the Alar Rim

The alar lobule can be used as a composite graft to lower an alar rim. This is a nice technique because, by using available local material, the ear can be spared.

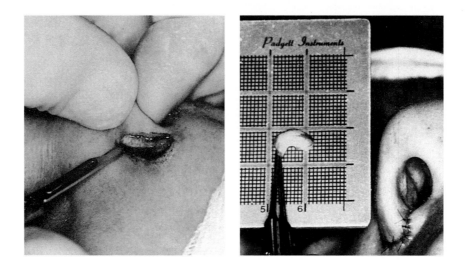

A type I alar resection (cutaneous) is done. The composite lobular graft is shown.

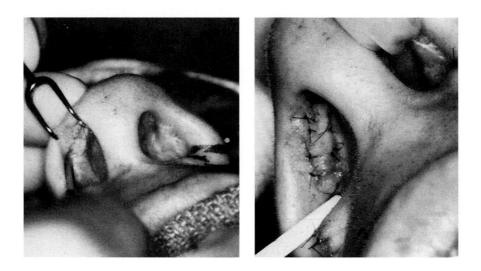

An incision is made parallel to the rim of the nostril. The graft is carefully sutured in place with 7-0 chromic suture.

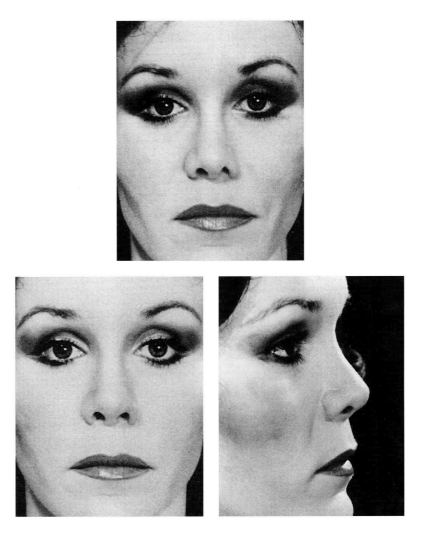

The patient is shown 1 year postoperatively. Following placement of a composite graft from the right lobule the left alar rim was lowered to a more symmetric position relative to the right. The scar remains visible after 1 year.

■ KEY POINTS

■ Nostril–alar lobule disproportion and visible scarring or distortion of the nostril are the most frequent complications of alar resection.

■ The cutaneous or lobular surface and the vestibular surface must be managed independently with different types and amounts of resection.

■ Preserving a small triangle of skin at the medial edge of the incision using a back cut can prevent surgical distortion of the nasal sill.

■ Alar resection must take into account the position of the vertical plane of the alar lobule relative to the horizontal plane of the nasal base.

BIBLIOGRAPHY

1. Fomon S, et al. Physiologic surgery of the nares. Arch Otolaryngol 47:608, 1948.
2. Hage J. Collapsed alae strengthened by conchal cartilage: The butterfly cartilage graft. Br J Plast Surg 18:92, 1964.
3. Hardin JC Jr. Alar rim reconstruction by a dorsal nasal flap. Plast Reconstr Surg 66:293, 1980.
4. Joseph J. Joseph's Rhinoplasty and Facial Plastic Surgery. Phoenix: Columella Press, 1987, p 111.
5. Michelson LN. Rhinoplasty. Ancillary procedures. Clin Plast Surg 15:139, 1988.
6. Millard DR Jr. Adjuncts in primary rhinoplasty. In Millard DR Jr, ed. Symposium on Corrective Rhinoplasty. St. Louis: CV Mosby, 1976.
7. Millard DR Jr. Alar margin sculpting. Plast Reconstr Surg 40:337, 1967.
8. Millard DR Jr. External excisions in rhinoplasty. Br J Plast Surg 12:340, 1960.
9. Peck GC. Techniques in Aesthetic Rhinoplasty. New York: Gower, 1984, pp 100-105.
10. Rees TD. Aesthetic Plastic Surgery. Philadelphia: WB Saunders, 1980.
11. Rees TD. Current concepts of rhinoplasty. Clin Plast Surg 4:131, 1977.
12. Regnault P, Daniel RK. Septorhinoplasty. In Regnault P, Daniel RK, eds. Aesthetic Plastic Surgery. Boston: Little, Brown, 1984.

Alar Base Surgery

Bahman Guyuron, M.D.

*I*mproper correction of alar base abnormalities can have prodigious aesthetic and functional consequences. The resultant deformity from poor surgical planning during alar base surgery can be difficult and sometimes impossible to correct. It is therefore crucial to evaluate the alar base abnormality prudently and plan the surgical correction with utmost thought.

ANATOMY AND PATHOLOGY

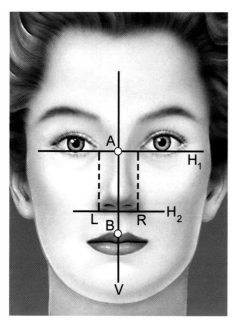

Analysis of alar base position
on the frontal view

Proper analysis and treatment of alar base abnormality depend on an understanding of the normal alar base relationship. Horizontally, the distance from one lateral alar base to the opposite one is approximately 2 mm wider than the intercanthal distance as long as the latter is deemed optimal (normally 31 to 33 mm). Should the intercanthal distance be judged abnormal, the orbital fissure (distance from the medial to lateral canthus) can be used as a reference. Vertically, the caudal limits of the alar base are approximately 2 mm cephalad to the junction of the middle two thirds and caudal one third of the distance from the medial canthus to the stomion. The intercanthal distance is bisected (point *A*) and a vertical line (*V*) is drawn to pass the philtrum dimple (point *B*) on an otherwise symmetric face. Two parallel lines (lines *L* and *R*), symmetrically positioned in relation to the vertical midline starting at the medial canthi, should pass 1 mm medial to the outer boundary of the alar base on a congruous alar base relationship in a patient who also has a normal intercanthal distance.

913

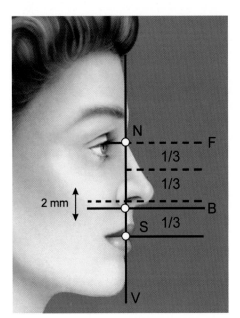

Analysis of vertical alar base disharmony
on the profile view

Point *N* (nasion) is connected to point *S* (stomion) and divided into three equal lengths. The caudal border of the alar base is located 2 mm caudal to the junction of the middle and lower thirds.

The following classification of alar base deformities is based on either horizontal excess or deficiency or vertical malposition, which is either caudal or cephalad. An excess can be the result of either a wide alar base, a thick alar base, or a wide nostril sill. A combination of these conditions may also exist. An alar base deficiency is often more conspicuous and may be traumatic, iatrogenic, or congenital in origin. Some horizontal abnormalities are secondary to tip projection or maxillary abnormalities (protrusion/retrusion). Correction of those underlying skeletal anomalies will improve the appearance of the alar base without direct surgery on this site.

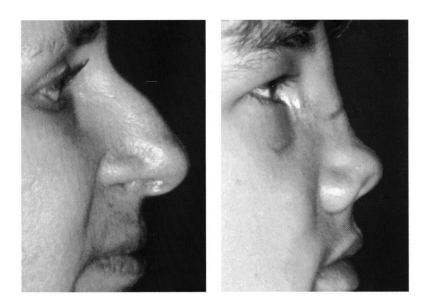

Cephalic malposition of the alar base gives the appearance of a longer nose and a more exposed columella. A caudally malpositioned alar base causes hooding of the base, decreased columellar show, and a nose that often appears shorter. Either condition may be unilateral or bilateral.

GENERAL OPERATIVE TECHNIQUES

The procedure may be conducted under general anesthesia in conjunction with a more extensive rhinoplasty, although minor alar base surgery could be performed under local anesthesia with or without intravenous sedation.

Horizontal Deformities
Wide Nostril Sill

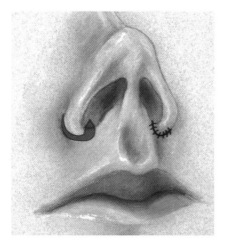

Careful analysis of the alar base may prove the nostril sill wider than ideal, the most common abnormality. The excess nostril sill to be excised is marked by two points. Two lines are commenced from these points and are connected with a horizontal line placed at the junction of the nostril sill and the upper lip and extended laterally along the alar-facial crease using a No. 10 blade. Adequate tissue is left laterally to avoid violation of the junction between the alar base and the nostril sill. The incision is continued with a microneedle electrocautery, releasing the soft tissue to facilitate medial transposition of the alar base tripod. This type of incision maintains the graceful transition from the alar-facial crease to the nostril sill, thus avoiding the "fixed" alar base appearance with an undesirable augmentation. The incision is then repaired using 6-0 plain catgut.

Excess Nostril Sill and Wide Alar Base

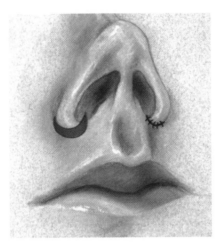

The excised area includes a combination of nostril sill and alar base in varying proportions, depending on the degree of excess. The technique is similar to the excision of a wide nostril sill except that the shape of the excised area is more of a wedge. Furthermore, the excised area may be more lateral, and a very small segment is removed from the nostril sill.

Thick Alar Base

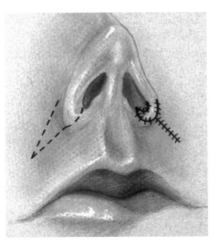

An L-shaped excision is made where the anteroposterior limb of the L reduces thickness, and the cephalocaudal excision will narrow the nostril. A mirror image of the incision is made on the left nostril. The thickness can also be reduced by removal of the excess soft tissue between the skin and intranasal lining through an incision along the alar rim.

Combination of Wide Nostril and Thick Alar Base

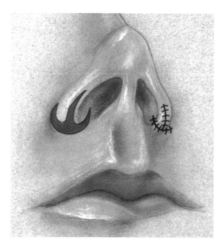

To narrow the nostril and thin the alar base simultaneously, the surgeon may use an inverted T resection. An incision is made at the alar-facial crease and continued around the base of the nostril. Another anteriorly oriented incision is designed to reduce the thickness of the alar rim and the base. The excess tissue is removed and the margins are reapproximated.

An inverted T resection is used to narrow the nostril and thin the alar base simultaneously.

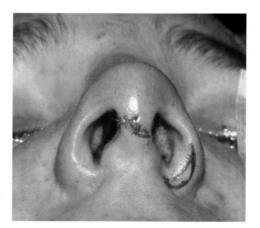

An elliptical excision along the vestibular aspect of the alar base can be used to correct a faceted alar base. The intraoperative view of excision of an elliptically shaped skin flap from a faceted alar base on the left side of the patient's nose is shown above. The right side has been left intact for comparison.

Secondarily Widened Alar Base

Depending on the cause, whether an altered projection or maxillary advancement, the surgeon should use a nostril sill excision, a lateral excision, or both to harmonize the nasal base.

Narrow Nostrils

Constricted nostrils are either secondary to maxillary retrusion or excess tip projection and are rarely encountered. Reducing the nasal base projection can usually reverse the condition. If the problem is maxillary retrusion, a LeFort-type maxillary advancement will resolve the alar base problem. Iatrogenic narrow nostrils can be corrected by transposition of a subcutaneous-based skin flap from the lateral alar base to the medial base.

Vertical Deformities
Cephalically Malpositioned Alar Base

If the alar base is wide as well as cephalically malpositioned, narrowing the alar base results in medial and caudal translocation of the base. Otherwise removal of an elliptically shaped area of skin from the upper lip at the junction of the alar base and the lip is planned. The incision is made in the alar-facial crease and continued around the base to the nostril sill. The size of the resected skin is determined by preoperative facial analysis. It is essential to release the soft tissue contained in the alar thickness completely so that the alar base can be advanced. Otherwise this procedure may result in elevation of the upper lip rather than the alar base being transposed caudally.

If the soft tissue in the alar thickness is not completely released, the upper lip may be elevated instead of the alar base being caudally transposed.

Caudally Malpositioned Alar Base

A caudally malpositioned alar base is less common and more difficult to correct. An incision is made in the vestibular lining just above the alar rim, and a strip of the lining is resected and repaired to reposition the alar base.

ALAR BASE DYNAMICS

The most significant dynamic changes occur in the alar base when the projected caudal nose is altered. When the overprojection is reduced, the extra soft tissue will extend caudally and laterally, thus necessitating a maneuver to narrow the base. Conversely, a wide alar base will be automatically corrected if caudal nasal projection is increased. The alar base is widened by maxillary advancement and narrowed by retraction of the maxilla. Lengthening the maxilla will transpose the alar base caudally and reduce the distance between the alar bases. Intrusion of the maxilla will result in cephalic displacement and widen the alar base.

Narrowing the alar base also affects other facets of nasal base appearance. The alar rim is repositioned caudally, which reduces the columellar-alar vertical discrepancy. In most patients this improves nasal aesthetics; however, it will be detrimental to the nasal balance in patients with a caudally positioned alar rim or a retracted columella.

Narrowing the alar base will be detrimental to the nasal balance in patients with a retracted columella or a caudally positioned alar rim.

Prior to any alar base resection the columella base has to be adjusted if necessary. Excess footplate divergence may ostensibly render the nostrils narrow, and repositioning the footplates may unveil the alar base excess.

■ KEY POINTS

- ■ Alar base pathology can vary, and successful correction mandates a careful analysis and masterful execution of the surgical plan to achieve a pleasing alar base.

- ■ Alar base harmony is judged by comparing the interalar distance to either the intercanthal distance or the orbital fissure width.

- ■ The position of the alar base should be assessed and corrected while considering all three dimensions.

- ■ Alar base surgery is planned so that there is a graceful and pleasing transition from the ala to the nostril sill following correction of the disharmony.

- ■ Narrowing the alar base will result in caudal transposition of the alar rim.

BIBLIOGRAPHY

1. Conley JJ, Von Fraenkel PH. The principle of cooling as applied to the composite graft in the nose. Plast Reconstr Surg 17:444, 1956.
2. Constantian MB. An alar base flap to correct nostril and vestibular stenosis and alar base malposition in rhinoplasty. Plast Reconstr Surg 101:1666, 1998.
3. Giberson WG, Freeman JL. Use of free auricular composite graft in nasal alar/vestibular reconstruction. J Otolaryngol 21:153, 1992.
4. Guyuron B. Precision rhinoplasty. Part I: The role of life-size photographs and soft tissue analysis. Plast Reconstr Surg 81:489, 1988.
5. Rees TD, et al. Composite grafts. In Transaction of the Third International Congress of Plastic and Reconstructive Surgery. Washington: Excerpta Medica, 1963.
6. Sheen JH, Sheen AP. Aesthetic Rhinoplasty, 2nd ed. St. Louis: Quality Medical Publishing, 1998 (reprint of 1987 ed.).
7. Guyuron B. Alar base abnormalities: Classification and correction. Clin Plast Surg 23:263, 1995.

53

The African-American Patient*

Rod J. Rohrich, M.D. ▪ Arshad R. Muzaffar, M.D.

*R*hinoplasty has become increasingly popular among African-American patients. This challenging surgical endeavor requires an appreciation of ethnic concepts of beauty and of the unique anatomic characteristics of the African-American nose. These general anatomic characteristics are compounded by the wide-ranging variations in individual anatomy and the relationship of the nose in the context of the African-American face. Attaining consistent aesthetic results is significantly more complicated in African-American rhinoplasty patients than in Caucasians. A pragmatic, systematic analysis of the African-American nose and the techniques commonly used to modify the African-American nose while maintaining or achieving facial aesthetic harmony will be discussed.

Ethnic concepts of beauty and the anatomic characteristics of the African-American nose are unique considerations.

---

*Excerpted in part from Rohrich RJ, Muzaffar AR. Rhinoplasty in the African-American patient. Plast Reconstr Surg (in press).

NASAL AESTHETICS IN THE AFRICAN-AMERICAN PATIENT

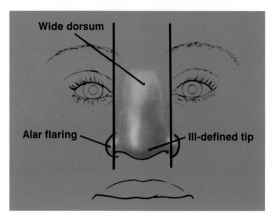

Harmony and symmetry are universal elements of beauty and are the ultimate objectives of any surgical plan regardless of the patient's ethnicity.[1,2] In general, the African-American nose is characterized by a wide, depressed dorsum, inadequate tip projection, ill-defined tip, excess alar flaring and/or increased interalar width, a diminished nasal length and height, an acute columellar-labial angle, and a low radix.[3-12]

As emphasized by Sheen[13] and Gunter,[14] standards of beauty in our society have been influenced by the mass media and reflect the idealized Northern European characteristics, which in respect to the nose include a straight, narrow bridge, a well-defined projecting nasal tip, refined alae, and a nasolabial angle of approximately 90 to 95 degrees in men and 95 to 100 degrees in women. In contrast to the traditional African-American concepts of beauty, Millard[15] described the aesthetic Caucasian female face as having clear, pale, and smooth skin, large, widely spaced soft eyes with long lashes, a small, slim nose, high cheek bones, and a medium-sized mouth with gentle lips that are not too thick.

Ethnic groups may feel that their "nonstandard" appearance sets them apart. An African-American patient who seeks rhinoplasty usually has one of two aesthetic objectives: to achieve a more "accepted standard of beauty" or to attain a more attractive nose that retains its ethnic character. It is imperative that the surgeon understand this distinction in the preoperative assessment of an African-American rhinoplasty patient to avoid any postoperative problems due to patient misunderstanding. Furthermore, clarification of this objective will help establish preoperatively whether the patient is attempting to transform or erase his ethnic features, which may be impossible and is usually undesirable based on anatomic limitations. Patients who have unrealistic goals will seldom be satisfied with the postoperative result, and the prudent surgeon will decline to proceed with treatment.

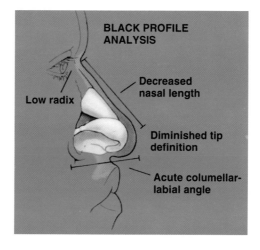

The African-American nose typically has a short columella, broad, flat dorsum, slightly flaring alae, and a rounded tip with ovoid nares. The upper lip is highlighted by the prominent Cupid's bow and fullness over the lips. Bimaxillary protrusion is common. It is obvious from this description that it would be an error to apply the standards of Caucasian beauty to the African-American patient. Therefore the plastic surgeon managing the African-American rhinoplasty patient must understand and appreciate what constitutes African-American facial aesthetics.

As Farkas[16] has delineated, the aesthetic face is not divided into equal thirds or fourths. Rather the lower face has a greater vertical dimension that the midface, which in turn has a greater vertical dimension than the upper face.[17,18] These proportions are amplified in African-American facial features. African-American patients commonly have bimaxillary protrusion. However, it is important to identify any underlying skeletal disproportion and point this out to the patient preoperatively. The treatment plan should not be based on a frontal photograph alone. According to Byrd and Hober,[19] the ideal nasal length measured from the radix to the tip-defining points should approximate the distance from the stomion to the menton. The nasal length measurement should be derived from a clinical examination and a profile view of the patient. Nasal projection is defined as the distance from the alar-cheek junction to the nasal tip and is approximately $0.67 \times$ the ideal nasal length in Caucasians. Nasal projection is usually inadequate in the African-American patient and is approximately $0.5 \times$ the nasal length.

Ideal nasal length measured from the radix to the tip-defining points should approximate the distance from the stomion to the menton, whereas nasal projection should be 0.67 × the ideal length.

Proper nasal alignment will help maintain ethnicity in African-American rhinoplasty patients. Broadbent and Matthews[20] described the ideal nasal alignment as a lateral attachment of the ala to the cheek that lies within a vertical line drawn through the medial canthus. Nasal features can be improved without altering ethnic appearance by bringing the elements of the nose closer to this boundary. In conclusion, an appreciation of African-American nasal-facial aesthetics is essential for obtaining consistent aesthetic results in the African-American patient.

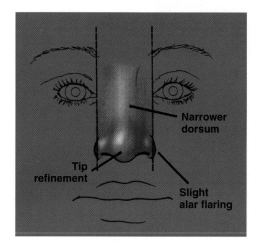

The overall goals in African-American rhinoplasty are to achieve:
- Nasal-facial harmony and balance
- A narrower, straight dorsum
- Enhanced tip projection and definition
- Slight alar flaring
- Normal interalar distance

Narrowing the interalar distance or correcting alar flaring can improve nasal appearance without disturbing the ethnic character of the nose.

ANATOMIC VARIATIONS

Descriptions of anatomic distinctions between the Caucasian nose and the African-American nose abound in the literature. Among them are a number of myths. As Ofodile and associates[8-11] have described, the many variations in African-American nasal anatomic features can be attributed to the tri-ethnic background of African-Americans in the United States: African, Caucasian, and Native American. Thus individualized anatomic diagnosis and surgical planning are as essential for African-American patients as for other patients. Anatomic variations in Caucasian and African-American patients may be summarized as follows:

	Caucasian	African-American
Skin	Thin	Thick
Alar cartilage		
Size	Large	Large
Support	Strong	Strong
Alar base	Slight alar flaring	Excess alar flaring; increased interalar distance
Nasal pyramid		
Nasal bones	Long	Long but flattened
Base	Narrower	Wide
Dorsum	Thin	Broad/depressed

African-American nasal anatomic features may exhibit considerable variation.

Skin

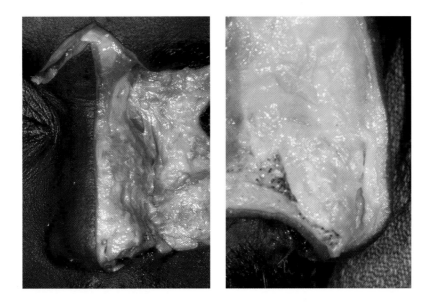

The skin, especially in the tip area, is notably thicker in the African-American patient. The tip is usually flattened, bulbous, and ill-defined. The skin is thick, sebaceous, and relatively inelastic with increased subcutaneous fibrofatty tissue present above the lower lateral cartilages, obscuring tip definition. This fibrofatty layer often measures 2 to 4 mm in thickness.

The skin and fibrofatty layer are generally quite thick.

Alar Cartilages

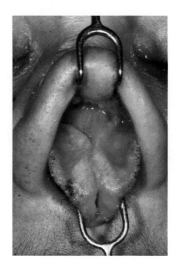

Previously the alar cartilages were thought to be thin and weak, affording little support to the overlying heavy skin and fibrofatty unit. However, our own anatomic studies[21] as well as those of Ofodile and James[11] have demonstrated that the alar cartilages in African-American patients are similar in size to those of Caucasian patients. The medial and lateral projections of the alar cartilages are not shorter and weaker than in Caucasians as previously thought but are quite well developed. The angle between the medial and lateral crura (the "soft triangle") is obtuse, and the space is filled with a relative abundance of fat and skin. The nasal spine is underdeveloped in many cases, contributing to the paucity of tip projection.

The alar cartilages are not typically weak and underdeveloped as once thought.

Alar Base

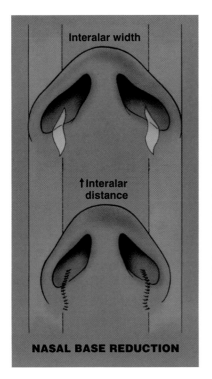

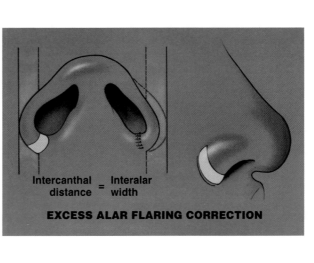

Alar base abnormalities in the African-American patient can be defined as one of three entities:

1. Increased interalar distance with the alar bases being lateral to the medial canthal lines
2. Excessive alar flaring, which is characterized by a portion of the ala extending lateral to the alar attachment of the cheek (>2 mm)
3. A combination of alar flaring and increased interalar distance, making the correction more difficult

---

The alar bases may exhibit increased interalar distance, alar flaring, or both.

The columella is short and rounded and often hidden on the profile view by heavy overlying alar rims.

Nasal Pyramid

The base of the bony pyramid is widened and the dorsum is depressed, broad, and often saddlelike. There is a deepened nasofrontal angle that exaggerates the flattened look. The nasal bone's dimensions are similar in height and width.

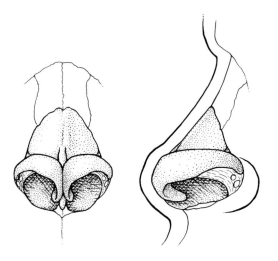

The striking characteristic is the splaying and lack of vertical projection of the ascending process of the maxilla, which contributes to the low and widened nasal base.[22-24] However, the flat external appearance of the nose is usually secondary to a lower dorsal bridge rather than a wide base. For this reason osteotomies and infractures are frequently not necessary and may be contraindicated. Rather dorsal augmentation alone is frequently required. It is important to note that the bony base in African-Americans is wider than in Caucasians.

The dorsum is usually broad and low with a wide bony pyramid and splayed and shortened ascending processes of the maxillae.

OPERATIVE TECHNIQUE

With growing experience in rhinoplasty techniques, advancements in technology, and the increased use of autologous tissue for grafting, consistently reproducible results in the aesthetic African-American rhinoplasty have become attainable. By applying the principles of augmentation rhinoplasty to correcting the characteristic deformities noted in the African-American nose, the following techniques have evolved:

A. Increasing tip projection
1. Midcolumellar autologous cartilage strut
2. Suture plication of medial crura using interdomal and transdomal sutures (see Chapter 18)
3. Tip grafts: infratip lobular (Sheen), onlay (Peck), and combined infratip lobular/onlay grafts (Gunter)
B. Increasing tip definition
1. Transdomal suture technique
2. Multiple tip grafts, particularly infratip lobular grafts
C. Dorsal augmentation
1. Autologous tissue (see Chapter 57)
2. AlloDerm (see Chapter 49)
D. Alar base surgery
1. Correction of alar flaring by alar base resection
2. Decrease of interalar distance by nostril sill excision and advancement

An organized approach to rhinoplasty is essential in attaining consistent results. The following six principles are respected to ensure consistent functional and aesthetic results in African-Americans[22-24]:

1. External transcolumellar approach
2. Accurate intraoperative anatomic diagnosis
3. Meticulous hemostasis
4. Routine use of autologous tissue or allografts for dorsum/tip augmentation
5. Minimum skin defatting
6. Meticulous wound closure

It should be emphasized that before entering the operating room the surgeon must define the deformity, determine the etiology of the deformity, establish realistic surgical goals, and formulate a treatment plan (see Chapter 4). Once these preparatory steps have been completed, the following technique is employed. An external approach is advocated since accurate anatomic diagnosis under direct binocular vision is essential for achieving pleasing and reproducible modifications of the challenging African-American nasal anatomy. With the patient under general anesthesia the external nose and septum are injected with 10 ml of 0.5% lidocaine with 1:200,000 epinephrine, and the internal nose is packed bilaterally with 3½-inch neuropledgets moistened with oxymetazoline (Afrin).

Accurate preoperative analysis and diagnosis are essential to formulating a realistic surgical plan.

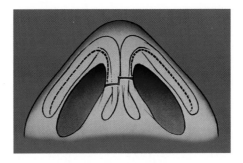

Bilateral infracartilaginous incisions along the caudal edge of the lower lateral cartilages are terminated medially at the narrowest portion of the columella and connected via a transcolumellar stair-step incision. This allows for precise wound closure, and the splinting supplied by the underlying cartilages via the medial crura aids in preventing scar contracture.

The external approach is optimal for correction of the African-American nose.

Methylene blue dots are placed with a 25-gauge needle on both sides of the infracartilaginous incision at the midpoint of the caudal portion of the lateral crura prior to skin elevation. These marks allow more accurate approximation at final wound closure. The skin elevation is begun by dissecting the thin columellar skin off the caudal edges of the medial crura and intervening subcutaneous tissue. Great care must be taken to avoid transecting the fragile medial crural cartilages. Dissection proceeds from inferiorly to superiorly, to the level of the infratip lobule, and then laterally over the lateral crura to medially, stopping at the soft triangle. The soft triangle is dissected last, affording optimal visualization to avoid damage to the vulnerable genu of the lower lateral cartilage. Accurate anatomic dissection is achieved by hugging the perichondrium of the lower lateral cartilage. No subdermal defatting is done, but the prominent supratip globular fibrofatty tissue can safely be removed.

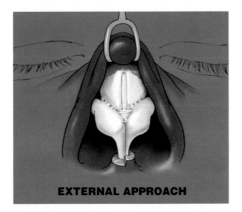

EXTERNAL APPROACH

The dissection subsequently is continued over the upper lateral cartilages and the cartilaginous and bony dorsum up to the root of the nose. This enables retraction of the undermined area, exposing the entire nasal framework.

> *Initial exposure of the alar cartilages is best performed in the*
> *supraperichondrial plane by dissecting from inferiorly to superiorly*
> *and laterally to medially, exposing the genu of the alar cartilages last.*

The soft tissues are elevated from the nasal framework, and the tip cartilages are evaluated and correlated with the preoperative diagnosis. The extent of the nasal tip deformity and paucity of nasal projection are then determined based on direct visualization and the preoperative analysis. Usually tip projection needs to be increased. The desired tip projection will dictate the dorsal height; therefore any alteration of the dorsum should be performed with the final tip projection in mind.

After the desired tip projection is determined, the dorsum is evaluated. Usually dorsal augmentation is required in the majority of African-American rhinoplasty patients. However, rasping may be necessary to remove any irregularities and provide a smooth bed on which to place the autologous dorsal graft. Lateral osteotomies are infrequently performed. When augmentation is indicated, it is performed after septal reconstruction or septal graft harvest. The dorsal height should be reevaluated after final tip projection is achieved to determine whether further dorsal augmentation is necessary and if osteotomies are needed.

> *The desired tip projection dictates the appropriate dorsal height.*
> *Dorsal augmentation should be performed after septal graft harvest*
> *and prior to setting the final tip projection.*

If septal work is required, either to straighten the septum or for harvesting autologous cartilage grafts, the septum can be approached either from the anterior septal angle through the open approach or through a separate transfixion incision. We prefer to approach it from the anterior septal angle through the open approach. This approach necessitates separating the medial crura to gain adequate exposure. The septum proper is separated from the upper lateral cartilages in a component fashion (see Chapter 26). There need be no hesitation in doing this in the African-American rhinoplasty patient since the tip structures need to be reconstructed to establish increased projection. Submucous resection of the anterior inferior turbinates is usually performed at this time since inferior turbinate hypertrophy is quite common in the African-American nose (see Chapter 36).

The septum is ideally approached from the anterior septal angle via the open approach by separating the lower and upper lateral cartilages from the septum in a component fashion.

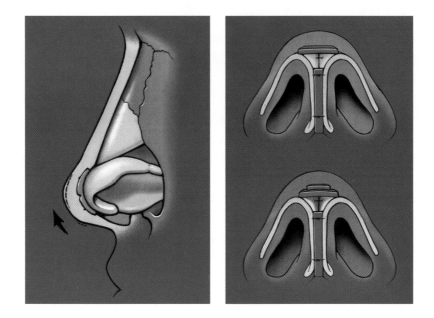

After the septal cartilage is harvested, infrequently osteotomies are performed in African-American patients to properly align or narrow the nasal base prior to dorsal augmentation and final tip reconstruction. Attention is directed to the tip for final modification of the tip cartilages and establishment of tip projection. To establish and enhance tip projection and/or definition, a graduated approach is used (see Chapter 18).[25] Initially a columellar strut is secured with intercrural sutures; then, interdomal and transdomal sutures are used to unify the tip and increase tip projection. These suture techniques are followed by a combined infratip lobular/onlay tip graft (Gunter type) and additional double- and even triple-layer onlay cartilage grafts as required to attain final tip definition/projection.[25]

A graduated approach to increasing tip projection should be used that employs a three-step suture technique and cartilage grafting as dictated by the preoperative nasal analysis.

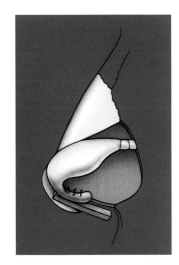

A strong, long bowie knife–shaped strut in the columella both increases the tip projection and augments the columellar-labial angle since African-American patients usually have a retracted columella as well as decreased tip projection. This graft is placed in a pocket within soft tissue in front of the nasal spine between the feet of the medial crura. The strut and the medial crura are advanced until the desired tip projection is achieved. The medial crura are secured to the strut using intercrural sutures of 5-0 clear PDS. Next interdomal and transdomal sutures are routinely used due to the thick skin and the need for increased tip refinement and projection in African-American patients. Prior to establishing final tip projection *only* the excess fibrofatty tissue over the dome area of the lower lateral cartilages is removed. As it is removed, the subdermal plexus must be preserved to prevent postoperative nasal tip necrosis. This maneuver enhances tip definition by decreasing the thickness of the overlying soft tissue envelope. Tip definition is optimally accentuated by the use of a combined Sheen (infratip) and Peck (onlay) tip cartilage graft (see Chapter 11).[25] To increase tip projection and definition, multiple Gunter-type combined grafts can be fashioned from septal cartilage and are suture stabilized with 5-0 clear PDS to the middle crura and domal cartilages. However, if more infralobular definition is needed, a Sheen-type graft is used in a similar fashion. These combined grafts give the optimal projection and definition to the African-American nose with thick skin.

The columellar strut is the foundation for tip reconstruction and enhanced projection.

Meticulous technique must be employed when removing excess fibrofatty tissue from the domal area to preserve the subdermal plexus blood supply and thereby prevent tip skin necrosis.

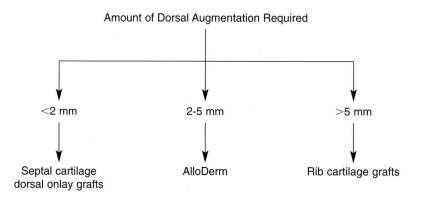

Once the final tip projection is established, dorsal augmentation is usually required in the African-American patient. When <2 mm dorsal augmentation is required, septal cartilage dorsal onlay grafts are preferred (see Chapter 27).[26] For 2 to 5 mm of dorsal augmentation we prefer to use AlloDerm placed in multiple layers on the dorsum (see Chapter 49). Finally, when >5 mm of dorsal augmentation is required, an anatomically contoured rib cartilage graft should be used (see Chapter 28).

A graduated approach to dorsal augmentation is used, progressing from septal cartilage onlay grafts for minimal augmentation (<2 mm) to AlloDerm onlay grafts for moderate augmentation (2 to 5 mm) and costal cartilage grafts for significant dorsal augmentation (>5 mm).

The skin is redraped after a final inspection of the nasal framework, the external appearance is evaluated, and all incisions are closed. The infracartilaginous incisions are closed with 5-0 chromic catgut, and the transcolumellar incisions are closed meticulously with 6-0 nylon in an interrupted fashion. Next the final dorsal appearance of the nose on the profile view is inspected, and attention is directed to the basal view for correction of any alar base abnormality (i.e., either increased alar flaring or increased alar base distance or a combination of both).[7]

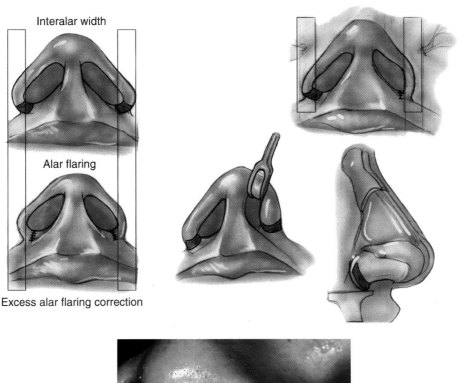

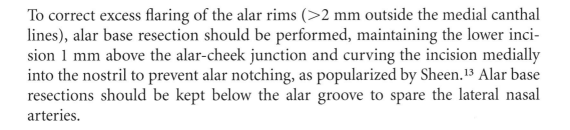

To correct excess flaring of the alar rims (>2 mm outside the medial canthal lines), alar base resection should be performed, maintaining the lower incision 1 mm above the alar-cheek junction and curving the incision medially into the nostril to prevent alar notching, as popularized by Sheen.[13] Alar base resections should be kept below the alar groove to spare the lateral nasal arteries.

Alar base resection or nostril sill resection is performed after closure of the nasal incisions. Carrying alar base resections above the alar groove will jeopardize the nasal tip blood supply by transecting the lateral nasal arteries.

After the required resection of the alar base there is always an increased width of the base of the alar-cheek junction. This is corrected by using a buried 5-0 Vicryl suture followed by closure of the alar base resection with 6-0 nylon. These sutures are removed in 3 to 4 days.

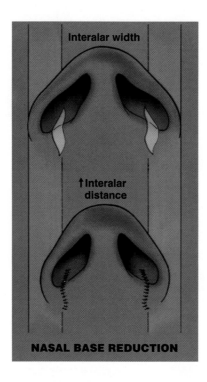

If there is an increased interalar distance, a Millard-type alar nostril sill resection and advancement are performed in a similar fashion to decrease interalar distance.[27-29]

After alar base surgery is completed and the result inspected from the basal view for complete symmetry, the nasal splints and dressing are applied (see Chapter 5). This is a critical portion of the procedure since there appears to be prolonged postoperative edema in the African-American rhinoplasty patient. Therefore, if septal work has been performed, bilateral septal splints are placed and sutured into place anteriorly with through-and-through 3-0 nylon sutures. Nasal packing is avoided. An external dressing of Steri-Strips and a conforming metal splint (Denver type) is placed on the dorsum of the nose for a period of at least 1 week. Postoperatively the patient is instructed to keep ice on the periorbital and nasal area for a period of 2 days as well as to maintain 40-degree elevation of the head to decrease postoperative swelling. Activities are restricted for 2 weeks, and the patient is given appropriate medication to alleviate anxiety. The importance of keeping the splint on is reemphasized. All patients receive perioperative antibiotics (preoperative cefazolin and cephalexin for 2 to 3 days postoperatively) as well as steroids (dexamethasone, 8 mg, preoperatively and methylprednisolone dose pack postoperatively). Silicone sheeting is also used postoperatively in thick-skinned patients for 3 months as tolerated to accelerate the resolution of edema.

A conforming external nasal splint is critical to counteract the increased postoperative edema seen in the African-American rhinoplasty patient.

Preferential Use of Autologous Tissue (see Chapter 28)

Septal Cartilage	Ear Cartilage	Rib Cartilage	Cranial Bone
Tip graft	Alar cartilage	Dorsal onlay	Dorsal onlay
Dorsal onlay	Dorsal onlay	Columellar strut	Columellar strut
Columellar strut	Tip graft		
Spreader graft			

In most cases we prefer autologous tissue primarily. However, we have been using AlloDerm on the dorsum for over 2 years with remarkably good results and essentially no resorption (see Chapter 49).

Septal Cartilage

When dorsal augmentation, columellar struts, or tip grafts are needed, autologous septal cartilage is preferred. Septal cartilage is the material of choice because it provides rigid support that does not have the convolutions found in auricular cartilage. In our hands it has proved excellent for dorsal onlay, columellar strut, spreader, and tip grafts.

Ear Cartilage

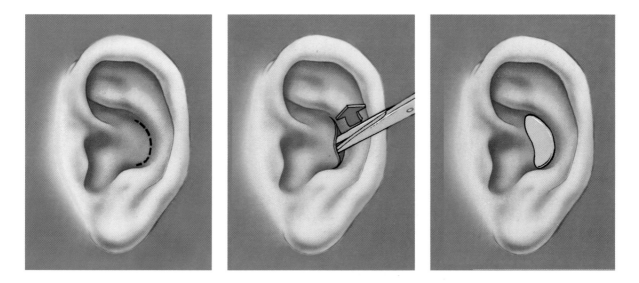

The auricle can provide a large amount of material for cartilage reconstruction. Because of its flaccidity and convolutions, auricular cartilage is best used when these characteristics are desired, especially when reconstructing the lower lateral cartilages.

Rib Cartilage

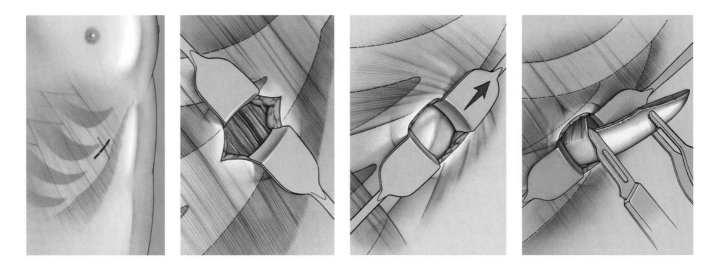

Rib cartilage is excellent when support is a major consideration. Access is obtained via a small incision over the anterior portion of the ninth rib, and the cartilaginous portion is removed. The key element in rib grafts is to have a straight piece of cartilage to begin with; postoperative warping of the graft can then be avoided in many cases. This cartilage is ideal for a midcolumellar strut, and it can be fashioned for use in dorsal augmentation. If a large amount of cartilage is needed, an incision should be made over the junction of the seventh and eighth ribs where a large block of rib cartilage can be harvested, especially when needed for dorsal augmentation. The principles of balanced cross-sectional carving established by Gibson and Davis[30] must be respected in that the cartilage must be carved so that equal amounts are removed from both sides to prevent warping or bending. End slices of rib cartilage have a tendency to curl and can be used for lower lateral cartilage replacement or selective onlay grafts.

Use of the ninth rib cartilage, which is relatively straight, minimizes the incidence of postoperative graft warping.

Other Grafts/Alloplastic Material

As we prefer primarily autologous material or AlloDerm for long-term safety and to minimize resorption and especially extrusion, we do not advocate the use of silicone, Gore-Tex, or other alloplastic materials in the nose (see Chapter 49).

CASE ANALYSES

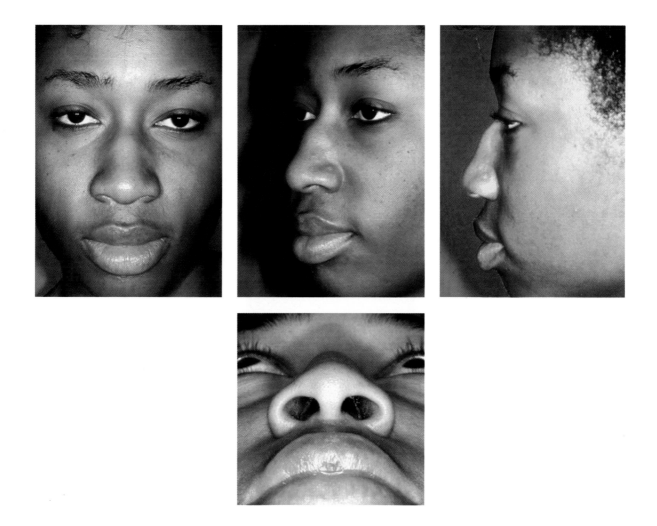

This primary rhinoplasty patient complained of her dorsal hump and wide, poorly defined nose. The frontal view demonstrated wide bony and alar bases with poor tip definition. On the lateral view the high dorsal hump was evident as well as the hanging ala/hidden columella. The basal view confirmed the alar flaring and bulbous appearance of the nasal tip with columellar-lobular disproportion. The intranasal examination showed no abnormality.

The operative goals included:
- Reduction of the dorsal hump
- Narrowing of bony pyramid
- Correction of alar flaring
- Refinement of tip

The surgical plan called for:
- An open approach with a stair-step transcolumellar incision and bilateral infracartilaginous incisions
- Component reduction of dorsum
- Cephalic resection of lower lateral cartilages
- Columellar strut stabilized with intercrural sutures (5-0 PDS)
- Multiple tip suturing techniques using interdomal and transdomal sutures
- Onlay tip graft × 3 suture stabilized to tip with 5-0 PDS
- Lateral osteotomies (low to high)
- Alar base resections (9 mm alar base resection)

The preoperative analysis and diagnoses were confirmed intraoperatively on direct visualization of the nasal framework via the open approach.

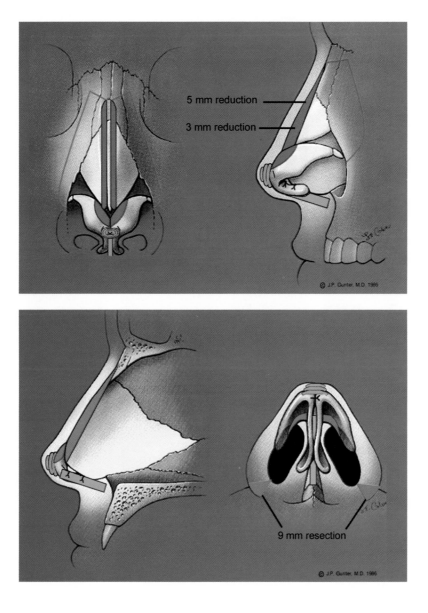

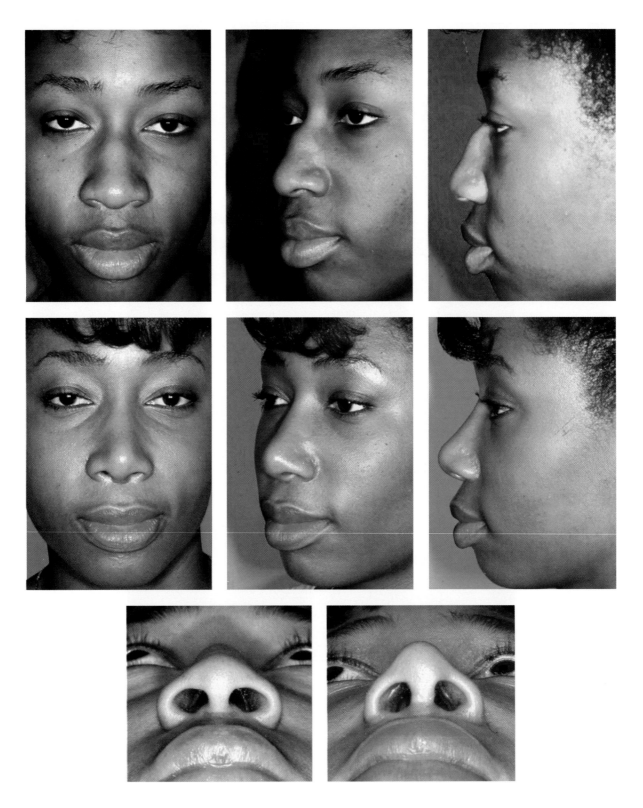

The 2-year postoperative result demonstrates good correction of these deformities.

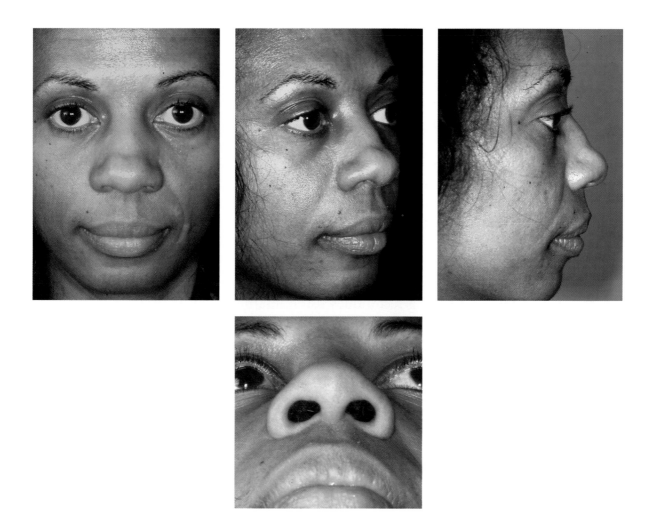

This primary rhinoplasty patient described her nose as large and unrefined. On the frontal view a wide bony base, wide dorsal aesthetic lines, and a poorly defined and bulbous tip were apparent. The lateral view revealed a small dorsal hump and alar-columellar disharmony. The basal view demonstrated the characteristic alar flaring and columellar-lobular disproportion with a bulbous tip. The findings on intranasal examination were normal.

The operative goals included:
- Reduction of dorsum
- Narrowing of bony base
- Correction of alar flaring
- Refinement of tip

The surgical plan called for:
- An open approach with a stair-step transcolumellar incision and bilateral infracartilaginous incisions
- Component reduction of high proximal dorsum
- Cephalic resection of lower lateral cartilages (preserve 6 mm of lower lateral cartilage)
- Columellar strut stabilized with 5-0 PDS intercrural suture
- Multiple tip suturing techniques using interdomal and transdomal sutures
- Three stacked onlay tip grafts (Peck type) suture stabilized to domal cartilages
- Lateral osteotomies and medial osteotomies
- Alar base resection with preservation of nostril (9 mm resection bilaterally)

The preoperative analysis and diagnoses were confirmed intraoperatively on direct visualization of the nasal framework via the open approach.

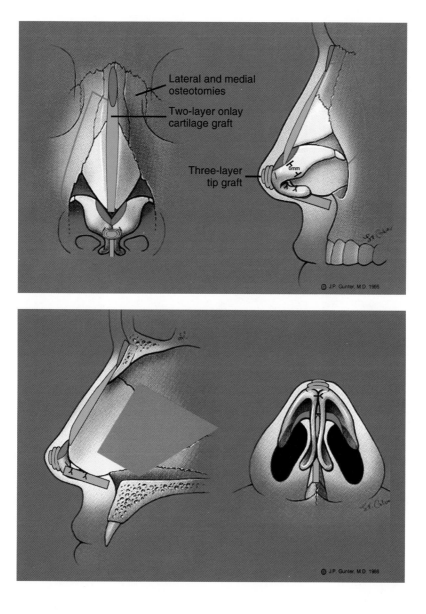

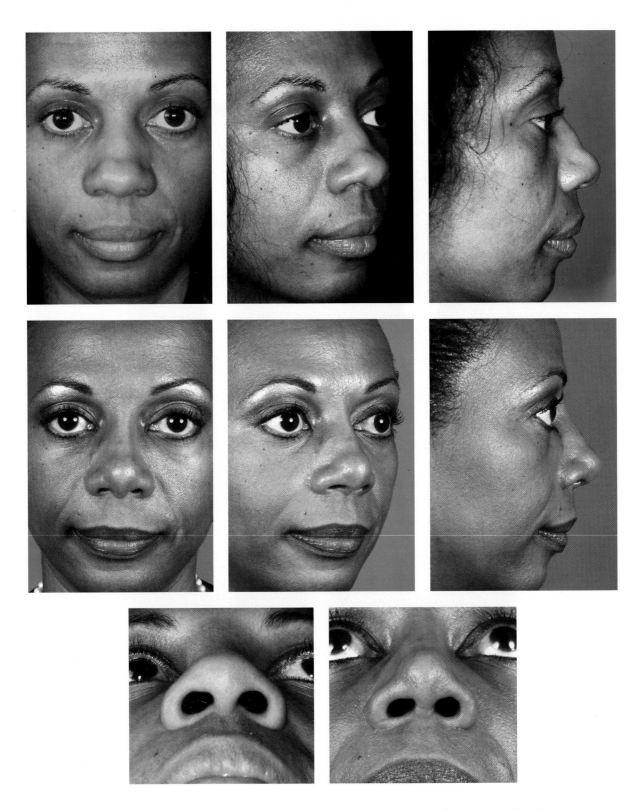

The 2-year postoperative results demonstrate a narrowed, more refined nose with improved tip definition and projection and maintenance of racial nasal-facial balance and harmony.

COMPLICATIONS

Unsatisfactory results following rhinoplasty have been previously described by several authors, and complications in the African-American rhinoplasty patient are no different.[31,32] However, several are worth emphasizing. The African-American rhinoplasty patient may be more prone to certain complications. Matory and Falces[7] plan a secondary procedure routinely, and their patients are counseled accordingly. We do not routinely plan a secondary procedure. In fact, our revision rate in African-American rhinoplasty patients is similar to that for Caucasian patients. However, the patient is certainly told of the possibility, as are all rhinoplasty patients. Certain sequelae are more apt to occur in the African-American rhinoplasty patient.

Protracted Edema

Edema may last up to 12 months because of the thick skin inherent to the African-American nose, the multiple incisions, as well as the external approach. However, this can be ameliorated somewhat by meticulous intraoperative hemostasis and prolonged postoperative splinting as well as the use of perioperative steroids. Prolonged postoperative use of silicone gel sheeting applied to the nose further accelerates resolution of edema. Mucosal preservation when possible during alar base resection has sometimes been advocated to minimize lobule edema.

Excess External Scarring/Keloid Formation

Scarring obviously is of great concern in the African-American patient because of the increased propensity for keloid and hypertrophic scar formation. However, this has not been our experience using meticulous wound closure and early suture removal at 3 to 4 days after alar base resections and at 6 to 7 days after the transcolumellar incision. We have never seen a keloid scar of the nose in any of our African-American rhinoplasty patients.

Asymmetry

Asymmetries are noted especially after alar base resections and are due to inadequate preoperative planning and operative execution of alar base resection or nostril sill excision. Any degree of asymmetry can be noted intraoperatively and can be easily corrected at that time to minimize or prevent postoperative alar base asymmetry.

Nasal Tip Necrosis

Nasal tip necrosis has not occurred in our experience. However, it is of concern, especially using the external approach, when extensive alar base resections are undertaken. Alar base resections must not transgress the alar groove, as we have emphasized in our studies delineating the nasal tip blood supply.[33] Onlay tip grafting may apply excessive nasal tip skin tension, which can either compromise blood supply or cause dehiscence or separation of the transcolumellar incision.

Racial Incongruity

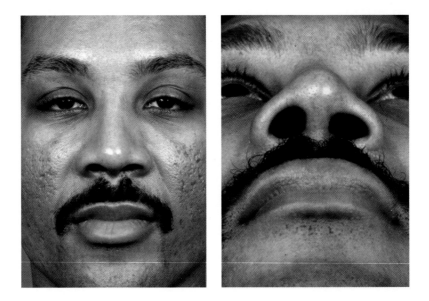

Racial incongruity is the most ominous complication in the African-American rhinoplasty patient. In these patients nasal infracture accompanied by excessive alar base resection or nostril sill resection creates a disproportionate narrowing of the dorsum with respect to the lobule because the alar base resection does not significantly narrow the alar and lobular width. This disproportion can be avoided by one of three methods:

1. Adjusting the infracture proportionate to the lobule size or avoiding nasal pyramid infracture in the majority of African-American noses
2. Performing alar base and/or interalar sill reduction at the end of the operative procedure or at a subsequent stage if in doubt about the necessity for this procedure (If there is any doubt about the need for alar base resections, they should not be done at the primary procedure.)
3. Simultaneous use of a columellar strut and a cartilaginous tip graft so that the increased tip height and definition will lessen the accentuation of the alar width/alar flaring

Care should be taken to ensure that alar base resections do not compromise the lateral nasal artery blood supply to the nasal tip; if necessary, alar base resections can be performed secondarily as an outpatient procedure. The dorsum and lobule should be kept in proportion to avoid racial incongruity. Alar base resections should not be done at the primary procedure if there is any doubt as to whether or not they are necessary.

■ KEY POINTS

- ■ The African-American nose is characterized by a wide and depressed dorsum, inadequate tip projection, an ill-defined tip, excess alar flaring and/or interalar distance, diminished nasal length and height, an acute columellar-labial angle, and a low radix.

- ■ An appreciation of ethnic concepts of beauty and nasal-facial harmony and aesthetic balance is a prerequisite for success in treating the African-American rhinoplasty patient.

- ■ A detailed, systematic preoperative evaluation of the nasal deformity, including a comprehensive nasal history and nasal-facial analysis, is critical in determining the goals of the procedure. The patient's aesthetic aims must be clearly verbalized. An accurate internal and external nasal examination is essential. An individualized, organized, and realistic operative plan can then be formulated.

- ■ The external approach is advocated for accurate intraoperative anatomic diagnosis under direct binocular vision and precise correction of the deformity. The external technique permits more options in the modification of the native tissues, allowing for precise application of suturing techniques and better utilization of cartilage grafts, specifically midcolumellar struts and tip grafts to increase tip projection and dorsal onlay grafts to enhance the dorsal profile in the African-American patient.

- ■ Dorsal augmentation is routinely required in the African-American patient; in contrast, infracture of the bony nasal pyramid is infrequently necessary and may be contraindicated in many patients.

- ■ Harmony between the width of the bony nasal pyramid and of the lobule must be maintained; failure to respect this principle results in racial incongruity.

- ■ The use of autologous cartilage grafts is advocated if possible; the use of alloplastic materials is not recommended.

- The combined infratip lobular/onlay tip cartilage graft is an extremely powerful and useful technique for enhancing tip refinement and projection in the African-American patient.

- The blood supply of the nasal tip skin must be respected at all times; therefore care should be taken when removing excess fibrofatty tissue and when performing alar base excisions to preserve the subdermal plexus and lateral nasal arteries, respectively.

- Alar base resections should be done at the end of the procedure and should not be performed at the initial procedure if there is any doubt as to whether they are required.

- Protracted postoperative edema is controlled with postoperative ice, prolonged postoperative splinting, elevation, perioperative steroids, and postoperative application of silicone gel sheeting.

- Revisions or secondary procedures are not required more frequently in the African-American patient; however, if they are necessary, they should not be done for at least 12 to 15 months after the initial procedure.

REFERENCES

1. Bernstein L. Esthetics in rhinoplasty. Otolaryngol Clin North Am 9:705, 1975.
2. Converse JM. Corrective rhinoplasty. In Converse JM, ed. Reconstructive Surgery, 2nd ed. Philadelphia: WB Saunders, 1977, pp 1040-1163.
3. Falces E, Wesser D, Gorney M. Cosmetic surgery of the non-Caucasian nose. Plast Reconstr Surg 45:317, 1970.
4. deAvelar JM. Personal contribution to the surgical treatment of Negroid noses. Aesthetic Plast Surg 1:81, 1976.
5. Rees T. Nasal plastic surgery in the Negro. Plast Reconstr Surg 43:13, 1969.
6. Snyder GB. Rhinoplasty in the Negro. Plast Reconstr Surg 47:572, 1971.
7. Matory WE Jr, Falces E. Non-Caucasian rhinoplasty: A 16-year experience. Plast Reconstr Surg 2:239, 1986.
8. Ofodile FA, Bokhari FJ, Ellis C. The African-American nose. Ann Plast Surg 31:209, 1993.
9. Ofodile FA, Bokhari F. The African-American nose: Part II. Ann Plast Surg 34:123, 1995.
10. Ofodile FA. Nasal bones and pyriform apertures in African-Americans. Ann Plast Surg 32:21, 1994.
11. Ofodile FA, James EA. Anatomy of alar cartilages in African-Americans. Plast Reconstr Surg 100:699, 1997.
12. Rohrich RJ, Kenkel JM. The definition of beauty. In Matory WE Jr, ed. Ethnic Considerations in Facial Aesthetic Surgery. Philadelphia: Lippincott-Raven, 1998.
13. Sheen JH, Sheen AP. Aesthetic Rhinoplasty, 2nd ed. St. Louis: Quality Medical Publishing, 1998 (reprint of 1987 ed.).
14. Gunter JP. Facial analysis for the rhinoplasty patient. Dallas Rhinoplasty Symp 14:45, 1997.
15. Millard DR. Adjuncts in mentoplasty and rhinoplasty. Plast Reconstr Surg 36:48, 1965.
16. Farkas LG. Anthropometry of the Head and Face in Medicine. New York: Elsevier, 1981.
17. Patterson CN, Powell DG. Facial analysis in patient evaluation for physiologic and cosmetic surgery. Laryngoscope 84:1004, 1974.

18. Rogers BO. The role of physical anthropology in plastic surgery today. Clin Plast Surg 1:439, 1974.
19. Byrd HS, Hobar PC. Rhinoplasty: A practical guide for surgical planning. Plast Reconstr Surg 91:642, 1993.
20. Broadbent TR, Matthews UL. Artistic relationships in surface anatomy of the face: Application to reconstructive surgery. Plast Reconstr Surg 20:1, 1957.
21. Rohrich RJ, Schwartz R. Alar cartilage anatomy in the African-American nose—a cadaver study (in preparation).
22. Rohrich RJ. Rhinoplasty in the black patient. In Daniel RK, ed. Aesthetic Plastic Surgery, 2nd ed. Boston: Little, Brown, 1993.
23. Rohrich RJ, Friedman RM. Black male. In Marchac D, Granick MS, Solomon MP, eds. Male Aesthetic Surgery. Boston: Butterworth-Heinemann, 1996.
24. Rohrich RJ. The African-American Rhinoplasty. Dallas Rhinoplasty Symp 11:229, 1994.
25. Rohrich RJ. Graduated approach to tip projection in rhinoplasty. Dallas Rhinoplasty Symp 14:129, 1997.
26. Gunter JP, Rohrich RJ. Augmentation rhinoplasty: Dorsal onlay grafting using shaped autogenous septal cartilage. Plast Reconstr Surg 86:39, 1990.
27. Millard DR. External excisions in rhinoplasty. Plast Reconstr Surg 36:48, 1965.
28. Millard DR. Alar margin sculpturing. Plast Reconstr Surg 40:337, 1967.
29. Ship AG. Alar base resection for IVSP flaring nostrils. Br J Plast Surg 28:77, 1975.
30. Gibson T, Davis B. The distortion of autogenous cartilage grafts: Its cause and prevention. Br J Plast Surg 10:257, 1958.
31. Davis PKB, Jones SM. The complications of Silastic implants. Br J Plast Surg 24:405, 1971.
32. Klabunde EU, Falces E. Incidence of complications in cosmetic rhinoplasties. Plast Reconstr Surg 34:192, 1964.
33. Rohrich RJ, Gunter JP, Friedman RM. Nasal tip blood supply: An anatomic study validating the safety of the transcolumellar incision in rhinoplasty. Plast Reconstr Surg 95:795, 1995.

54

The Non-Caucasian Patient

Fernando Ortiz-Monasterio, M.D.

*A*ccepted standards of beauty universally promoted through journals, the cinema, and TV reflect the "ideal" characteristics of the European nose, also referred to as Caucasian or, according to ethnologic terminology, as Indo-European. Thus the ideal nose is depicted as a straight narrow nose with a moderately projecting tip covered by thin skin. The alar cartilages protruding under the skin produce an effect of angularity. The radix is located at the level of the upper lid tarsus when the patient is looking straight ahead. The width of the nasal base is the same as the intercanthal distance. On the lateral view the columella shows below the alar rim, and the nasolabial angle is about 90 to 100 degrees. The nose of other races, however, has thicker skin, a wider bony pyramid, and a smaller and weaker cartilaginous structure. The facial features differ as well.

The innumerable ethnic combinations have led to the development of many different rhinoplasty techniques. My personal experience has largely involved nasal correction in a group of people that represent a mixture of European immigrants and the native population of the American continent.[1-3] Because of the origin of the Amerindians in northeast Asia there is a strong Mongoloid component in their facial features, making rhinoplasty techniques successful in this group also applicable to Orientals. Because of some other anatomic characteristics such as skin thickness and weak cartilaginous support, the basic technical concepts for the mestizo nose can also be used for nasal correction of some people of Mediterranean and African origin.[4-6]

ANATOMIC FEATURES
Skin

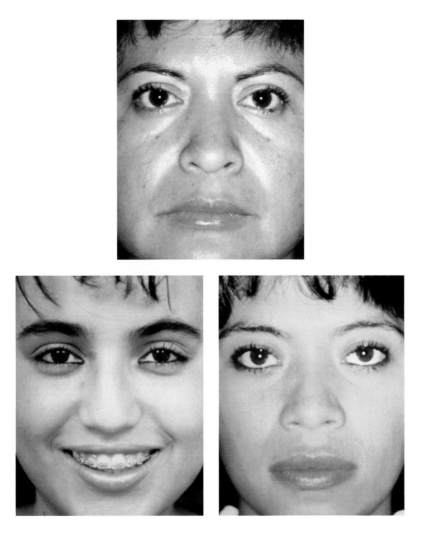

The skin of the mestizo population of many areas of Latin America and the Orient is moderately thick. The thickness of the skin cover is produced by the presence of a thin layer of subcutaneous fat and is also related to a slightly larger number of sebaceous glands than in the Indo-European nose. The presence of this fat layer is evidenced by the gliding of the skin over the alar cartilages as compared with the firmly adherent skin found in other groups.

The skin of the mestizo nose is moderately thick as a result of a thin layer of subcutaneous fat.

Dorsum

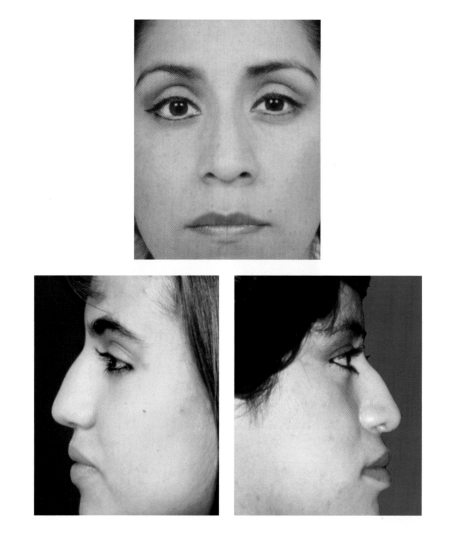

The nasal pyramid is small and relatively narrow. The visual impression of broadness is related to the limited height more than the actual width of the bony structure. The radix is often located below the level of the free margin of the upper lid, which accounts for the dorsal convexity. The dorsal convexity is usually discrete but may also be exaggerated by the limited projection of the tip.

The apparent broadness of the nose is more an attribute of limited height rather than actual width of the bony structure.

Tip

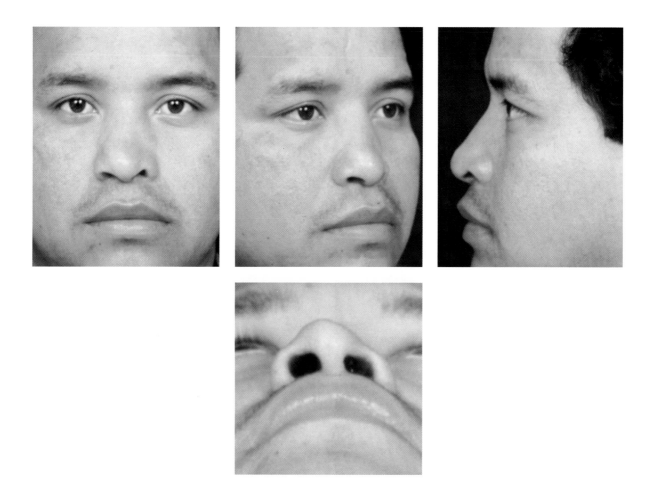

The alar cartilages are small and rather thin, which accounts for the under-projected tip; the short medial crura are responsible for the caudal rotation of the tip. Because of the skin thickness and the weak cartilaginous framework the nasal tip is round and poorly defined.

Nasolabial Angle

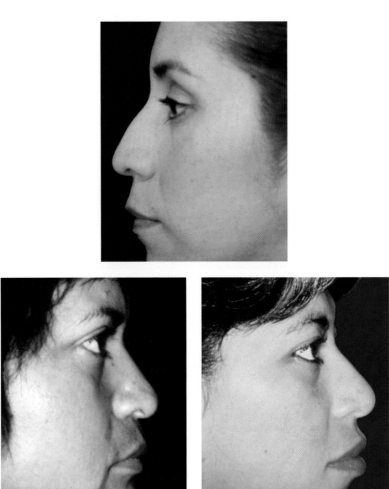

The nasolabial angle aperture varies from 60 to 80 degrees. This is the result of the caudal rotation of the tip and the position of the upper lip supported by a protruding maxillary dental arch.

Nasal Base

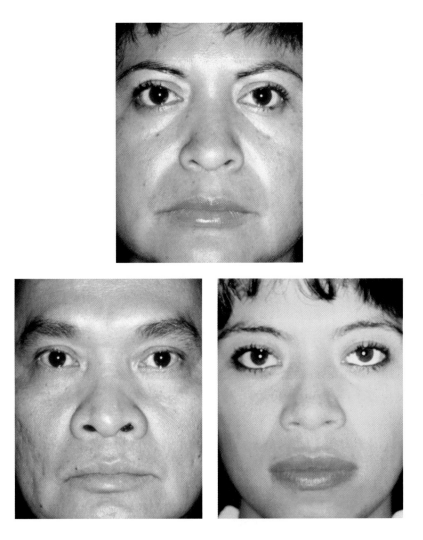

The nasal base is wide in some patients. The alar-cheek junction may be located more than 2 mm lateral to a vertical line extended from the medial canthus. In many others the impression of excessive width is related to the limited projection of the tip, that is, the relationship between the height and the width of the triangle when the nose is examined on the basal view.

Facial Skeleton

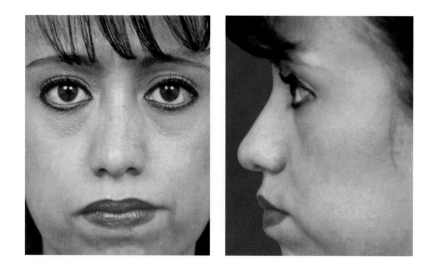

One of the most common features of the mestizo face is the procidence of the dental arches. This projects the upper lip anteriorly automatically, resulting in an acute nasolabial angle. The nasal spine, which is usually located in a prominent position, appears receded because of the prominence of the upper dental arch. The paranasal area may be slightly depressed, and the effect is also exaggerated by the prominence of the dental arch.

The procidence of the dental arches projects the upper lip anteriorly.

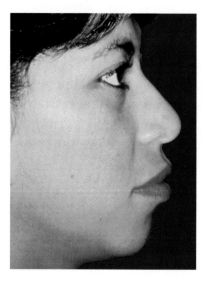

The chin is usually located in a good position, but it may appear to be receding because of the biprocident dental arches, which altogether enhance the facial convexity.

OPERATIVE TECHNIQUE

We use the closed approach in all of our patients. Intracartilaginous incisions are extended along the caudal edge of the septum on one side when septal work or graft harvesting is necessary.

Skin

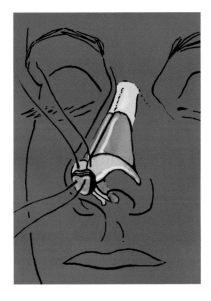

No substantial alteration of the skin thickness can be achieved. A small amount of the interdomal subcutaneous fat can be resected by an experienced surgeon, but more extensive defatting may result in circulatory compromise and skin necrosis. Visual alterations of the skin cover are obtained by augmentation of the structural support, which automatically stretches the skin. Cartilage grafts inserted subcutaneously are also used to further project the skin in certain areas such as the tip. Tip cartilage grafts are placed in front of the domes in a pocket dissected between the dermis and the superficial layers of the superficial musculoaponeurotic system. Sutures passed through the skin to maintain the position are fixed only with tape.

Extensive defatting may compromise the circulation and result in skin necrosis.

Dorsum

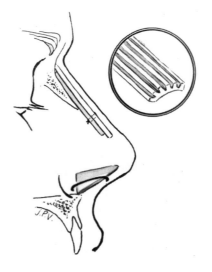

Minimal rasping of the dorsal convexity is necessary in most cases. It is also useful to provide an adequate bed for grafting. Dorsal augmentation is often necessary. Septal cartilage is the optimal material; a double or triple layer is used at the level of the radix to place the frontonasal groove in a more cephalic position.[1,2,7] Single- or double-layered septal cartilage grafts are applied to the dorsum, as shown above. A double layer is usually necessary at the radix. Longitudinal scoring of the graft is necessary to produce a smooth curvature that conforms to the dorsum (see inset).

Dorsal augmentation is generally needed.

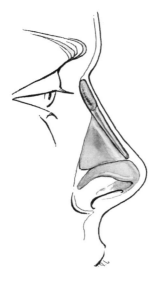

I use chondrocostal grafts when more augmentation is necessary.[3] A small section of cartilage (about 6 to 8 mm) is left on one end to achieve more projection at the radix.

Tip

The weak alar cartilages require minimal trimming. Minor resection of the cephalic border of the lateral crura and section of the intercartilaginous ligament are useful to allow rotation of the tip cephalad. Simultaneously the interdomal fat is resected. It is necessary to insert a cartilage strut to elongate the central leg of the tripod corresponding to the columella. Increased tip support is achieved by this maneuver. Triangular cartilage grafts are used to increase tip projection and to give an impression of angularity.[3,8,9] Septum and ear concha are the preferred donor areas. Two or more layers of cartilage may be used when necessary. The grafts are introduced through a small rim incision into a pocket dissected between the dermis and the superficial layers of the superficial musculoaponeurotic system.

Nasolabial Angle

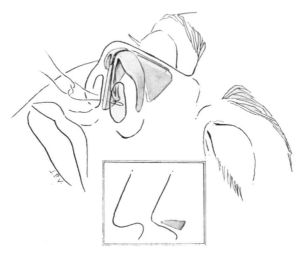

The nasolabial angle is partially corrected by cephalic rotation of the tip. To camouflage the prominence of the maxillary dental arch, a triangular cartilage graft is carved measuring about 14 to 20 mm long and 5 to 9 mm at the base. A pocket is dissected between the two medial crura to the base of the columella. The graft is inserted in a sagittal position with the base of the triangle located at the base of the columella. In this manner the vertex of the nasolabial angle is obliterated, camouflaging the acute nasolabial angle. The cartilage is fixed with a through-and-through absorbable suture at the base of the columella. This graft also increases the length and the structural support of the medial crura.[1-3]

Cephalic rotation of the tip helps correct the nasolabial angle.

Alar Base

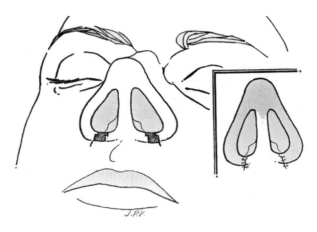

Wedge excisions of the floor of the nostrils are made to correct excessive width of the nasal base and flaring of the alae. The shape of the resection is determined by the width of the sill and the perimeter of the nostril. Care must be taken so that the final scar is located at the base of the nostril medial to the curvature of the alae.

Wedge excisions of the nostril floor are needed to correct the excessive width of the nasal base and flaring of the alae.

Chin

The relative microgenia may be corrected by the insertion of a Silastic implant on the anterior aspect of the mandibular symphysis immediately above the inferior margin of the bone. When an increase of more than 4 mm is necessary, I prefer to perform a sliding genioplasty. The horizontal osteotomy of the inferior mandibular margin is made through a small incision on the inferior buccal sulcus. The insertion of the suprahyoid muscles is maintained on the advanced free segment to improve the neck angle.

Skeleton

Depressed perialar areas are corrected by the insertion of costal cartilage grafts. The grafts are carved in a semilunar shape to conform to the piriform aperture and introduced into a snug subperiosteal pocket through a 1 cm buccal vestibular incision. A third graft shaped as a bar about 25 to 30 mm long and 5 mm in diameter may be inserted at the nasal base in front of the nasal spine to complement the correction of the depressed paranasal area.

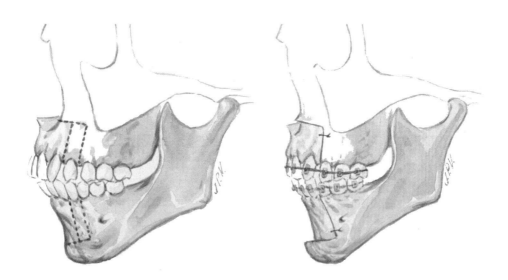

Segmental maxillary and mandibular osteotomies are necessary when the procidence of the alveolar arches is very exaggerated. One premolar on each side is extracted from the upper arch, and a section of bone is resected from the alveolar arch and from the palatine process to displace the premaxilla to the desired position. The segments are immobilized with an orthodontic bar fixed to the dental bands. The same technique is used for the mandibular arch.

CASE ANALYSES

This 29-year-old woman had a medium-size nose with medium-thickness skin, a minimal osseocartilaginous hump, an underprojected tip, an acute nasolabial angle, and moderate protrusion of the dental arches. The surgical plan included minimal dorsal resection, trimming of the cephalic edge of the lateral crura, and medial and lateral osteotomies. A septal cartilage graft was placed on the columella. The postoperative result is shown at 3 years.

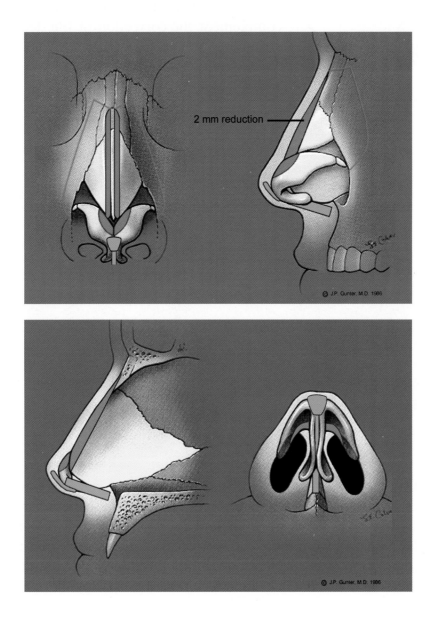

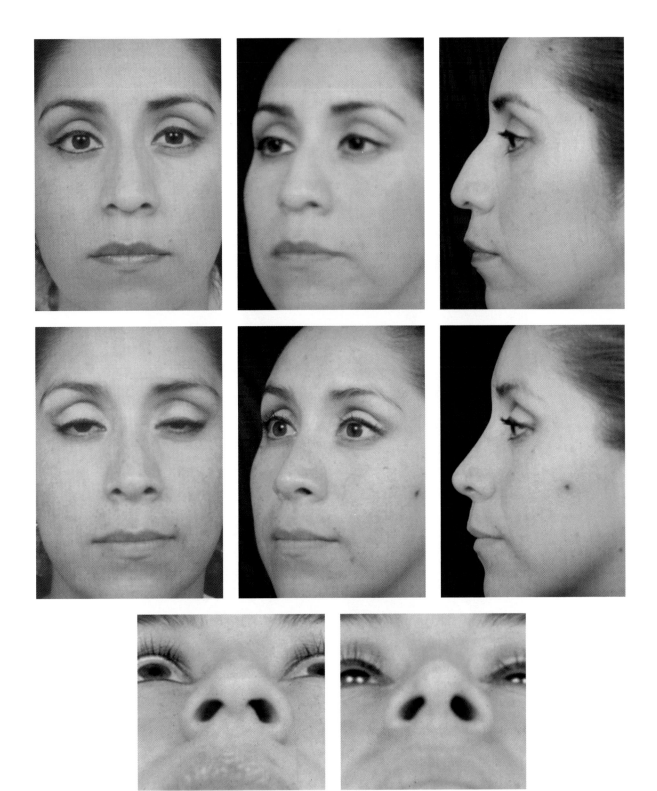

This 26-year-old woman had a small-size nose with medium-thickness skin, small hump, underprojected tip, acute nasolabial angle, wide nasal base, and procident dental arches. The surgical plan included minimal trimming of the lateral crura, no osteotomies, wedge resection of the nostril base, and insertion of a septal cartilage graft on the dorsum, costal cartilage grafts on the columellar base and the tip, and costal cartilage grafts on the paranasal area and nasal base in front of the nasal spine. The postoperative result is shown at 1 and 5 years.

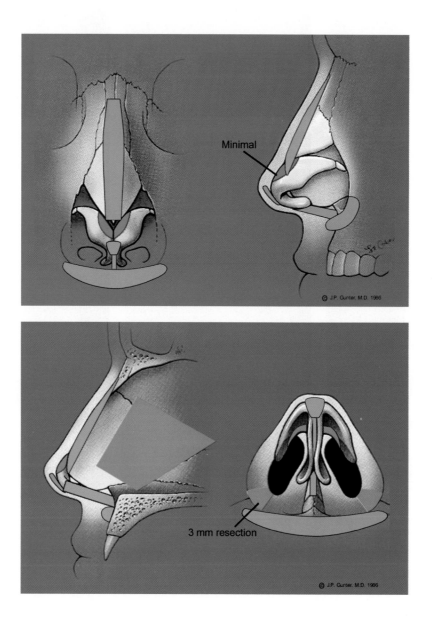

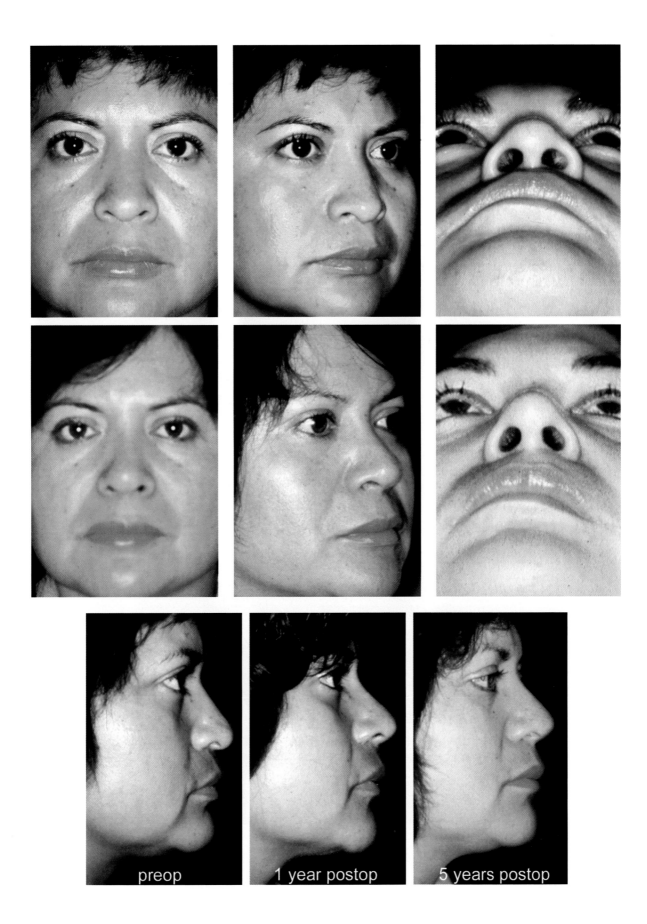

preop   1 year postop   5 years postop

This 18-year-old woman had a small nose with moderately thick skin, small dorsal hump, wide bony pyramid, underprojected tip, and acute nasolabial angle. The surgical plan included a 2 mm dorsal resection, medial and lateral osteotomies, and placement of septal cartilage grafts on the columella and nasal tip. The postoperative result is shown at 2 years.

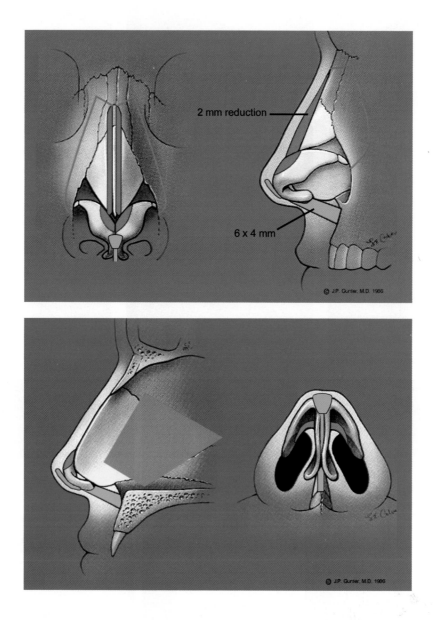

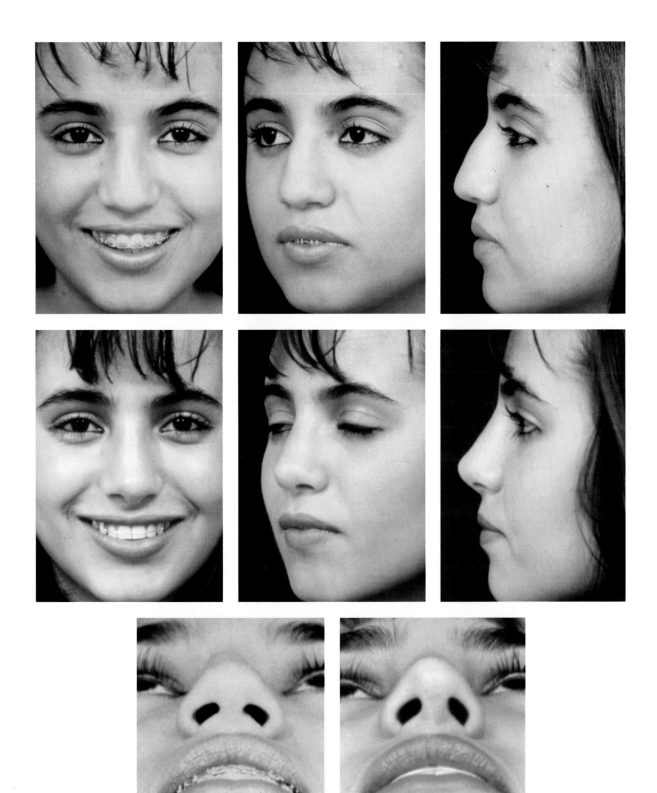

This 25-year-old man had a small nose, deviation of the bony pyramid resulting from trauma, underprojecting tip, acute nasolabial angle, and moderate biprocidentia. The surgical plan included septoplasty, medial and lateral osteotomies, repositioning of the left side of the bony pyramid, and placement of septal cartilage grafts on the dorsum, columella, and tip. The postoperative result is shown at 1 year.

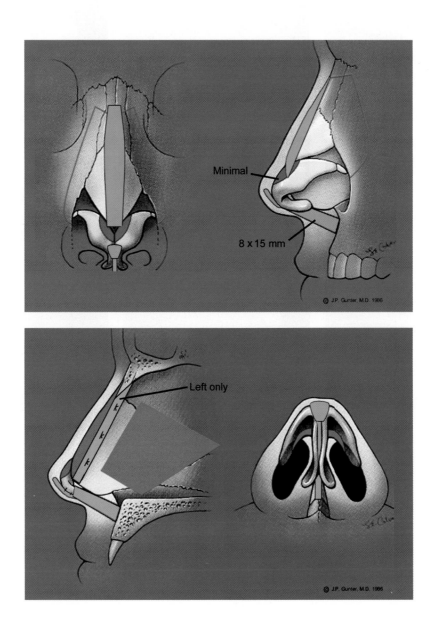

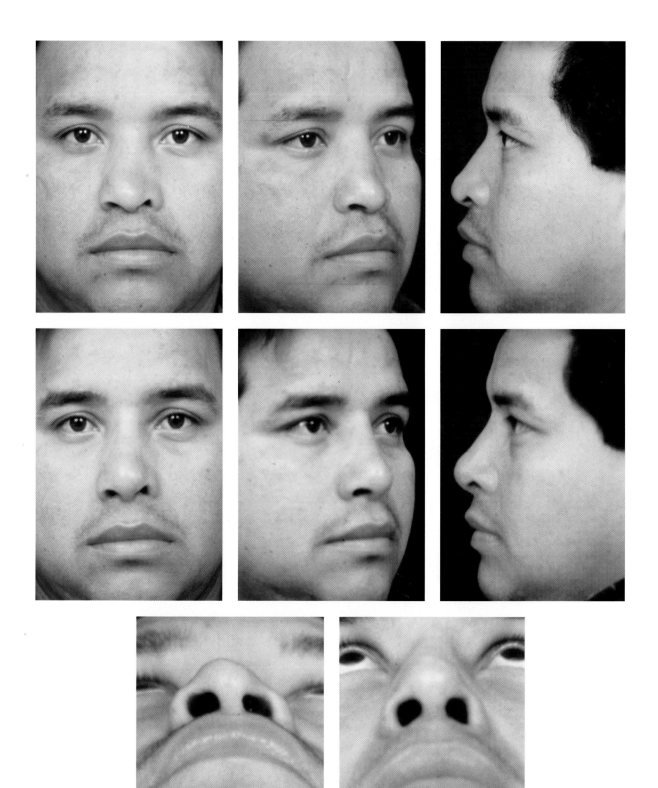

This 51-year-old Oriental man had a small nose with a concave dorsum, low radix, underprojected tip, and wide nasal base. The surgical plan included placement of a rib cartilage graft on the dorsum and columella that extended to the tip, forming an L with the dorsal graft, and wedge resection of the base of the nostrils. The postoperative result is shown at 1 year.

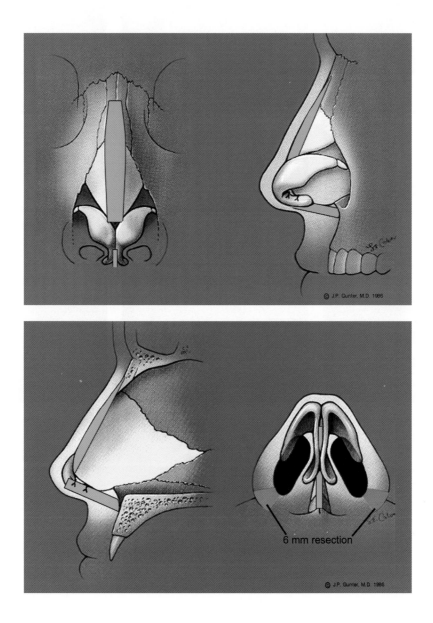

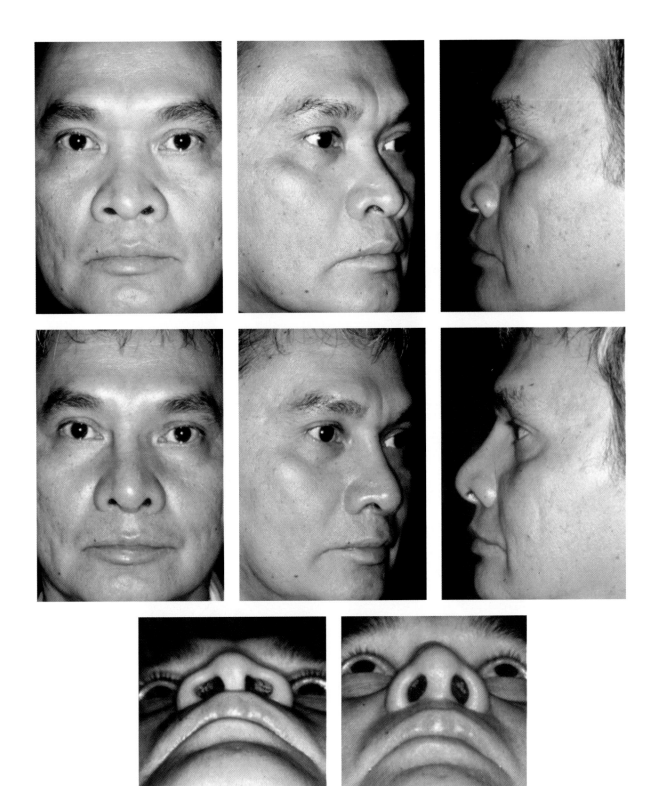

This 25-year-old woman had a relatively small nose, moderately thick skin, minimal osseocartilaginous hump, underprojecting tip, acute nasolabial angle, wide nasal base, marked protrusion of the dental arches, and apparent microgenia relative to the facial convexity. The surgical plan included minimal dorsal resection, no osteotomies, trimming of the cephalic edge of the lateral crura, wedge resection of the nostril base, and placement of septal cartilage grafts on the columella and the tip and a Silastic chin implant. The postoperative result is shown at 2 years.

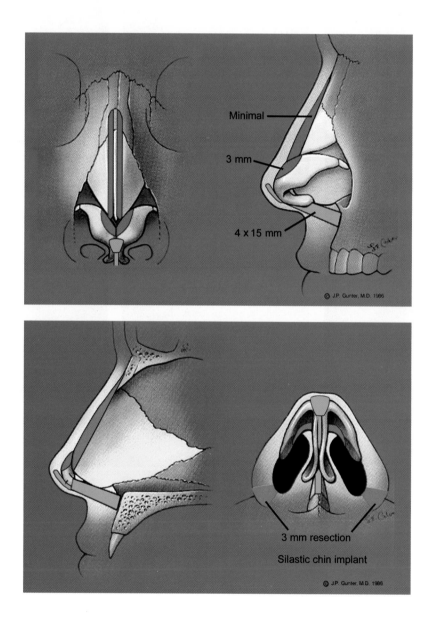

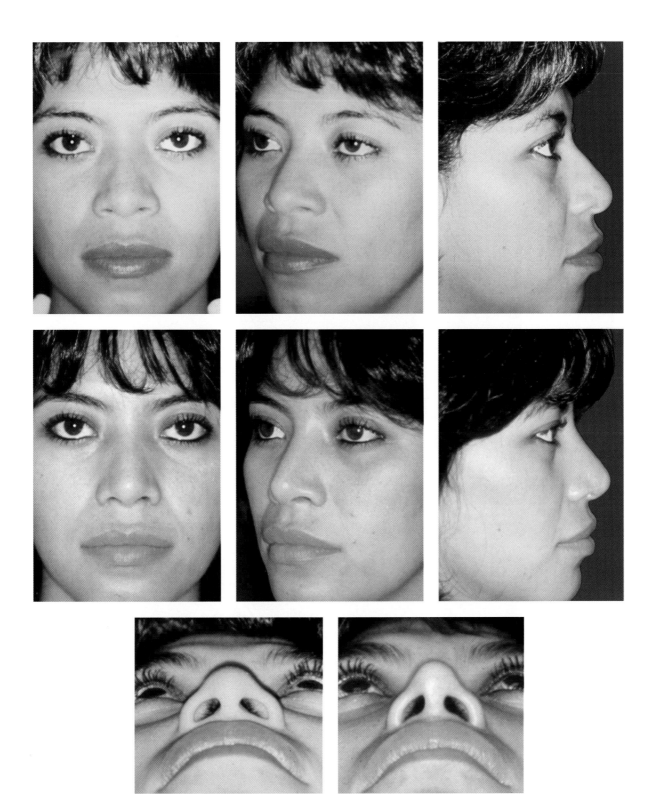

This 23-year-old woman had a small nose with a convex dorsum, underprojecting tip, acute nasolabial angle, procidentia of both dental arches, and a depressed paranasal area. The surgical plan included minimal dorsal resection, minimal trimming of the cephalic edge of the lateral crura, section of the intercartilaginous ligament, and placement of costal cartilage grafts on the anterior aspect of the maxillae around the piriform fossa, transversely in front of the nasal spine, on the columella, and on the nasal tip and paranasal region. The postoperative result is shown at 1 and 8 years.

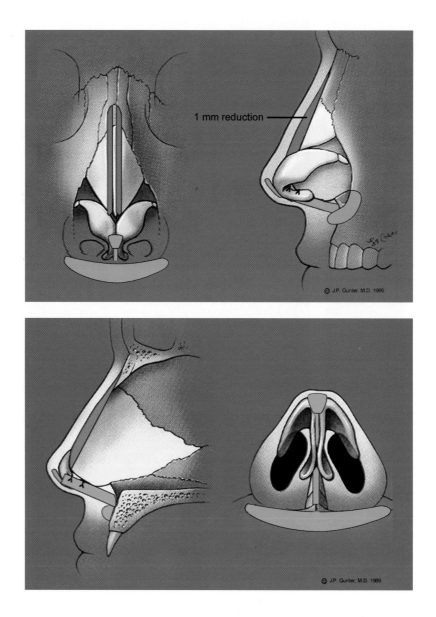

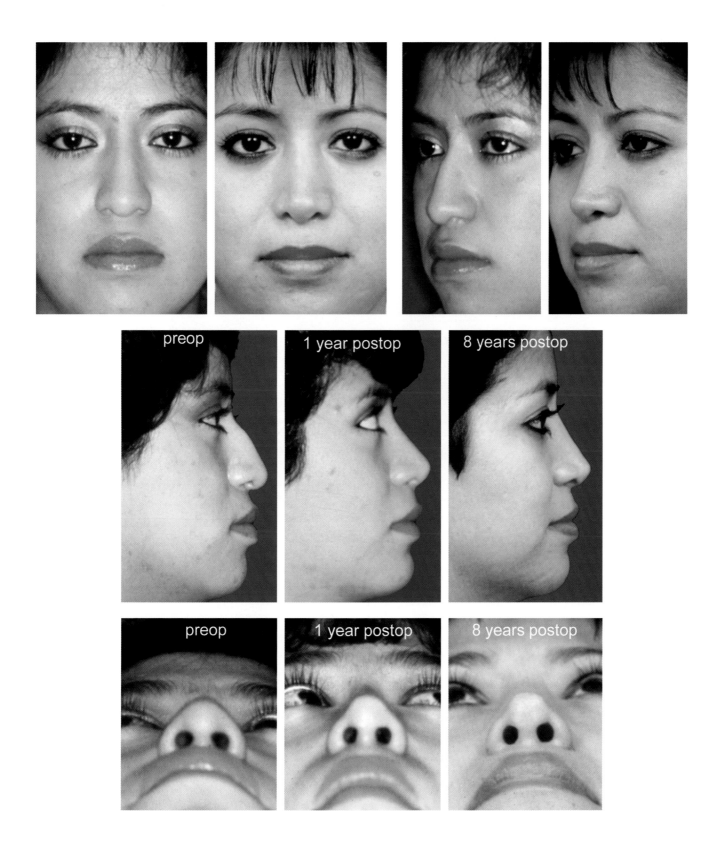

This 20-year-old woman had an exaggerated facial convexity with a small nose, moderately thick skin, caudal rotation of the nasal tip, acute nasolabial angle, and overprojecting dental arches that produced a gummy smile and lip strain when her mouth was closed. The surgical plan included segmental maxillary and mandibular osteotomies, trimming of the cephalic edge of the crura, and placement of septal cartilage grafts on the columella and tip. The postoperative result is shown at 2 years.

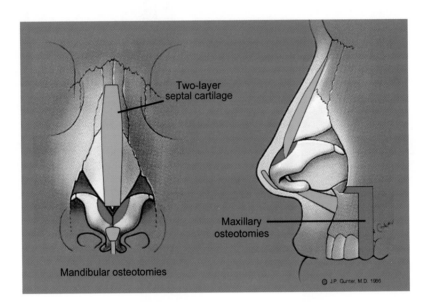

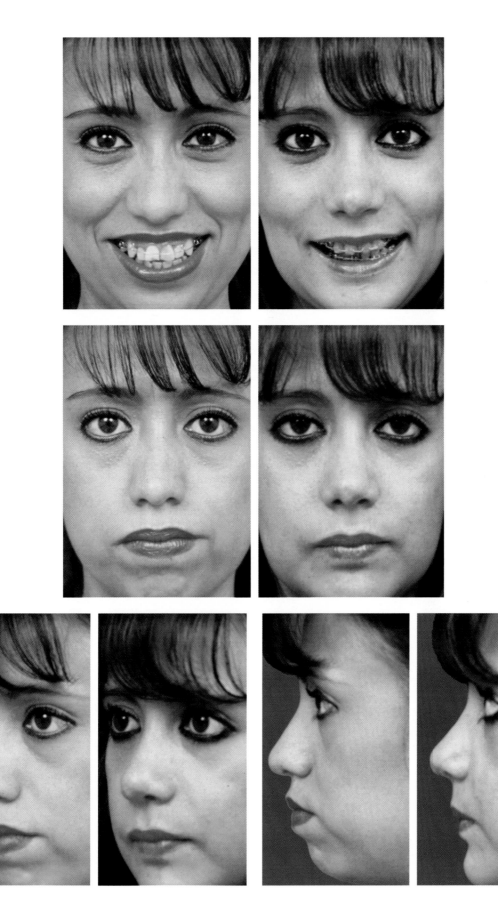

■ KEY POINTS

- ■ The small size plus the skin thickness of the mestizo nose is a contraindication to conventional reduction rhinoplasty.

- ■ Minimal hump resection, limited trimming of the cephalic edge of the lateral crura, and wedge excision of the nostril sill may be needed.

- ■ Dorsal, tip, columella, or paranasal augmentation or a combination of these grafts is necessary to increase nasal projection and shape definition.

- ■ Segmental maxillomandibular osteotomies and sliding genioplasty may be necessary to achieve optimal overall aesthetic results.

REFERENCES

1. Ortiz-Monasterio F, Olmedo A. Rhinoplasty on the mestizo nose. Clin Plast Surg 4:1, 1977.
2. Ortiz-Monasterio F, Michelena J. The use of augmentation rhinoplasty techniques for the correction of the non-Caucasian nose. Clin Plast Surg 15:57, 1988.
3. Ortiz-Monasterio F. Rhinoplasty. Philadelphia: WB Saunders, 1994.
4. Flowers RS. The surgical correction of the non-Caucasian nose. Clin Plast Surg 4:69, 1977.
5. Matory WE, Falces E. Non-Caucasian rhinoplasty: A 16-year experience. Plast Reconstr Surg 77:239, 1986.
6. Rees TD. Nasal plastic surgery in the Negro. Plast Reconstr Surg 43:13, 1969.
7. Gunter JP, Rohrich RJ. Augmentation rhinoplasty: Dorsal onlay grafts using shaped autogenous septal cartilage. Plast Reconstr Surg 86:39, 1990.
8. Sheen JH, Sheen AP. Aesthetic Rhinoplasty, 2nd ed. St. Louis: Quality Medical Publishing, 1998 (reprint of 1987 ed.).
9. Sheen JH. Achieving more nasal tip projection by the use of a small autogenous vomer or septal cartilage graft. A preliminary report. Plast Reconstr Surg 56:35, 1975.

The Aging Nose

Rod J. Rohrich, M.D. • Larry H. Hollier, Jr., M.D. • Jack P. Gunter, M.D.

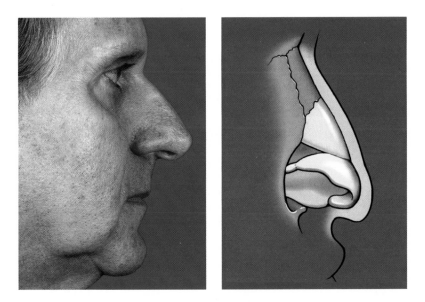

*T*he appearance of the nose progressively changes with age. These age-related changes are primarily characterized by drooping of the nasal tip complex and increasing prominence of the dorsal hump. Since rhinoplasty in older patients differs from rhinoplasty in younger patients in many aspects, these differences must be understood prior to embarking on any surgical procedure. The motivation of these patients must be carefully evaluated during the initial consultation. Rees[1] has pointed out that older patients frequently have unrealistic expectations, having desired changes in the appearance of their nose since they were very young. Often major life stressors in this age group will precipitate the consultation for rhinoplasty. It is clearly better to avoid surgery during these stressful times in a patient's life.

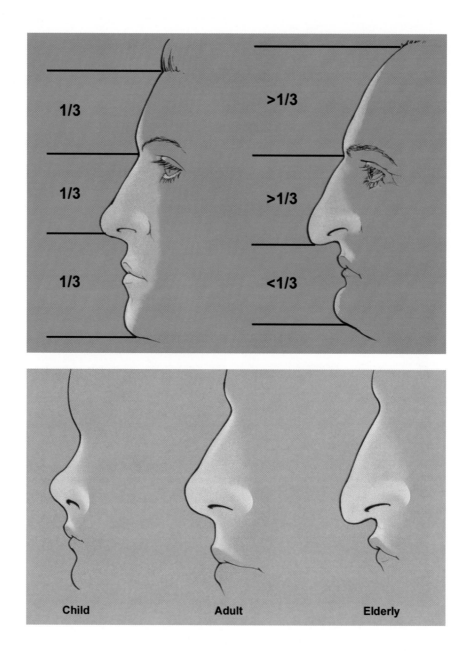

The surgeon must also appreciate the generalized changes seen in the face and nose as a consequence of aging. There is a relative shortening of the lower third of the face, primarily as the result of alveolar, maxillary, and mandibular resorption characteristics of the edentulous state of many patients. This contributes to a relative lengthening of the nose, giving the appearance of a drooping tip and accentuating any dorsal convexity.[2-5] Additionally, dermal changes accompany the aging process, including diminished skin elasticity with a reduction in the amount of dermal collagen and a disorganization of the elastic tissue.[2,6] There is also an increase in sebaceous gland concentration in the skin, particularly in the region of the nasal tip, that may lead to significant fullness in this region. At the extreme end of the spectrum this may result in rhinophyma. The generalized skin redundancy and lack of elasticity conceal minor surgical changes in the underlying nasal skeleton. Consequently, wide skin undermining is necessary to allow for redraping of the skin, and a more significant structural alteration may be necessary to create the desired result.[1]

In evaluating the older patient for rhinoplasty differences in motivation and anatomy must be thoroughly understood before surgery.

ANATOMY
Tip Complex/Dorsum

The most consistent change seen in the aging nose occurs within the nasal tip complex. Progressive descent results in the appearance of a drooping, elongated tip complex. To some degree, this is a relative change resulting from the reduction in height of the lower third of the face. However, there is also an intrinsic loss of support of the lower lateral cartilages.[2,4,7-8]

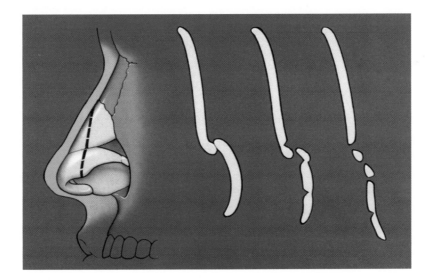

The fibroelastic support in the scroll area between the upper and lower lateral cartilages may attenuate, fragment, or even ossify in older patients,[2-3,7] resulting in inferior migration of the lateral crura. This is exacerbated by the thickening of the skin and subcutaneous tissues, which add bulkiness and weight to the tip. Concomitantly, there is loss of support for the nasal base and medial crura as a result of alveolar hypoplasia,[1-2,4] causing a relative shortening of the columella and an increase in the columellar-lobular angle that further rotates the nasal tip down.

> *The nasal tip rotates inferiorly with age due to extrinsic and intrinsic loss of support of the lower lateral cartilages, resulting in a drooping, elongated tip complex.*

As a consequence of the descent of the tip, any preexisting dorsal convexity is exaggerated. This may be manifest as an apparent prominent dorsal hump. However, great care must be taken in addressing this problem in the older patient. Once the drooping nasal tip has been corrected, the nasal dorsum will become less prominent. Any dorsal hump reduction should be accomplished after tip rotation to avoid overresection.

> *The dorsal hump in the aging nose is accentuated by the drooping tip and should be corrected only after repositioning the tip complex to minimize the resection necessary.*

Bony Vault

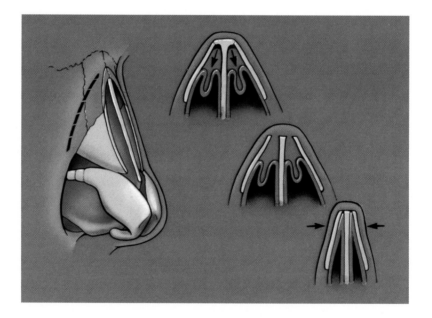

The bony pyramid in the older patient tends to be thinner and more brittle. Osteotomies are prone to comminution, and resulting irregularities are not camouflaged as well because of the changes in the overlying skin.[2,4,6,9] Osteotomies should be avoided if at all possible. However, when necessary, they should be performed in a low-low fashion. Complete osteotomies are preferred over greenstick fractures to control the fracture pattern and minimize the chance of comminution.

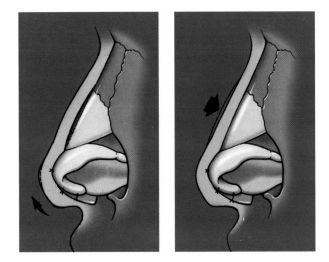

The need for osteotomies to correct open-roof deformities following hump reduction is minimized by correcting tip rotation initially to minimize the relative prominence of the dorsal convexity.

Osteotomies should be avoided in the older patient because of the brittle nature of the nasal bones that predisposes them to comminution.

Nasal Airway

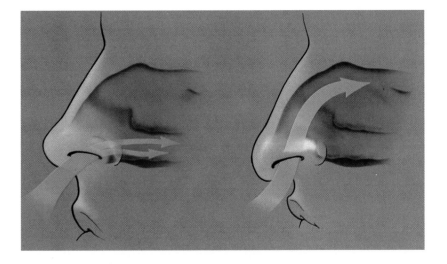

The nasal airway is affected in several ways by the aging process. Most prominently, the descent of the nasal tip may alter the flow of air into the nasal vestibule, resulting in obstructive airway symptoms.[1,4,10] Cephalic rotation of the tip may allow normal airflow into the vestibule, correcting the obstructive symptomatology. There may also be loss of support of the internal nasal valve area since collapse of the scroll area and atrophy of the nasal musculature may allow the caudal border of the upper lateral cartilages to collapse on maximal inspiration.

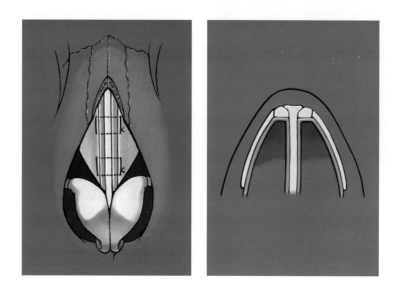

Consideration should be given to the placement of dorsal spreader grafts at the time of rhinoplasty to correct this problem or prevent its development postoperatively.[11-13]

Deformities of the septum or hypertrophy of the inferior turbinates should also be corrected at the time of rhinoplasty. However, the mucoperichondrium attenuates and becomes more fragile with age, and great care must be taken during septal dissection to prevent tearing. Hypertension is not uncommon in this patient population, and postoperative elevations in blood pressure may lead to bleeding from raw areas within the nose. Therefore inferior turbinate reduction is best performed extramucosally to minimize postoperative bleeding.

The descent of the nasal tip and the collapse of the internal nasal valve may result in obstructive airway symptoms that can be corrected by tip rotation and the placement of spreader grafts.

CONSULTATION

Careful consideration must be given to the motivation of the older patient seeking rhinoplasty. Why after so many years is the patient seeking surgical intervention? Appropriate motivational factors include midlife career change, worsening airway obstruction, previous failed rhinoplasty, or the desire to enhance economic potential. However, significant life stressors such as divorce or a death in the family are not uncommon in this age group. The history should clarify such events, and rhinoplasty should be deferred until these situations have been resolved.[1,14-15]

There is also a tendency for older patients to develop unrealistic expectations regarding the outcome of rhinoplasty.[1] These patients may have desired a change in the appearance of their nose since adolescence. A frank discussion with the patient is imperative to define realistic goals for the procedure.

OPERATIVE TECHNIQUE

Operative goals for rhinoplasty in the older patient include increased tip projection, cephalic tip rotation/refinement, reduction in nasal length, correction of the dorsal hump, and restoration of the internal nasal valve. Several operative principles that should be followed to achieve these goals:

1. Wide skin undermining to accommodate the diminished skin elasticity
2. The use of nondestructive tip-refining techniques (suture techniques and conservative cephalic trim)
3. Conservative dorsal hump removal
4. Use of spreader grafts to maintain the internal nasal valve
5. Minimal use of osteotomies using a low-low technique to control the medial movement when necessary
6. Rotation of the nasal tip using columellar struts and septal spanning of sutures

Special attention must be given to the rotation of the nasal tip using the above-mentioned techniques. Frequently this will minimize the perceived problem of the dorsal hump and the exaggerated nasal length. Reduction of the dorsal convexity before tip rotation may result in overresection.[16] Otherwise the operative sequence is similar to that for standard rhinoplasty using the open approach and general anesthesia.

In the older patient special attention must be given to the unique anatomy, cephalic tip rotation, conservative hump reduction, and minimal use of osteotomies.

CASE ANALYSIS

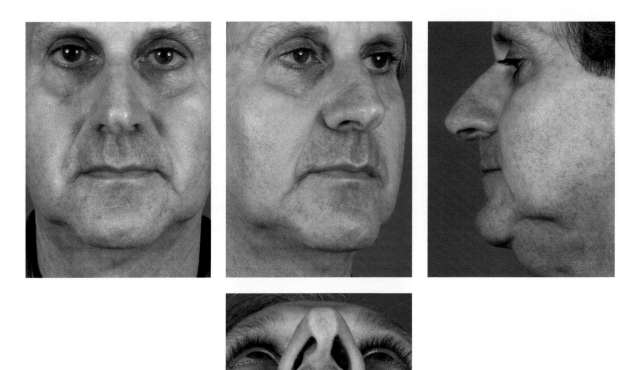

This 54-year-old man complained of a drooping nasal tip, a dorsal hump, and nasal airway obstruction (greater on the right than left side) that had been progressive over the preceding 5 years. He also desired concomitant rhytidectomy. Nasal analysis demonstrated thick sebaceous nasal skin, a nasolabial angle of less than 85 degrees, a normal radix position, adequate tip projection with a drooping tip, a dorsal hump with increased nasal length, a narrow midvault area, right caudal septal deviation, and left posterior septal deviation and compensatory right inferior turbinate hypertrophy.

The operative goals were:
- Upward tip rotation and definition
- Nasal shortening
- Dorsal hump reduction
- An increase in the nasolabial angle to 90 degrees
- Septal reconstruction with correction of caudal septal deviation with a swinging door flap
- Bilateral anterior inferior submucosal turbinate resection (greater on the right than left side)
- Avoidance of osteotomies

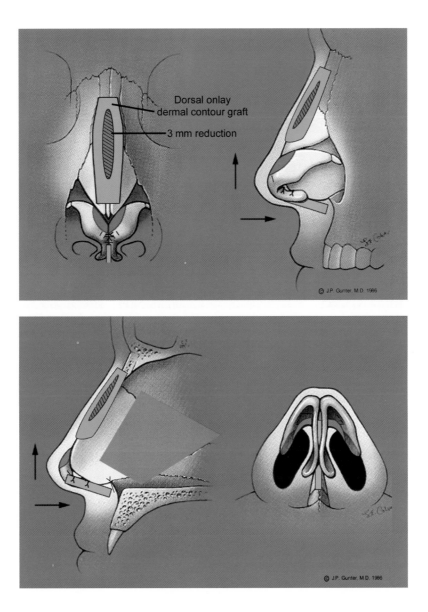

The operative plan included:

- Open rhinoplasty with a transcolumellar stair-step incision
- Left hemitransfixion incision for septal dissection and correction of the caudal deviation with a swinging door septal flap and a 5-0 PDS suture to secure the caudal septum to the nasal spine
- Bilateral submucosal inferior turbinate resection anteriorly
- Cephalic trim of lower lateral cartilages with medial crural, interdomal, and transdomal 5-0 PDS for tip definition
- Columellar strut and medial crural septal spanning sutures to rotate tip and increase nasolabial angle
- Incremental (3 mm) hump reduction and dorsal onlay contour dermal graft
- Silastic septal splints and application of external metal contouring splint

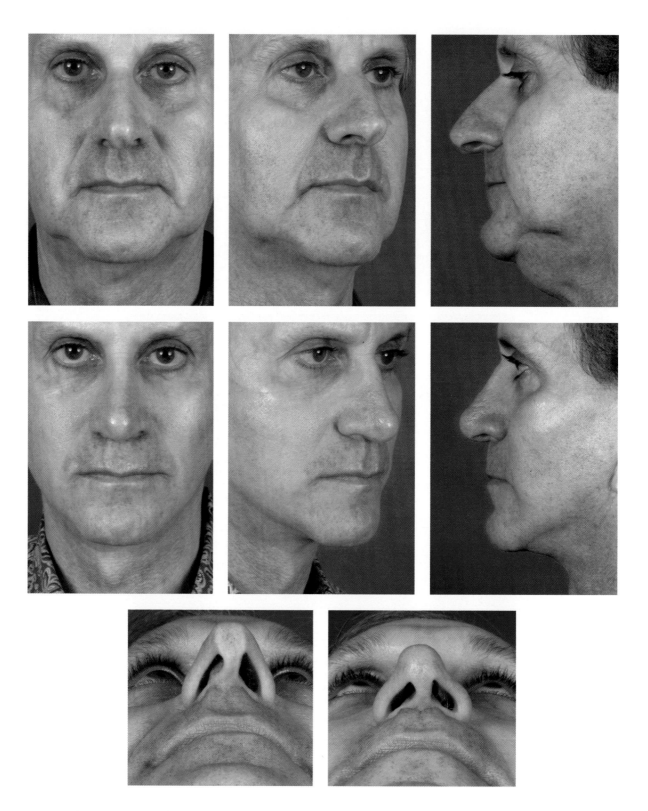

The patient is shown 15 months following rhinoplasty and rhytidectomy. The nasal-facial balance as well as correction of the dorsal hump and tip rotation has been well maintained.

■ KEY POINTS

■ Loss of support of the lower lateral cartilages results in a drooping nasal tip complex with an apparent increase in nasal length.

■ Nasal tip descent accentuates preexisting dorsal deformities.

■ Changes in the nasal skin with age result in a loss of elasticity and do not allow the skin to redrape over the altered nasal framework as well as in younger patients.

■ Descent of the tip and loss of support in the internal nasal valve region may result in nasal obstructive symptoms that should be addressed at the time of rhinoplasty.

■ The nasal bony pyramid in older patients is thinner and more brittle and consequently osteotomies should be avoided if at all possible.

■ The motivation of older patients seeking rhinoplasty must be carefully evaluated to screen for significant life stressors such as death of a loved one or divorce.

■ Operative techniques for correction of the nasal deformity in older patients should emphasize upward tip rotation, conservative dorsal hump reduction, and the avoidance of nasal osteotomies.

■ The nasal tip position should be corrected prior to dorsal hump reduction to avoid overresection.

REFERENCES

1. Rees TD. Rhinoplasty in the older patient. Ann Plast Surg 1:27, 1978.
2. Krmpotic-Nemanic J, Kostovic I, Rudan P, Nemanic G. Morphological and histological changes responsible for the droop of the nasal tip in advanced age. Acta Otolaryngol 71:278, 1971.
3. Parkes ML, Kamer FM. The mature nose. Laryngoscope 83:157, 1973.
4. Patterson C. The aging nose: Characteristics and correction. Otolaryngol Clin North Am 13: 275, 1980.
5. Powell N, Humphries B. Proportions of the Aesthetic Face. New York: Thieme & Stratton, 1984.
6. Gilchrist B. Age-associated changes in the skin. J Am Geriatr Soc 30:139, 1982.
7. Beekhuis GJ, Collin JJ. Nasal tip support. Arch Otolaryngol 112:726, 1986.
8. Gunter JP. Anatomical observations of the lower lateral cartilages. Arch Otolaryngol 89:599, 1969.
9. Rohrich RJ. Dorsal reduction and osteotomies. Dallas Rhinoplasty Symp 12:209, 1995.
10. Bridger GP. Physiology of the nasal valve. Arch Otolaryngol 92:543, 1970.
11. Rohrich RJ. Correction of the dorsally deviated nose: Dual use of internal spreader grafts. Presented at the American Society of Aesthetic Surgeons Meeting, Dallas, May, 1994.
12. Rohrich RJ. Versatility of spreader grafts in rhinoplasty. Presented at the Rhinoplasty Society Meeting, San Francisco, May, 1995.

13. Sheen JH. Spreader grafts: A method of reconstructing the root of the middle nasal vault following rhinoplasty. Plast Reconstr Surg 73:230, 1984.
14. Goin MK. Psychological understanding and management of rhinoplasty patients. Clin Plast Surg 4:3, 1977.
15. Thomson HS. Preoperative selection and counseling of patients for rhinoplasty. Plast Reconstr Surg 50:174, 1972.
16. Rohrich RJ. The aging nose—management principles. Presented at the Aesthetic Surgery Symposium, Washington University Medical Center, St. Louis, 1991.

56

Male Rhinoplasty

Rod J. Rohrich, M.D. ▪ Jeffrey M. Kenkel, M.D. ▪ Jack P. Gunter, M.D.

*P*lastic surgeons are somewhat more cautious when evaluating a male patient who requests rhinoplasty or any aesthetic procedure for that matter. In general, men are regarded to be less attentive during the consultation and to be more demanding. This, however, is a stereotype that we have not confirmed in our practice. It is essential to recognize the specific characteristics unique to the male rhinoplasty patient. The male rhinoplasty patient must be approached cautiously so that masculine features are preserved, resulting in facial harmony.[1] Excessive dorsal reduction and/or tip refinement produce unsatisfactory results. This chapter will focus on how to properly evaluate the male nose as well as surgical planning and intraoperative techniques that will produce a balanced, harmonious nose in relationship to the rest of the face.

CONSULTATION

As with any patient seeking consultation for cosmetic surgery, it is imperative to identify those rhinoplasty patients that may pose potential problems and have unrealistic expectations. Gunter[1] identified the following 13 "danger signs" that should alert the physician to possible underlying psychiatric disturbances.

1. Minimal disfigurement
2. Delusional distortion of body image
3. An identity problem or sexual ambivalence
4. Confused or vague motives for wanting surgery
5. Unrealistic expectations of change in life situations as a result of surgery
6. History of poorly established social and emotional relationships
7. Unresolved grief or a crisis situation
8. Present misfortunes blamed on physical appearance
9. Older neurotic man who is overly concerned about aging

10. Sudden anatomic dislike, especially in older men
11. A hostile, blaming attitude toward authority
12. History of seeing physicians and being dissatisfied with them
13. Indication of paranoid thoughts

Gorney[2] describes potentially problematic patients using the acronym SIMON: single, immature males who are overly expectant and narcissistic. Unfortunately men tend to have a poorer understanding of their deformity and are more reluctant to discuss aesthetic improvements than women, who generally are specific about their deformity and the changes they feel are needed.[1,3] Therefore during the initial consultation the patient's goals must be determined and evaluated as to whether they are in fact realistic.

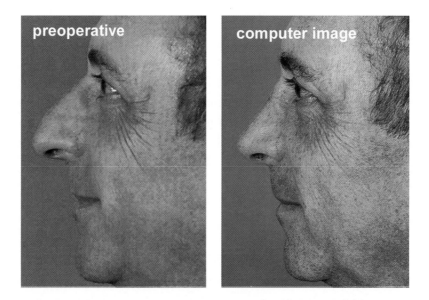

Standardized anterior, lateral, oblique, and basal photographs are imperative for proper preoperative evaluation by the surgeon. They assist the patient in understanding the perceived deformity and how he thinks this could be improved. The use of computer imaging allows the surgeon to simulate potential nasal changes after rhinoplasty. It is particularly useful in the male patient who is contemplating major reduction rhinoplasty for demonstrating the importance of balanced facial harmony. It also allows the surgeon to establish realistic goals with the patient and confirm the surgical plan. Although computer imaging can be time consuming, it may help alleviate anxiety in the male patient and allows the patient to play an active role in determining the final surgical outcome.[4] It is important for patients to understand that computer images are for educational use only and do not imply or guarantee results. Each patient must sign an informed consent confirming that they understand the goals of imaging as such.

Proper patient selection of male patients can be difficult. Computer imaging helps establish realistic expectations and verifies the importance of facial harmony.

Facial Analysis

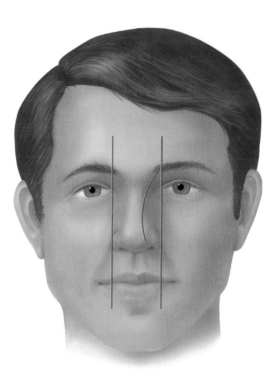

Proper evaluation of the entire face during rhinoplasty consultation is essential to ensure that facial harmony and balance are maintained. The details of proper facial analysis are discussed in Chapters 7 and 8. The differences between the male and female patient will be highlighted here.

In general, the male face tends to be more pronounced, squarer, and heavier than a woman's.[1,5] Whereas the female dorsum is outlined by two slightly curved, divergent lines, the male dorsum tends to be wide and straight with less concavity at the superciliary ridges.[1,4] The bony base width should remain 75% to 80% of the alar base, which typically is equal to the intercanthal distance.[4]

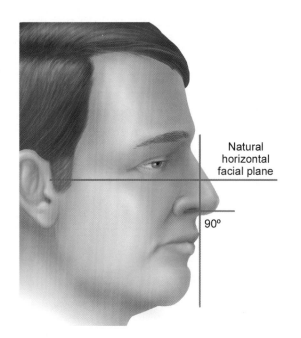

The nasal tip in males is broader and more bulbous than that in females. The tip-defining points may be difficult to appreciate because of the thick overlying soft tissues. On the lateral view the nasal frontal angle is more recessed in men due to the prominence of the brows. The male nasal dorsum should lie along a line drawn from the nasal frontal angle to the tip-defining points. There should be no supratip break.[4] Tip projection in males is increased due to the length of the nasal dorsum, resulting in less nostril show and a more acute nasolabial angle (90 to 95 degrees) than seen in females.[1,4] The quality of the skin is typically thickened, which limits the amount of change that can be achieved.[1,6]

It is imperative to evaluate the lip-chin relationship when assessing nasal aesthetics. Byrd[7] determines ideal chin projection by dropping a vertical line from a point one half the ideal nasal length tangential to the vermilion of the upper lip. The chin should project to this line in males, whereas in woman the chin is ideally 2 to 3 mm posterior to this line.[4,7]

OPERATIVE GOALS AND PRINCIPLES OF TREATMENT

Overall the change produced in the male nose should be quite subtle and natural appearing. Deformities of the male nose are classified as either aesthetic or traumatic in nature.[1] Correction of aesthetic deformities include reduction of a prominent dorsal hump, narrowing the nasal base, refinement of the tip complex, and correction of the aging nose and ethnic nose. Traumatic deformities are either acquired or iatrogenic. The reduction of a large nose, especially in males, must be performed with the goal of maintaining facial harmony. In other words, a small nose on a male face is generally inappropriate.

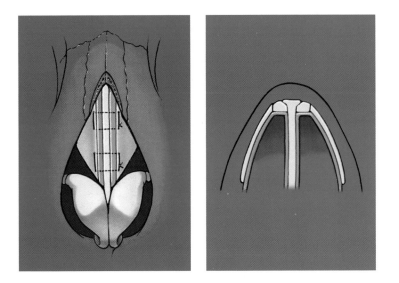

Males frequently require dorsal hump reduction, modification of the tip, and osteotomies. The extent of modification of each one of these nasal areas is adjusted accordingly to fit the remainder of the face. Although smaller dorsal hump reductions can be accomplished with simple rasping, larger reductions (>2 mm) should include the creation of submucous tunnels and sharp release of the upper lateral cartilages from the septum to avoid injury to the cartilage and/or mucoperichondrium.[8-10] Failure to preserve the middle vault can result in deformities and/or internal valve dysfunction. Stabilization of the middle vault is best accomplished with the use of spreader grafts.[11,12] These grafts will help maintain the internal valve, stabilize the septum to prevent a saddlenose deformity, and preserve dorsal aesthetic lines.[12-14]

Spreader grafts help preserve the middle vault, stabilize the septum, and preserve the dorsal aesthetic lines.

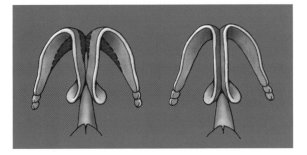

Males typically have thick nasal skin, which limits tip modification and definition. Resection of the cephalic margins of the lower lateral cartilages will permit medialization of the tip-defining points.

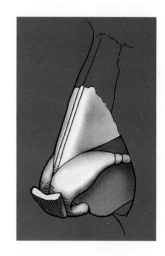

Further definition can be accomplished with a graduated suture technique as described in Chapter 18.[15] The incorporation of intercrural, interdomal, and transdomal sutures allows unification and refinement of the nasal tip.[15] Tip grafts can accentuate the tip-defining points and enhance tip projection in males with especially thick skin. However, caution must be used to avoid an overrefined tip that will feminize the nose.

Management of the nasal pyramid in the male patient must also be approached with caution. Osteotomies should be planned so that the bony base is proportionate (75%) to the alar base. As with the aging nose, we prefer to avoid greenstick osteotomies because they are less precise than complete osteotomies.

Functional and cosmetic deformities are typically seen after traumatic injury to the nose. Long-lasting correction of the deformity depends on appropriate management of the septum (see Chapter 21). Traumatic injuries to the nose may require osteotomies to reshape the nasal bones. Medial and lateral osteotomies may be required to reposition the nasal bones. Periosteum is left over the lateral nasal bones to control and prevent comminution. Traumatic injuries are covered in more detail in Chapter 43.

POSTOPERATIVE MANAGEMENT

Postoperative management is similar to that described in Chapter 5. The patient should be aware that prolonged swelling is more common in males, and this should be documented on the informed consent. Steri-Strips are used for at least 2 weeks to help reduce edema in males.

CASE ANALYSES

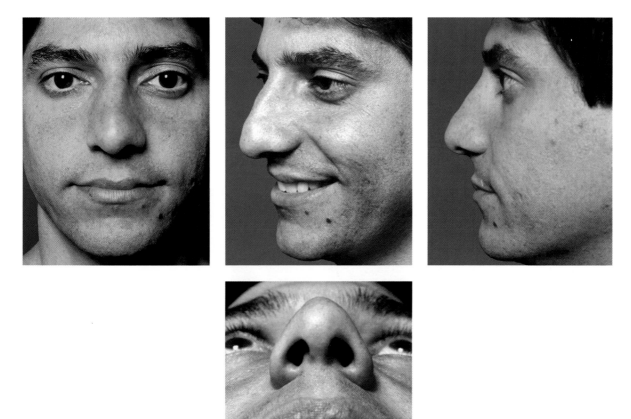

This 31-year-old man had a history of preexisting nasal trauma to the left side of his nose. His priorities in order of importance were straightening of the nose, correction of nasal airway obstruction, improvement of the bulbous asymmetric tip, correction of the wide nasal base, augmentation of his small chin, and correction of the dorsal hump.

The analysis revealed adequate facial proportions with microgenia and a class I occlusion on the frontal view. His nose was deviated to the left and exhibited a C-shaped deformity; the left middle vault had collapsed. He had a wide bony base with a bulbous and asymmetric nasal tip. He had thick Fitzpatrick type II skin. Slight alar flaring (more on the left than the right) was noted. The lateral and oblique views demonstrated moderate dorsal irregularity and a dorsal hump in the keystone area as well as angularity with some tip ptosis. His nasal length was slightly increased, but tip projection was adequate. Some alar base overhang was observed. The nasolabial angle was 90 degrees. The basal view confirmed that he had more tip fullness and deviation on the left with some caudal septal deviation on the right. The internal examination revealed a septal deviation internally in the right anterior inferior turbinate that was obstructing his right nasal airway and inferior hypertrophy on the left.

The operative goals included:
- Correction of nasal airway obstruction
- Dorsal hump reduction
- Correction of nasal deviation
- Correction of dorsal hump
- Improvement of nasal tip symmetry
- Osseous advancement genioplasty to correct microgenia

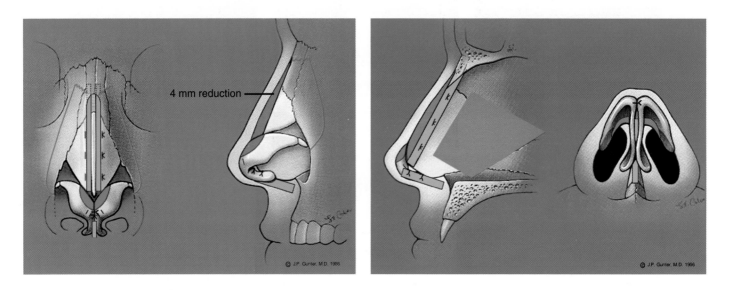

The surgical plan called for:
- External approach with a transcolumellar incision and infracartilaginous extension
- Exposure of the nasal framework
- Compartment dorsum reduction (dorsal hump reduction of 3 mm)
- Exposure of the nasal septum and harvest of septal cartilage graft
- Bilateral inferior turbinate submucosal resection
- Bilateral placement of the dorsal spreader graft (secured with three 5-0 PDS horizontal mattress sutures) to correct the dorsally deviated nose that was straightened by the septal reconstruction and separation of the upper lateral cartilages from the septum
- Cephalic trim to retain 6 mm of lower lateral cartilage
- Columellar strut fashioned and secured with intercrural sutures
- Interdomal and transdomal sutures (5-0 PDS)
- Scoring of the caudal septum and creation of swinging door flap with a figure-of-eight suture to the contralateral periosteum of the anterior spine and 5-0 PDS to maintain the caudal septum deviation
- External percutaneous osteotomies

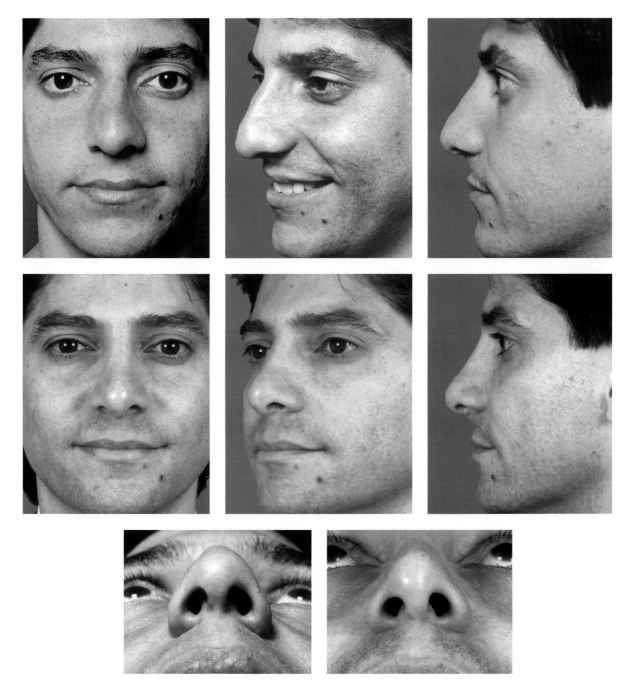

The frontal view 8 years postoperatively shows a straight nasal dorsum with improved dorsal aesthetic lines and tip refinement. Slightly more alar convexity and some increased infratip lobular projection can still be observed. The oblique and lateral views exhibit a normal radix and minimal supratip break, nasolabial angle of 95 degrees, and improved nasolabial/alar–columellar relationship and tip refinement. The alae and nasal base are in better proportion and the general facial proportions are good after correction of the microgenia. The tip is symmetric. The basal view revealed improved triangularity of the straight nasal tip and an improved columellar–infratip lobular projection. Some asymmetry of the nostrils and slight alar convexity bilaterally (more on the right than the left) remain. The nasal airway obstruction is improved.

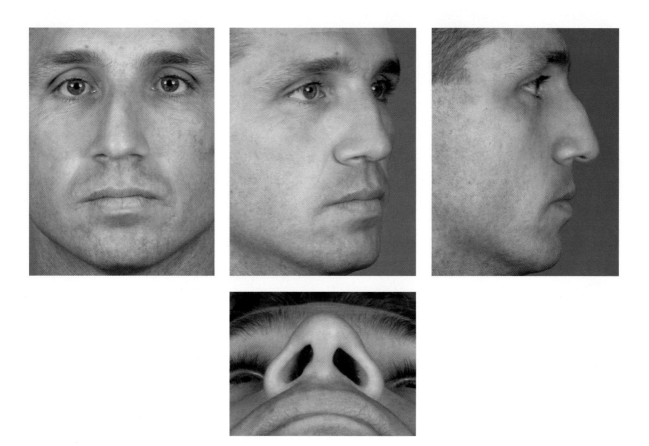

This 35-year-old with thin Fitzpatrick type II skin also had a history of nasal trauma and nasal airway obstruction (more on the right than the left). His major complaints were nasal airway obstruction, high dorsal deviation, and dorsal convexity osseonasal hump.

The frontal view revealed adequate facial proportions with a C-shaped deformity of the septum and collapse of the left middle vault. The dorsal aesthetic lines ended at the midvault area. His tip deviated to the left. The oblique and lateral views demonstrated a normal radix with slightly decreased tip projection and adequate nasal length. He had a high dorsum (more bony than cartilaginous hump) with a nasolabial angle of approximately 85 degrees. On the basal view his nose could be seen deviating to the left with columellar splaying of the right medial crural footplates. The internal examination revealed a thick mucosa with a caudal septal deflection to the right as well as postero-inferior septal deviation obstructing 85% of his airway and inferior turbinate hypertrophy on the left.

The operative goals included:
- Correction of nasal airway obstruction
- Dorsal hump correction
- Correction of deviated septum
- Correction of tip asymmetry

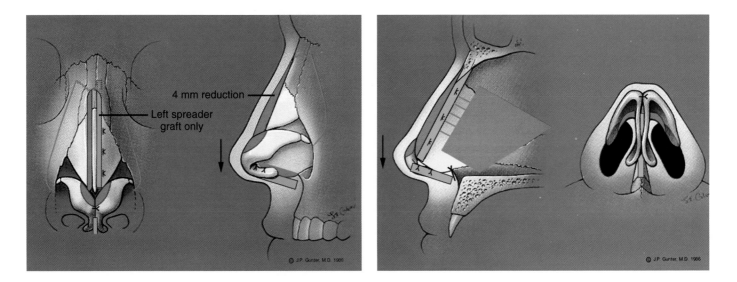

The surgical plan called for:
- External approach with columellar incision and infracartilaginous extension for exposure of the nasal framework
- Component dorsal reduction (dorsal hump reduction of 4 mm)
- Correction of septal deviation and harvesting of septal cartilage grafts posteriorly and inferiorly
- Scoring of the caudal septum and creation of a swinging door flap after 2 mm of dorsal caudal septal reduction and correction of the caudal septal deflection with a figure-of-eight suture to the contralateral periosteum of the anterior nasal spine and 5-0 PDS to correct the septal deviation caudally
- Left spreader graft to correct dorsal deviation after full-thickness inferior cuts through 50% of the septum to correct the deviated septum
- Cephalic trim leaving 6 mm of lower lateral cartilage followed by application of intercrural sutures and a columellar strut and interdomal sutures only
- External percutaneous osteotomies

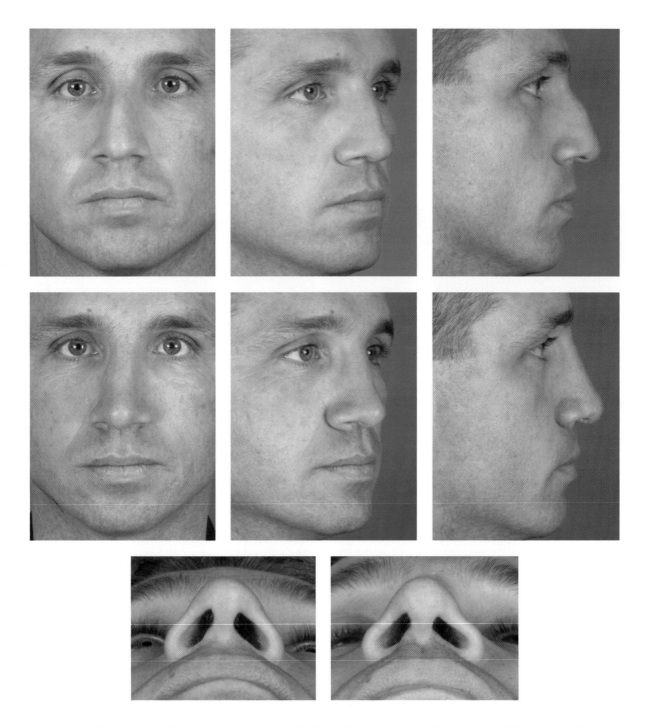

He is shown 1½ years postoperatively. The straight dorsum and improved dorsal aesthetic lines can be seen on the oblique view. The tip is more refined and in balance with the nasal base. The oblique and lateral views confirm that the radix is normal and the dorsum is straight with a slight supratip break. His nasolabial angle is about 85 degrees. The basal view shows that the caudal septum has been straightened. Some slight deflection of the right medial footplate remains, but the columella–infratip lobular area is straight. There is slight alar notching and alar convexity bilaterally. The nasal airway problems have improved.

■ KEY POINTS

- ■ Certain "danger signs" suggest that a patient may have underlying psychiatric disturbance.

- ■ Proper facial analysis is crucial to ensuring appropriate facial harmony and balance.

- ■ Rhinoplasty in males typically produces more subtle results.

- ■ The most common deformities seen in males include a prominent dorsal hump, widened nasal bones, poor definition of the tip complex, and ethnic noses.

- ■ Thick nasal skin typical of males limits tip modification and definition.

- ■ Avoid feminizing the male nose.

REFERENCES

1. Gunter JP. Rhinoplasty. In Courtiss EH, ed. Male Aesthetic Surgery, 2nd ed. St. Louis: CV Mosby, 1990.
2. Gorney M. Criteria for patient selection: An ounce of prevention. Presented at the Senior Resident's Conference Risk Management Course, Dallas, 1996.
3. Wright MR. The male aesthetic patient. Arch Otolaryngol Head Neck Surg 113:724, 1987.
4. Loomis A. Drawing the head and hands. New York: Viking Press, 1956.
5. Byrd HS, Hobar PC. Rhinoplasty: A practical guide for surgical planning. Plast Reconstr Surg 91:642, 1993.
6. Daniel RK. Rhinoplasty and the male patient. Clin Plast Surg 18:751, 1991.
7. Rohrich RJ, Gunter JP, Shemshadi H. Facial analysis for the rhinoplasty patient. Dallas Rhinoplasty Symp 13:67, 1996.
8. Robin IL. Extramucosal method in rhinoplasty. Aesthetic Plast Surg 3:171, 1979.
9. Converse JM. Corrective rhinoplasty. In Converse JM, ed. Reconstructive Plastic Surgery, 2nd ed. Philadelphia: WB Saunders, 1977.
10. Jost G. Posttraumatic nasal deformities. In Regnault P, Daniel RK, eds. Aesthetic Plastic Surgery. Boston: Little, Brown, 1984.
11. Rohrich RJ, Hollier LH. Uses of spreader grafts in the external approach to rhinoplasty. Clin Plast Surg 23:281, 1996.
12. Sheen JH. Spreader grafts: A method of reconstructing the root of the middle vault following rhinoplasty. Plast Reconstr Surg 73:230, 1984.
13. Rohrich RJ. Correction of the dorsally deviated nose: Dual use of internal spreader grafts. Presented at the American Society of Aesthetic Surgeons Meeting, Dallas, May, 1994.
14. Rohrich RJ. Versatility of spreader grafts in rhinoplasty. Presented at the Rhinoplasty Society Meeting, San Francisco, May, 1995.
15. Tebbetts J. Shaping and positioning the nasal tip without structural disruption: A new systemic approach. Plast Reconstr Surg 94:61, 1994.
16. Gunter JP, Rohrich RJ. Management of the deviated nose—the importance of septal reconstruction. Clin Plast Surg 15:43, 1988.

57

Harvesting Cartilage Grafts

Rod J. Rohrich, M.D. ▪ Larry H. Hollier, Jr., M.D.

*R*hinoplasty techniques once focused on reduction of the nasal structures. Today, however, the emphasis is on conservation and augmentation of nasal anatomy. Consequently, there is a growing need for donor sites that provide consistent and effective autologous supportive tissue. Although bone can be used for nasal augmentation, the variable resorption of these grafts tends to pose problems. Most rhinoplasty surgeons prefer to use autologous cartilage for grafting material.

There are three potential donor sites for cartilage grafts: septum, ear, and rib. The septum has become the preferred site for harvesting grafts for several reasons. Since it is already within the operative field, no separate incisions are necessary. In addition, there is no significant donor site morbidity, and indeed, if the harvest is performed on a deviated segment of septum, the patient's airway may be improved postoperatively.

Ear cartilage can provide a surprisingly large volume of graft material. However, because of the flaccidity and convolutions inherent in its structure, it is best used for reconstructing the lower lateral cartilages. It is not useful when structural support is mandatory.

Donor Sites for Cartilage Grafts

Septal Cartilage	Ear Cartilage	Rib Cartilage
Tip graft	Alar cartilage graft	Dorsal onlay graft
Dorsal onlay graft	Dorsal onlay graft	Columellar strut
Columellar strut	Tip graft	Tip graft
Spreader graft		Spreader graft
		Alar cartilage graft

Rib provides the most abundant source of cartilage for grafts. It is the graft material of choice when structural support is needed. However, its drawbacks include potential warping of the graft as well as the donor site scar.

We will discuss the specific technique for harvesting cartilage from each of these donor sites with minimal morbidity.

SEPTAL CARTILAGE

Septal cartilage is our primary choice for all grafts used in rhinoplasty with the exception of those situations requiring reconstitution of the lower lateral cartilage. Its location within the operative field and the absence of donor site morbidity when properly performed make it particularly useful. However, in secondary rhinoplasties previous septal harvest may necessitate the use of other donor sites. A record should be kept at the time of rhinoplasty of the amount of graft material harvested from the septum and any excess material replaced for use during any subsequent procedures.

Technique

The cartilaginous septum is quadrangular in shape and bounded by three bones: the perpendicular plate of the ethmoid, the vomer, and the nasal crest of the maxilla. Access for harvest can be obtained by a hemitransfixion incision, a Killian incision, or the open technique. If the rhinoplasty is being performed in an open fashion, then septal harvest is best performed by separating the medial crura and upper lateral cartilages from the septum with the dissection performed from above. Either the Killian or the hemitransfixion incision can be used during a closed rhinoplasty. A full transfixion incision is to be avoided since 2 to 3 mm of tip projection can be lost, particularly when the dissection is carried down over the anterior nasal spine.

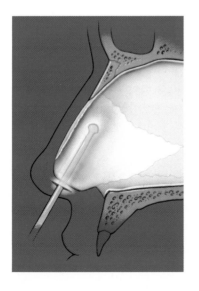

After the initial incision is made, a sharp Cottle elevator is used to dissect the subperichondrial plane on one side of the septum.

The proper plane of dissection can be recognized by the distinct gray-blue appearance of the cartilage and by the relative ease of dissection. If this color is not apparent or if the dissection is not proceeding easily, the dissection must be carried deeper to ensure entry into the subperichondrial space.

This dissection should be continued over the entire surface of the cartilage. At the junction of the cartilaginous septum with the bony septum dissection becomes more difficult, and care should be taken not to perforate the mucoperichondrial flaps. A similar dissection should be accomplished on the contralateral side of the septum after making a small incision along the caudal septum using the Cottle elevator. This should be made approximately 10 mm up from the inferior border of the caudal septum to preserve an adequate strut. Visualization can be facilitated at this point by using the tips of a long Vienna speculum on either side of the septum to elevate the dissected mucoperichondrial flaps.

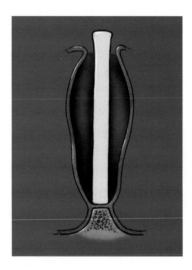

The dissection is continued inferiorly and posteriorly over the posterior vomer. The junction of the perichondrium with the periosteum overlying the vomer is particularly difficult to dissect and should be done with great care. It may be helpful to dissect two separate tunnels, one subperichondrial and one subperiosteal, and divide the junction sharply to help avoid tears in this region.

At this point the septum is ready for harvest. One should only harvest that amount of cartilage necessary for the reconstructive needs of the patient. In the event that a large amount of cartilage is necessary, the quadrangular cartilage can be harvested in its entirety, preserving a dorsal and caudal strut. The previous cartilaginous incision is extended posteriorly and anteriorly parallel to the nasal floor. Anteriorly, it turns 90 degrees at a point approximately 10 mm from the dorsal border of the septum. It then parallels the nasal dorsum up to the level of the perpendicular plate of the ethmoid.

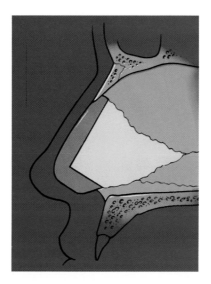

This creates a 10 mm L-shaped strut of septal cartilage. It is necessary to maintain this strut for support of the nasal soft tissues. Angled septal scissors are used to disarticulate the cartilage from its junction with the ethmoid plate. The cartilage is then removed from its position by gently rocking a long, straight hemostat back and forth. Once the septal cartilage graft has been removed, any deviated portions of the ethmoid and vomer can be further dissected in a subperiosteal fashion and rongeured. This removes any bony interference that might prevent the septum from moving into the midline. Unless there is an intrinsic deformity of the septal cartilage or its attachment to the anterior nasal spine, the septum should be easily positioned in the midline. Silastic nasal splints (Xomed) are placed and stabilized using sutures of 3-0 nylon anteriorly. Nasal packing is not routinely performed.

An L-strut 10 mm in width should be maintained to preserve dorsal support. Failure to do so may result in a saddlenose deformity.

EAR CARTILAGE

Because of the irregular shape and flaccidity of auricular cartilage the ear is most frequently used when the septum has previously been harvested. However, it is ideal for lower lateral cartilage reconstruction. In addition, it can provide a surprisingly large volume of cartilage for graft material, and the scar resulting from its harvest is very well concealed, even when placed anteriorly within the conchal bowl.

Technique

One of two methods is used to harvest the auricular cartilage, depending on the intended use of the ear cartilage graft.

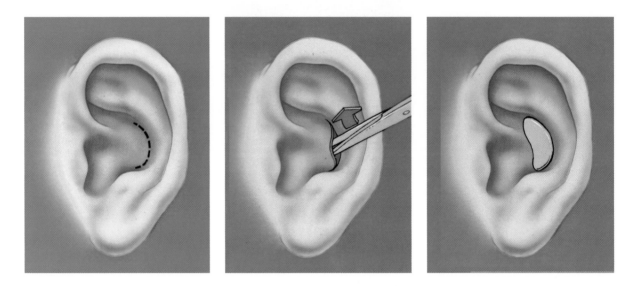

If a graft is needed for lower lateral cartilage or tip grafting only, then an anterior approach is preferred. The incision is placed approximately 3 mm inside of the conchal bowl both to camouflage the incision and to preserve the rim of the concha. Prior to the incision the concha is infiltrated with 2 to 3 ml of 1% lidocaine with epinephrine. In addition to hemostasis, this tends to hydrodissect the proper plane of dissection. The initial incision is made with a No. 15 blade, and after a single hook is placed for traction on the skin edge, the remaining dissection is performed with a sharp scissors. Once the skin has been elevated from the anterior aspect of the conchal bowl, a full-thickness cut is made 3 mm inside of the conchal bowl and extending through the posterior perichondrium. Scissors are used to dissect the posterior perichondrium off the postauricular skin. The harvest is then completed by incising the cartilage medially. Hemostasis is obtained and closure accomplished using a running 5-0 plain gut suture. A tie-over cotton and Xeroform bolster is used to obliterate the dead space created and prevent formation of a hematoma. This is secured by placing a 3-0 chromic suture through the anterior and posterior skin. It is removed in 3 days.

If a longer piece of auricular cartilage is necessary, a postauricular approach should be used for graft harvest. As with the anterior approach, the postauricular skin is infiltrated with 1% lidocaine with epinephrine. The postauricular incision is made through skin only, and the skin is dissected from the conchal bowl using scissors.

To preserve the conchal rim and 3 mm of conchal bowl cartilage, it may be helpful to pass a 25-gauge needle from anterior to posterior full thickness through the cartilage. The point of exit of the needle from the conchal bowl posteriorly is then marked with methylene blue. This marks the line of cartilage incision, which is then performed with a No. 15 blade scalpel. With the use of a single hook for traction, the conchal bowl cartilage is dissected from the anterior skin. The resection is completed with another full-thickness incision through the medial conchal bowl, taking care not to perforate the anterior conchal bowl skin. Again, hemostasis is obtained and a closure is performed with a running 5-0 plain gut suture. As before, a tie-over bolster of cotton and Xeroform is applied.

A posterior approach is preferred for the harvest of larger auricular grafts.

RIB CARTILAGE

Rib cartilage is the graft material of choice when support is the primary consideration. As a donor site, the rib offers an abundant supply of cartilage for use in virtually every aspect of rhinoplasty. However, it does have several drawbacks. Foremost is the incision required to harvest this graft. It must be made anteriorly over the desired rib; thus the scar is noticeable. However, it can be kept to a very small size (2 cm) since the chest wall skin is mobile and can be manipulated to expose a large amount of cartilage. Another drawback of the donor site is the postoperative pain experienced by the patient as well as the potential for pneumothorax.

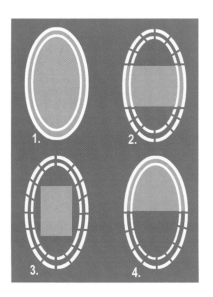

Although a problem with all cartilage, warping can be particularly problematic with rib cartilage. To minimize this distortion postoperatively, it is imperative that Gibson's principles of balanced cross-sectional carving be adhered to when fashioning the grafts.

*Warping of rib cartilage grafts may be minimized by balanced
cross-sectional carving according to the principles of Gibson.*

Technique

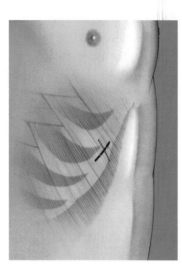

The optimal site for harvesting rib cartilage is
the lower chest wall at the level of the synchon-
drosis of the seventh, eighth, and ninth ribs.

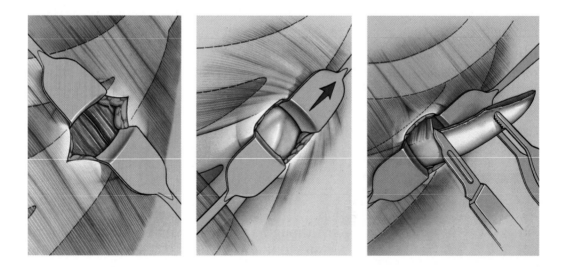

A 2 cm incision is made over the rib cartilage to be harvested, most frequently
the eighth rib. Since the chest wall skin is very mobile, with good lighting and
retraction a large segment of cartilage can be harvested through this minimal
incision.

*The length of the skin incision should be kept to a minimum
and manipulated to harvest the necessary volume of rib cartilage.*

The perichondrium is dissected out using a dental elevator, alternating with a Joseph elevator. A circumferential dissection is achieved, taking great care over the posterior aspect of the cartilage to prevent entry into the pleural space. The cartilage is then incised sharply with a scalpel and an appropriate size graft taken.

After hemostasis of the wound is ensured, the perichondrium is closed after ascertaining that no pneumothorax has occurred. This is best done by instilling saline solution into the wound and instructing the anesthesiologist to hold the patient in maximal inspiration. If no air bubbles are identified, the wound is closed in layers using deep Vicryl followed by a skin suture. If air bubbles *are* noted on maximal inspiration, this usually represents an injury only to the parietal pleura and not to the lung parenchyma itself. As such, this does not mandate chest tube placement. Rather, a red rubber catheter can be inserted through the pleural tear into the chest cavity. The incision is closed around the catheter as described above. As the patient is held in maximal inspiration, the red rubber catheter is placed on suction and removed.

At the termination of the procedure bupivacaine is injected into the operative site as well as into the intercostal spaces above and below the incision to provide prolonged postoperative analgesia and prevent chest wall splinting and atelectasis.

---

*Tears in the parietal pleura during harvest of rib cartilage grafts
can be managed by placing a red rubber catheter through the tear
and closing the incision. The catheter is removed while applying suction.
A postoperative chest x-ray film is mandatory.*

Rib cartilage grafts are ideal for dorsal onlay grafting and columellar struts. End slices of rib cartilage have more of a tendency to warp and are best used as lower lateral alar replacements or selective onlay grafts.

■ KEY POINTS

- ■ The septum is the most frequently used site due to its convenience and versatility as a graft material.

- ■ Rib cartilage is preferred when structural support is the primary concern.

- ■ Ear cartilage is best used for replacement of the lower lateral cartilages or as onlay graft material.

- ■ Regardless of its source, autologous material is preferred to alloplasts in all primary and secondary rhinoplasties.

BIBLIOGRAPHY

1. Chase S, Herndon C. The fate of autogenous and homogenous bone grafts: A historical review. J Bone Joint Surg 37A:809, 1955.
2. Gibson T. Cartilage grafts. Br Med Bull 21:153, 1965.
3. Gibson T, Davis WB. The distortion of autogenous cartilage grafts: Its cause and prevention. Br J Plast Surg 10:257, 1958.
4. Gibson T, Davis WB, Curran RC. The long term survival of cartilage homografts in man. Br J Plast Surg 11:177, 1958.
5. Gourney M. The ear as a donor site: Anatomic and technical guidelines. In Tanzer RD, Edgerton MD, eds. Symposium on Reconstruction of the Auricle. St. Louis: CV Mosby, 1974, p 106.
6. Gunter JP, Rohrich RJ. Augmentation rhinoplasty: Onlay grafting using shaped autogenous septal cartilage. Plast Reconstr Surg 86:39, 1990.
7. Gunter JP, Rohrich RJ. External approach to secondary rhinoplasty. Plast Reconstr Surg 80: 161, 1987.
8. Hagerty RF, Calhoon TB, Lee WH, Cuttino JT. Characteristics of fresh human cartilage. Surg Gynecol Obstet 11:3, 1960A.
9. Hoge J. Collapsed ala strengthening by conchal cartilage (the butterfly cartilage graft). Br J Plast Surg 18:92, 1965.
10. Mowlem R. Bone grafting. Br J Plast Surg 16:293, 1963.
11. Peer LA. Cartilage grafting. Br J Plast Surg 7:250, 1955.
12. Peer LA. The neglected septal cartilage graft. Arch Otolaryngol 42:384, 1948.
13. Sheen JH, Sheen AP. Aesthetic Rhinoplasty, 2nd ed. St. Louis: Quality Medical Publishing, 1998 (reprint of 1987 ed.).
14. Rohrich RJ. Rhinoplasty in the black patient. In Daniel RK, ed. Aesthetic Plastic Surgery. Boston: Little, Brown, 1993.

58

Selection of Cartilage and Bone Graft Donor Sites

Mark B. Constantian, M.D. • William P. Adams, Jr., M.D.

A NASAL MODEL AND THE RATIONALE FOR USING GRAFTS

One of the puzzles that has intrigued us for a number of years is why rhinoplasty is so difficult. We do not think that it is simply that the surgeon does not have binocular vision or cannot see skeletal asymmetries beneath the skin or that the surgeon has not made a proper preoperative diagnosis or did not sufficiently understand facial aesthetics. It may be that rhinoplasty is difficult because we have been thinking about it in the wrong way.

Reduction rhinoplasty is based on the simple principle that if the surgeon reduces the nasal skin to the desirable shape the soft tissue will contract to that skeletal shape. However, this model relies on two assumptions that may not always prove true. First is the assumption that the soft tissue has an infinite ability to contract to the shape of the underlying skeleton. But if that is true, why does supratip deformity occur? And why does augmentation correct supratip deformity? The second assumption of reduction rhinoplasty is that changes in the nose are purely regional; that is, when the surgeon changes the dorsum or tip, other areas are unaffected—each nasal part functions *independently,* not *interdependently.* But if that is true, why does the middle vault collapse when the dorsum is resected? Why does the size of the nasal base depend on the height of the bridge? Why does dorsal reduction usually shorten the nose and dorsal augmentation usually lengthen it? Why do all end-stage noses look the same?

Effects of Dorsal and Tip Grafts

Dorsal Grafts	Tip Grafts
Bridge contour	Tip contour
Nasal length—apparent and absolute	Tip support/projection
Nasal width—apparent and absolute	Nasal base size
Middle vault position (airflow)	Nostril/lobular proportion
Apparent nasal base size	Nasal length—apparent and absolute
Dorsum/tip relationships	Dorsum/tip relationships
Ethnicity	Ethnicity

Clearly, these two assumptions of reduction rhinoplasty are not always true. End-stage noses look the same and supratip deformity occurs because the vectors of soft tissue and skeletal contraction, while not identical, are consistent, but separate. Second, changes in one nasal area are not just regional, particularly in the dorsum and tip; surgical changes have "global" effects.

Limitations in the soft tissue envelope and interrelated effects of certain nasal regions on others influence rhinoplasty outcomes.

Therefore the pieces of the puzzle that must be considered are that the skin sleeve has only a limited ability to contract and the nasal areas are interdependent, with changes in one nasal area affecting others. These principles have a direct bearing on the use of cartilage and bone grafts because they justify the use of grafts. If the soft tissues can only contract to a limited degree and if nasal areas depend on each other for support or for proportion and balance, the surgeon must think in terms of redistribution and equilibration as much as reduction. We do not mean to imply that the rhinoplasty surgeon should never resort to reduction; however, soft tissues that are supported and skeletal segments that are balanced will remain balanced and equilibrated postoperatively.

When you control the postsurgical equilibrium, you control the postoperative result.

Both primary and secondary rhinoplasty are thus *rebalancing procedures* that take into account nasal function and balance in the context of a patient's aesthetic goals. Nasal reduction, nasal augmentation, and nasal grafts are common to both primary and secondary rhinoplasty.

PLANNING PARAMETERS

We use three parameters based on soft tissue morphology alone, not skeletal landmarks, to determine the rhinoplasty plan. Each one also influences the use of grafts and the technique selected. These parameters are:
1. Skin thickness and distribution
2. Tip-lobular contour
3. Balance between nasal base size and bridge height

The advantage of using soft tissue parameters is that they will be valid even when the skeleton does not influence surface contours (as in an overreduced secondary nose or in a thick-skin nose where soft tissues do not coapt to the preoperative skeletal shape).

I (Constantian) use grafts for two reasons: to augment an area so that contour can be altered and to correct an imbalance between soft tissue and skeleton (e.g., supratip deformity) or between skeleton and skeleton (e.g., middle vault collapse) that exists preoperatively *or that I create intraoperatively* (i.e., by resecting the middle vault roof).

Grafts are prioritized according to their:
1. Rigidity
2. Plasticity: Septum > ear > rib > cranial bone
3. Configuration needed
4. Special properties (i.e., composite graft)
5. Likelihood of survival (bed vascularity, crushed vs. solid)
6. Purpose: Function > dorsum > tip > columella > lateral walls

SPECIFIC DONOR SITES
Nasal Septum

It is important to harvest the septal segments long enough to serve the surgeon's needs. Leaving 15 mm dorsal and caudal struts at a minimum, I make my first cut with septal scissors 15 mm below the anterior dorsal edge and my second cut 10 mm posterior and parallel to the first through septal cartilage and ethmoid. When the segment is twisted with septal forceps, the ethmoid will break, usually producing a graft 25 mm or more in length. Additional graft material can be harvested toward the nasal floor and posteriorly. Septal cartilage makes excellent dorsal, spreader, tip, and columellar grafts. It can be shaved, beveled, or crushed so that it is either pliable or lacy. In a healthy bed it survives predictably and produces stable long-term results.

Summary of Surgical Aspects by Recipient Site

Radix
Source: Septum/ear
Technique: Narrow + crush
Fixation: By skeletonization

Dorsum
Source: Septum/ear/calvarial bone/rib
Technique: Layer—bevel or crush, not too narrow or wide, ± lateral wall grafts
Fixation: By skeletonization/ occasional wire or suture

Selection of Dorsal Graft Sources
Septum: First choice if available
Concha: Ideal for deep, asymmetric defect under thick soft tissue cover
Calvarial bone: Ideal for long, straight, shallow defect beneath medium or thin skin; graft surface is flat
Rib: Ideal for long, deep defect; graft surface is convex

Spreader Graft
Source: Cartilage or bone
Technique: Not too narrow or wide ± asymmetric
Fixation: Narrow pocket, caudal suture

Lateral Wall/Columellar Graft
Source: Ethmoid or cartilage— can use ear to recreate lateral crura
Technique: Not too much
Fixation: Pocket

Tip
Source: Cartilage, occasionally ethmoid
Technique: Always multiple—varied degrees of solid/crushed
Fixation: High pocket

Composite Graft
Source: Concha or alar wedge
Technique: Suit graft shape to defect; match cartilage/skin deficits
Fixation: Closure + percutaneous sutures if needed (remove in 24 hours)

The nasal septum is the premier donor site in terms of ease of harvesting and "plasticity" of the material yielded.

Ethmoid can be trimmed to provide underfill for dorsal grafts and makes excellent lateral wall grafts that are impalpable but supportive. Since ethmoid resorbs more readily than cartilage, it is not my first choice for solitary dorsal grafts. In addition, I would not place it alone at the root (where it may be palpable) or in the tip (where it will look artificially angular even if it survives). Ethmoid and vomer can both be used as so-called buttress grafts, as described by Sheen,[1] to prevent superior and posterior displacement of tip grafts placed caudal to them. Buttress grafts are primarily necessary in tightly scarred tips where the soft tissues are so unyielding that it would be otherwise difficult to maintain proper graft position. Irregular pieces of septal bone can often be crushed as well and used as filler. Pieces of septal cartilage that will not be needed for the reconstruction can be flattened and returned to the septal pocket to provide postoperative rigidity.

Ear Cartilage

Conchal cartilage removed from the cymba or cavum conchae (preserving the posterior conchal wall to avoid a change in ear contour) is a reliable and versatile graft material. Ear cartilage, however, is very different from septal cartilage and must be treated differently to avoid postoperative irregularities.

Solid or crushed cartilage can be used. Rolling the concha along its long axis, fixing it circumferentially with permanent sutures, and filling the open underside with scraps of trimmed cartilage, as described by Sheen,[1] create a dorsal graft that is perfect for a slightly asymmetric, relatively short (approximately 2 cm) dorsal defect beneath a thick soft tissue cover. Longer defects require longer grafts than the concha can usually supply; shallower defects will not lend themselves to a rolled graft, which is too bulky. Thin skin is likely to show the inevitable imperfections of the ear cartilage surface. Solid ear cartilage can also be used as tip grafts, although it is more difficult to achieve tips of varying contour until the surgeon becomes familiar with the graft material.

Ear cartilage can also be crushed, but it is more workable if the surgeon splits the cartilage tangentially before crushing rather than trying to crush the entire thickness of the concha. I (Constantian) have successfully used crushed conchal cartilage as a dorsal graft in situations where septal cartilage was not available, the defect was shallow (i.e., requiring a graft only 1 to 2 mm thick), and harvesting rib or calvarium did not appear justified. The chance of irregularities at the graft edges is always higher with crushed and split ear cartilage than it is with septal cartilage treated in the same fashion, and the patient should be so apprised beforehand and prefer this alternative to the other available possibilities. When used as lateral wall grafts it is important to be certain that the crushed ear cartilage is lying flat within the pocket so that it does not fold and curl, causing postoperative lumps.

When conchal cartilage has been thinned first, it will often crush almost like septal cartilage, becoming soft and then lacy with successive taps of a mallet. Solid ear cartilage often shatters when the surgeon attempts to crush it.

Calvarial Bone

I (Constantian) have used calvarial bone grafts with excellent success over the past 10 years. Early on my experience with the first two cases was not as good largely because of the use of higher speed orthopedic or neurosurgical air-driven drills.

Calvarial bone grafts must be harvested with an electric drill at low speed, keeping the bone surface cool. This is a tedious project, but if the graft is treated carefully, survival is virtually 100% in my experience with more than 50 patients followed up for 9 years.

The outer calvarial table is ordinarily 3 to 3.5 mm thick and provides a graft that can be thinned to 2 mm if necessary. This graft is perfect for a long, shallow defect beneath thin soft tissue cover in an otherwise symmetric nose. Calvarial bone can also be used for lateral wall or columellar grafts. We have been impressed with its survival in soft tissue pockets even where there was no bony contact. As with all dorsal grafts, it is important to roughen the surface of the bony vault to obtain graft adherence. Bony union is the rule, not the exception, and we ordinarily do not fix dorsal grafts unless the soft tissue is so distorted by prior trauma that it will dislodge the graft before it firmly unites to the orthotopic bone.

Costal Cartilage and Bone

I (Constantian) only recently began using rib grafts and therefore have only 6½ years of follow-up experience. Calvarial bone is the most difficult graft to obtain, but rib is the most difficult graft to shape because of its tendency to curl and warp even over the first few postoperative months. Nevertheless, rib does provide a long graft that will fill a deep symmetric or asymmetric defect; it thus fills defects that are too deep for calvarial bone and too long for folded ear cartilage. Nevertheless, it is important to minimize the chance for warpage by using the smallest rib needed for the defect and by splinting the rib internally with a Kirschner wire as necessary, a technique advocated by Gunter et al.[2] I ordinarily use the eighth or ninth rib if a dorsal graft, lateral wall grafts, maxillary augmentation, columellar grafts, and tip grafts are needed since these ribs will yield all of these products. If only a dorsal graft is necessary, the tenth rib gives a longer bony segment (and is therefore less likely to warp) and provides appropriately less donor material. It is important to "work both sides of the graft" to respect the "balanced cross-section" principle outlined by Gibson and Davis.[3] Rib cartilage slices can be crushed with some difficulty but will provide satisfactory lateral wall and columellar grafts. I have also used crushed costal cartilage for tip grafts successfully, although ear cartilage is easier to handle.

Composite Grafts

Composite skin/ear cartilage grafts supply excellent autologous units for correcting alar notches and replacing resected lateral crura in secondary rhinoplasty patients. Harvested from the cymba concha with its anterior overlying skin (the donor site is closed with a full-thickness retroauricular graft), the cartilaginous segment can be trimmed to recreate the lateral crus and the skin island used to replace the vestibular skin deficiency.[4] The graft is held in position by the pocket dissected for it and by fine absorbable sutures that inset the skin island to the vestibular incision made to accommodate it.

A WORD ABOUT ALLOPLASTICS AND HOMOGRAFTS

Many surgeons have reported success using alloplastics and homograft cartilage and employ them enthusiastically; we do not. It may certainly be true that in particularly favorable circumstances (e.g., as a dorsal graft in the primary thick-skinned nose) alloplastics may produce successful results in the short term. No one has reported any substantially long-term (10- to 20-year) experience with such materials in a large number of patients. Most of the studies, viewed critically, proclaim a success if a follow-up of 2 to 3 years has met with less than a 10% failure rate.

Although this data may be excellent for alloplastics, it is completely unacceptable for autografts. Even when the surgeon places the alloplast or homograft beneath a thick skin cover, it is impossible to protect it from the mucosal surface as well; the nasal layers are thin enough that the graft or implant must be close to one surface or another. If and when infection and/or extrusion occur, the patient will be worse off than if nothing had been done. Furthermore, the patient in whom one is tempted to use alloplastics or homografts is not ordinarily the patient with a primary unoperated nose and substantial septum. If these conditions were present, there would be no need to use alloplastics. The presenting circumstances are much more likely to be the tertiary rhinoplasty patient who has gone through a series of unsuccessful reconstructions and whose prior surgeons have exhausted multiple donor sites. This is the last type of patient that can (or should have to) face another temporary solution or surgical failure. We have not regretted the decision not to use alloplastics or homografts.

CONCLUSION

Rhinoplasty is indeed a puzzle. As the surgeon begins to understand the limits and interrelationships that exist, reduction and augmentation become compatible, not competing, strategies for balancing nasal structure, creating proper contours beneath a fixed skin volume, and achieving the patient's aesthetic and functional goals.

■ KEY POINTS

■ Soft tissue constraints and the effects that alteration of one rhinoplasty region has on others must be considered in rhinoplasty planning.

■ Nasal grafts can change contour and correct imbalances.

■ Nasal septum is the most versatile of all donor sites; however, auricular cartilage, calvarial bone, costal cartilage, and composite grafts have specific applications in rhinoplasty.

■ Effective use of nasal grafts enhances nasal balance.

REFERENCES

1. Sheen JH, Sheen AP. Aesthetic Rhinoplasty, 2nd ed. St. Louis: Quality Medical Publishing, 1998 (reprint of 1987 ed.).
2. Gunter JP, Clark CP, Friedman RM. Internal stabilization of autogenous rib cartilage grafts in rhinoplasty: A barrier to cartilage warping. Plast Reconstr Surg 100:162, 1997.
3. Gibson T, Davis WB. The distortion of autogenous cartilage grafts: Its cause and prevention. Br J Plast Surg 10:257, 1958.
4. Constantian MB. Functional effects of alar cartilage malposition. Ann Plast Surg 30:487, 1993.

59

Complications of Nasal Surgery

John F. Teichgraeber, M.D. • Ronald C. Russo, M.D.

*M*uch has been written on how to prevent and manage the untoward aesthetic and functional results of nasal surgery.[1-4] However, little information can be found in the literature on the disabling or life-threatening complications of nasal surgery and their appropriate management. This chapter will provide an overview of these complications and their treatment.

Severe complications after nasal surgery, although rare, do occur and can be divided into four categories: hemorrhagic, infectious, traumatic, and miscellaneous.[5] Although most reports of nasal surgery complications are anecdotal, there are several large series that report incidences of 1.7% to 18%.[6,7] Postoperative bleeding is the most frequently reported complication. Klabunde and Falces[6] reported postoperative hemorrhagic complications in 2% of 300 patients undergoing cosmetic rhinoplasty, whereas Miller[7] observed postoperative bleeding in 2.3% of 1150 patients undergoing rhinoplasties and septoplasties. Goldwyn[8] reviewed 780 patients undergoing rhinoplasty and septorhinoplasty and found the incidence of "excessive" bleeding to be 3.6% and "severe" bleeding to be 0.7%. More recently the incidence of hemorrhage after nasal surgery was reported to be 2%.[9,10] Infection, the next most common complication, was seen in 2.8% of the nasal reconstruction series of Miller[7] and in 17% of the cosmetic rhinoplasty series of Klabunde and Falces.[6] Yoder and Weimert[11] reported minor nasal infections in 0.48% of patients undergoing septal surgery. Septicemia and most recently toxic shock syndrome have been reported after septorhinoplasty.[12,13]

Most reports of traumatic complications after nasal surgery are anecdotal and include damage to the bony and soft tissues of the nose and adjacent structures. One series reported a 0.4% incidence of traumatic complications,[10] whereas Maniglia[4] reported 40 major traumatic complications, including 10 deaths, 10 cases of blindness, and 13 intracranial complications. Miscellaneous complications include anesthetic complications, psychiatric disturbances, and even asphyxiation from nasal packing.

The four main categories of severe complications after nasal surgery in order of frequency are hemorrhagic, infectious, traumatic, and miscellaneous.

HEMORRHAGIC COMPLICATIONS

Postoperative bleeding is the most common complication of nasal surgery.[6,8] Most early series reported the same incidence of bleeding after rhinoplasty with or without septal surgery.[7] However, a recent study reveals that postoperative bleeding is more frequently seen in rhinoplasty patients undergoing simultaneous septoplasty, turbinectomies, or both.[10] Bleeding may occur intraoperatively, but it is most frequently seen when the packing or splints are removed after surgery. Superficial mucosal ulceration and oozing from incision sites are the primary causes of mild bleeding problems. Silver nitrate sticks are used to treat superficial ulcerations, whereas judicious repacking with oxidized cellulose and petroleum jelly gauze impregnated with antibiotic ointment is used to stop incisional site bleeding. These "packs" are removed after 48 hours.

Severe postoperative hemorrhage usually occurs at the site of turbinate resection or osteotomy sites, although surgery on the premaxillary and maxillary crest can also cause profuse hemorrhage. When postoperative patients with epistaxis do not respond to conservative anterior packing or an intranasal balloon, they are returned to the operating room. With the patient under general anesthesia the nasal packing, splints, and remaining blood clots are removed and the nose irrigated. In addition to local hemostatic agents, the greater palatine foramen may be injected for temporary hemostasis. The foramen is located medial to the third maxillary molar and is injected with 3 ml of 2% lidocaine hydrochloride with 1:100,000 of epinephrine using a 27-gauge, 1.5-inch needle to a depth of 2.5 cm.[14,15] Bleeding sites are identified intranasally with a nasal speculum or a nasal endoscope and cauterized with a disposable malleable suction cautery.[16] Recently nasal endoscopy using a Karl Storz (Karl Storz Endoscopy–America, Culver City, Calif.) 30-degree, 4 mm scope with suction irrigation and a malleable suction cautery has been used in the treatment of epistaxis.[17-19] After the hemorrhage is stopped, an intranasal balloon or traditional anteroposterior packing is placed for 24 hours.

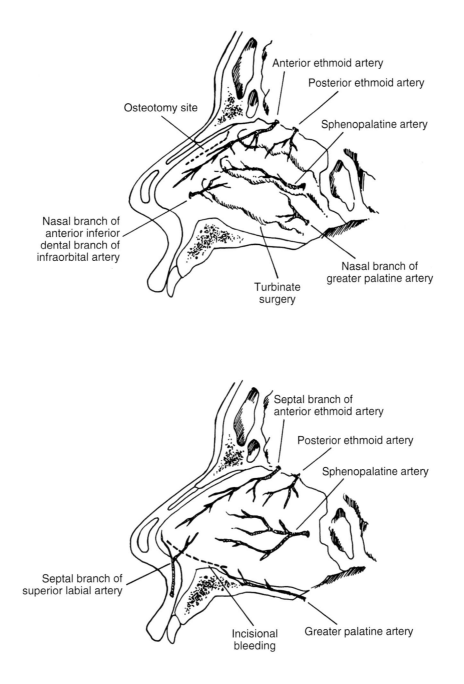

Anterior ethmoid artery

Posterior ethmoid artery

Osteotomy site

Sphenopalatine artery

Nasal branch of
anterior inferior
dental branch of
infraorbital artery

Nasal branch of
greater palatine artery

Turbinate
surgery

Septal branch of
anterior ethmoid artery

Posterior ethmoid artery

Sphenopalatine artery

Septal branch of
superior labial artery

Incisional
bleeding

Greater palatine artery

Angiography and embolization are used for epistaxis that does not respond to endoscopy and selective cauterization.[20] Embolization is used as a primary technique in patients with intractable epistaxis secondary to bleeding disorders, vascular abnormalities, tumors, or trauma and in patients who are poor surgical risks. Standard angiography or computerized digital subtraction angiography is used with Gelfoam or polyvinyl alcohol. The advantage of this treatment modality is that it identifies the bleeding site and can be performed rapidly with the patient under local anesthesia. However, it cannot be used to control anterior and posterior ethmoidal artery bleeding.[21-25]

If intranasal electrocoagulation, localized nasal packing, and embolization are unsuccessful in treating postoperative bleeding, specific vessel ligation is indicated. The internal maxillary artery is exposed transantrally and the ligation performed with neurosurgical clips.[26] There have also been reports of ligating the internal maxillary artery through an intraoral approach.[27] If this fails to stop the bleeding, the ethmoid vessels are exposed through an incision midway between the medial canthus and the middorsum of the nose. The anterior and posterior ethmoid vessels are electrocoagulated or doubly ligated with suture or self-locking neurosurgical clips.

The best way to manage postoperative epistaxis is to identify preoperatively those patients with "hemostatic defects" who are at risk for postoperative bleeding. Patients with a history of previous nasal surgery or craniofacial trauma and those patients having turbinate and septal surgery are at greater risk for preoperative and postoperative hemorrhage. Measures to prevent postseptorhinoplasty hemorrhage focus on the preoperative history and physical examination.[28] A personal family history for bleeding diastasis is taken, and specific inquiries are made for current medications that can affect hemostasis, that is, anticoagulants, aspirin, nonsteroidal anti-inflammatory drugs, and certain tranquilizers with a high antihistamine content. All patients are counseled to avoid aspirin and nonsteroidal anti-inflammatory drugs for 2 weeks before surgery. The physical examination focuses on evidence of ecchymosis, telangiectasia, splenomegaly, or Rendu-Osler-Weber syndrome. A preoperative laboratory workup includes complete blood count with platelets. Prothrombin times, partial thrombin times, and bleeding times are ordered only for patients at high risk for perioperative or postoperative hemorrhage. This battery identifies the most common hemostatic defects encountered in surgical patients, platelet dysfunction, and von Willebrand's disease. Intraoperative measures to prevent postoperative hemorrhage include meticulous closure of the intranasal incisions, the use of an interlocking horizontal septal mattress suture, and the use of a 2 mm osteotome to minimize trauma to the nasal mucosa during nasal osteotomies. In turbinate surgery only the anterior one third of the turbinate is resected, and a malleable suction cautery is used before and after the turbinates are incised.[28-31] Other postoperative measures to prevent bleeding include early removal of nasal packing (24 to 48 hours).

Bleeding after nasal surgery is most frequently seen in patients undergoing simultaneous septoplasty, turbinectomy, or both.

INFECTIOUS COMPLICATIONS

Because of the ubiquitous nasal flora and adjacent paranasal sinuses there is always the potential for infection after nasal surgery. Most infections are at the surgical site, but sinusitis and intracranial infections have also been reported. Local infections include cellulitis, abscesses, and granulomas that involve the overlying skin, columella, nasal vestibule, and septum.[32] Many of these infections can be prevented by meticulous irrigation and removal of bone dust, splinters, and blood clots after surgery. Most localized bacterial infections of the nose are caused by *Staphylococcus aureus*, *Streptococcus pneumoniae*, and *Haemophilus influenzae*, although localized *Pseudomonas aeruginosa* infections and actinomycosis have been reported after rhinoplasty.[33-36]

Localized infections respond well to antibiotic therapy and incision and drainage. The goal of treatment is to prevent contiguous spread to the orbit and cranium. The absence of valves in the facial, angular, ethmoidal, and ophthalmic veins and the extensive perineural drainage of the anterior cranial base make the involvement of these contiguous structures possible. Prompt treatment is critical, especially in septal abscesses where necrosis to the septal cartilage results in severe functional and aesthetic deformities.[37] The septum is approached along the floor of the nose, elevating a mucoperiosteal-mucoperichondrial pocket to drain blood clots and purulent material. Necrotic cartilage is excised and a silicone drainage tube is placed in the submucoperichondrial pocket.

The nose is lightly packed with Vaseline gauze placed in a finger cot (i.e., part of glove cut off in the shape of a finger) and irrigated with warm normal saline solution through the silicone tube for 24 hours. The silicone drainage tube is removed after 24 hours, and the remaining packing is removed after 48 hours.

Postoperative paranasal sinusitis results from chronic sinusitis or from nasal packing. Studies have shown that chronic inflammatory disease of the upper respiratory tract reduces mucociliary clearance, which in conjunction with nasal packing obstructs normal sinus oxygen content and facilitates bacterial overgrowth.[38,39]

In patients with postoperative sinusitis the nasal packing and splints are removed. The treatment consists of topical and systemic decongestants and sensitivity-directed antibiotic therapy. Antibiotic coverage of postsurgical sinusitis differs from that for routine acute sinusitis. The organisms implicated in acute sinusitis include *Streptococcus pneumoniae, Haemophilus influenzae,* and *Branhamella catarrhalis;* after nasal packing or instrumentation the most frequently implicated agents include *Klebsiella pneumoniae, Proteus mirabilis,* and *Staphylococcus aureus.*[40-41] The overall nasal carrier rate for *Staphylococcus aureus* has been reported to be 38%, although a carrier rate of 65% has been reported in patients with minor nasal abnormalities.[42,43] Semisynthetic penicillins, the first- and second-generation cephalosporins, and erythromycin are used for staphylococcal infections.[44]

Reports of intracranial infections after nasal surgery are frequently found in the preantibiotic era and are usually seen after septal surgery.[45] They include meningitis, cavernous sinus thrombosis (CST), and dural and brain abscesses. These infections begin in the nasal cavity or paranasal sinuses and spread through traumatic dehiscence, natural bony passages, and lymph and venous channels by retrograde thrombophlebitis. The vessels most likely to develop thrombophlebitis are those that penetrate the cribriform plate with the olfactory nerves and in rare instances vessels within the septal marrow. Typically the infection is rapid, progressive, and fatal.[46] Rosenvold[45] in 1944 reported 56 patients who had intracranial infections after submucous resections or septal abscesses, 52 of whom died.

Although there are still reports of meningitis and brain abscess after nasal surgery, reports of CST are becoming increasingly rare.[47-49] The cavernous sinus is a connective tissue space of anastomosing venous vessels that lies between the two dural layers on each side of the sella and contains the internal carotid artery and cranial nerves III, IV, V,[1,2] and VI. Anteriorly, it receives the valveless ophthalmic veins that anastomose with a succession of other valveless veins, which include the angular, frontal, supraorbital, and facial veins. Posteriorly, it terminates in the superior and inferior petrosal sinuses. CST results from thrombosis formation and has been reported after local infection, facial fractures, and surgery to contiguous structures. The thrombosis propagates in a retrograde fashion through the venous sinuses, cerebral veins, and the meninges. As a result, meningitis and septicemia are often a part of the syndrome, and brain abscess and pulmonary embolism are frequent complications. Signs and symptoms include conjunctival and eyelid edema, ophthalmoplegia, dilatation and fixation of the pupils, retinal vein dilatation, bilateral papilledema, and meningitis.

The treatment of CST involves prolonged anticoagulant therapy and sensitivity-directed antibiotic therapy. Although CST was uniformly fatal in the preantibiotic era, modern series report an 80% survival but with a high incidence of neurologic sequelae (77% to 88%).[50]

Septicemia and bacterial endocarditis have been reported after nasal surgery, as has toxic shock syndrome (TSS), which is a multisystem disease seen primarily in menstruating females who use tampons and are vaginal carriers of *Staphylococcus aureus*.[51,52] This syndrome is characterized by fever, rash, hypotension, mucosal hyperemia, vomiting, diarrhea, and laboratory evidence of multisystem dysfunction and desquamation during recovery. It is thought to be toxin mediated with a mortality rate of 5% to 10%. The incidence of TSS after nasal surgery has been reported to be 16.5/100,000 nasal operations and it occurs in patients with nasal packing as well as nasal splints. The treatment is symptomatic; the nidus of infection is eliminated by removing all nasal packing and splints and the surgical site cultured for *Staphylococcus*-producing toxin, TSS toxin number 1 (TSST-1). Aggressive fluid therapy and β-lactase–resistant antibiotics have been used as have corticosteroids in selected patients. Neither topical nor synthetic antibiotics have been shown to be effective in preventing TSS. Some authors advocate preoperative nasal cultures to identify TSST-1 *Staphylococcus aureus* and the use of povidone iodine to swab the nasal cavity. Nasal packing or splints should be avoided in carriers of TSST-1.[53-59]

Measures to prevent postoperative infections include a thorough history for underlying sinus disease and infectious skin disorders. Prophylactic antibiotics have been shown to significantly reduce the level of local bacteria contamination, particularly gram-negative forms.[60,61] *Staphylococcus*-sensitive antibiotics and decongestants are used when standard packing is used, and the packing is removed within 48 hours to prevent sinusitis.[62]

Infectious complications after nasal surgery are usually at the surgical site, but sinusitis and intracranial infections have also been reported.

TRAUMATIC COMPLICATIONS

Trauma to the nose and adjacent structures in rhinoplasty can result in significant complications. Trauma to the nose itself can cause anosmia and iatrogenic arteriovenous malformations (AVM). Most studies indicate that nasal surgery does not result in long-term deterioration of smell, although Stevens and Stevens[63] in a prospective study of 100 patients reported that one patient had permanent anosmia after septorhinoplasty.[64,65] Transient postoperative anosmia results from airway obstruction, ischemia from local anesthesia, mucous membrane injury, and psychological disturbances. Although the risk of developing anosmia after nasal surgery is small, it can be devastating to certain professionals such as perfumers, chefs, and wine tasters. The best treatment is prevention by avoiding damage to the cribriform plate.[66]

Although rare, iatrogenic AVM is a well-documented traumatic complication of nasal surgery. The mechanisms of injury include the intravascular injection of local anesthetic agents, surgical exposure, and osteotomies. Treatment is arteriography with embolization and excision.[67-68]

There have also been reports of injury to local dental structures. Osteotomies can damage the premaxilla and the vascular supply to the apices of the incisors, resulting in devitalized central incisors. Endodontic therapy and cosmetic dentistry are the treatment of choice.[69]

Orbital trauma during nasal surgery can result in bleeding epiphora and even blindness.[70,71] The epiphora is usually not from an actual surgical disruption of the lacrimal apparatus but is secondary to soft tissue edema and is self-limiting, resolving in 1 to 2 weeks. However, several authors have documented lacrimal sac injury during nasal osteotomies but only after subperiosteal tunneling, which was used in conjunction with a straight-line or saw osteotomy.[72,73] Recent studies demonstrate that the current technique of using low-curved osteotomies without subperiosteal dissection will not damage the lacrimal system.[74]

Blindness after nasal surgery is extremely rare. The mechanism of injury results from vascular damage or direct mechanical trauma to the optic nerve. Most reports of blindness associated with nasal instrumentation involve steroid injection of the nasal turbinates. Recently blindness after septorhinoplasty was reported that resulted from a retrograde flow of local anesthesia after an intra-arterial injection. Treatment is prevention.[75]

The most dramatic complication of nasal surgery is an iatrogenic intracranial injury.[4] The reported injuries include cerebrospinal fluid (CSF) rhinorrhea, pneumocephalus, and direct damage to the frontal lobes.[76] Injury to the anterior cranial fossa may result from direct injury with an osteotome, although this mechanism of injury is unlikely unless there is a congenital cranial floor abnormality or previous fracture. Direct injury to the frontal lobes has been reported to cause carotid cavernous sinus fistula, hematoma, and lacerations. The most likely mechanism of injury to the anterior cranial fossa is trauma to the septum, which fractures through the cribriform plate at its junction with the perpendicular plate of the ethmoid. If a small opening results, CSF rhinorrhea occurs, whereas a larger one permits the introduction of air into the subdural space (pneumocranium) or ventricles (pneumocephalus).[77] Prevention is the key to treating intracranial complications. Care is taken not to crack the cribriform plate when performing a septoplasty. The deviated portion of the perpendicular plate of the ethmoid is removed with double-action scissors. A rocking action to fracture the ethmoid plate is avoided.

If injury to the anterior cranial fossa does occur and a CSF leak is recognized, intraoperative repair is undertaken immediately.[78] The key to management of a CSF leak is precise localization, and intrathecal fluorescein with a Valsalva maneuver is helpful in this regard. Temporalis fascia, free and pedicled septal mucosal grafts, and an osteomucoperiosteal flap have all been used to repair the defect.[74,75,79-82] The repair may be done intranasally using a combination of headlight illumination, operating microscope, and endoscopic sinus surgery.[76,77] The graft or flaps are immobilized with microfibrillar collagen, Gelfoam, and antibiotic-impregnated gauze. Packing is removed after 7 to 10 days. If a CSF leak or pneumocephalus is diagnosed immediately postoperatively, the treatment is conservative.

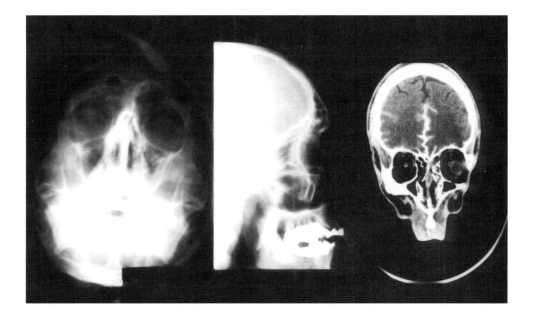

Plain radiographs, although of limited value, are used to localize the fracture, intracranial air, or opacified sinus. Currently CT scanning with metrizamide is the diagnostic study of choice in localizing a CSF fistula.[83-84] The patient is placed on bed rest in a semisitting position, avoiding physical strain. If the leak persists, repeated lumbar CSF puncture or an indwelling lumbar subarachnoid drain is used. Fortunately most traumatic CSF fistulas close spontaneously (70%), but a small percentage of patients (25% to 35%) develop meningitis.[85] The use of prophylactic antibiotics is controversial, and antibiotic therapy is reserved for symptomatic patients.

The infecting organisms in cases of meningitis are *Streptococcus pneumoniae* and *Haemophilus influenzae.* Surgical intervention is reserved for those patients in whom leaks persist after CSF drainage or those in whom leaks, though improved, persist after 2 weeks.[86]

The surgical approach may be extracranial or intracranial; there are numerous reports of successful endoscopic management. Free fascial or mucosa grafts, pedicled mucosa grafts from the septum or turbinates, and osteomucoperiosteal flaps all have been used.[87-89]

Iatrogenic trauma to the nose and adjacent structures can cause significant complications ranging from anosmia to intracranial injury.

MISCELLANEOUS COMPLICATIONS

Life-threatening anesthetic-related complications include malignant hyperthermia and cardiopulmonary collapse.[90] The newer anesthesia monitors can pick up changes in CO_2 saturation, an early indicator of malignant hyperthermia along with rapid temperature elevation. Early recognition, cessation of the anesthetic, and treatment with dantrolene sodium are the cornerstones for preventing complications from malignant hyperthermia.

The systemic effects of local anesthetics used for their hemostatic properties in nasal surgery result from elevated blood levels of the agent. Most deaths are directly related to overdoses.[91] The use of halothane and epinephrine should be avoided because of the risk of increased myocardial hyperactivity, arrhythmias, and even cardiopulmonary collapse. In addition, the use of "cocaine mud" should be avoided because the addition of epinephrine to cocaine can result in increased complications and mortality from the mixture.[92-94]

Psychiatric disturbances in the immediate postoperative period are more frequent in rhinoplasty than in any other elective cosmetic procedure. The percentage of patients requiring psychiatric supervision is directly proportional to the number of patients with existing psychiatric problems or the number of patients who seek nasal surgery for psychiatric reasons. A patient suspected of psychiatric disturbances may evidence a minimal physical defect and an inability to define the change desired from rhinoplasty. Moreover, the surgeon may be unable to establish a good relationship with this type of patient. Identification of these patients allows the surgeon to prevent sequelae by not operating on the patient or by seeking psychiatric support for help with preoperative and postoperative management.[95-96]

Finally, there have been two cases of asphyxiation as a result of nasal pack aspiration.[97] The patients' nasal cavities were packed with gauze strips that were aspirated in the recovery room. If gauze packing is used, a continuous strip, not individual pledgets, is recommended because a continuous strip is less susceptible to dislodgment. When individual pledgets are used, they are sutured transcolumellarly to prevent dislodgment.

Miscellaneous complications include malignant hyperthermia, cardiopulmonary collapse, and psychiatric disturbances.

CONCLUSION

The incidence of life-threatening complications after nasal surgery is low. Postoperative bleeding is the most common complication, but infectious complications and even intracranial traumatic complications have also been reported. This chapter has presented an overview of the complications and their treatment.

■ KEY POINTS

■ Severe complications after nasal surgery are classified in order of frequency as hemorrhagic, infectious, traumatic, and miscellaneous.

■ The reported incidences of nasal surgery complications range from 1.7% to 18%.

■ Postoperative bleeding is the most frequently reported complication (2%).

■ Infectious complications include local infections, sinusitis, intracranial infections, and toxic shock syndrome.

■ Traumatic complications are rare but include anosmia, blindness, and iatrogenic intracranial injury.

■ Miscellaneous complications are primarily anesthetic but may also stem from psychiatric disturbances.

REFERENCES

1. Gunter JP, Rohrich RJ. External approach for secondary rhinoplasty. Plast Reconstr Surg 80: 161, 1987.
2. Kamer FM, McQuown SA. Revision rhinoplasty. Arch Otolaryngol Head Neck Surg 114:257, 1988.
3. Rees TD, Krupp S, Wood-Smith D. Secondary rhinoplasty. Plast Reconstr Surg 46:332, 1970.
4. Maniglia AJ. Fatal and major complications secondary to nasal and sinus surgery. Laryngoscope 99:276, 1989.
5. Lawson W, Kessler S, Biller JF. Unusual and fatal complications of rhinoplasty. Arch Otolaryngol 109:164, 1983.
6. Klabunde EH, Falces E. Incidence of complications in cosmetic rhinoplasties. Plast Reconstr Surg 34:192, 1964.
7. Miller T. Immediate postoperative complications of septoplasties and septorhinoplasties. Trans Pacific Coast Otoophthalmol Soc 57:201, 1976.
8. Goldwyn RM. Unexpected bleeding after elective nasal surgery. Ann Plast Surg 2:201, 1979.
9. McKinney P, Cook JQ. A critical evaluation of 200 rhinoplasties. Ann Plast Surg 7:357, 1981.
10. Teichgraeber JF, Riley WB, Parks DH. Nasal surgery complications. Plast Reconstr Surg 85: 527, 1990.
11. Yonder MG, Weimert TA. Antibiotics and topical surgical preparation solution in septal surgery. Otolaryngol Head Neck Surg 106:243, 1992.
12. Tobin G, Shaw RC, Goodpasture HC. Toxic shock syndrome following breast and nasal surgery. Plast Reconstr Surg 80:111, 1987.
13. Coursey DL. Staphylococcal endocarditis following septorhinoplasty. Arch Otolaryngol 99: 454, 1974.
14. Stankiewicz JA. Greater palatine foramen injection made easy. Laryngoscope 98:580, 1988.
15. Williams WT, Ghorayeh BY. Incisive and pterygo-palatine fossa injection for hemostasis in septorhinoplasty. Laryngoscope 100:1245, 1990.
16. Andersen RG, Shannon DN, Schaeffer SD, Raney LA. A surgical alternative to internal maxillary artery ligation for posterior epistaxis. Otolaryngol Head Neck Surg 92:427, 1984.
17. Marcus MJ. Nasal endoscopic control of epistaxis—a preliminary report. Otolaryngol Head Neck Surg 102:273, 1984.
18. Sharp HR, Rowe-Jones JM, Biring GS, Mackay IS. Endoscopic ligation or diathermy of the sphenopalatine artery in persistent epistaxis. J Laryngol Otol 111:1047, 1997.
19. O'Leary-Stickney K, Makielski K, Wymuller EA Jr. Rigid endoscopy for the control of epistaxis. Arch Otolaryngol Head Neck Surg 118:966, 1992.
20. Pearson BW, Mackenzie RG, Goodman WS. The anatomical basis of transantral ligation of the maxillary artery in severe epistaxis. Laryngoscope 79:969, 1969.
21. Maceri DR, Makielski KH. Intraoral ligation of the maxillary artery for posterior epistaxis. Laryngoscope 94:737, 1984.
22. Struts J, Schemata M. Uncontrollable epistaxis. Arch Otolaryngol Head Neck Surg 116:697, 1990.
23. Schaitkin B, Strauss M, Houck JR. Epistaxis: Medical versus surgical therapy: A comparison of efficacy, complications and economic consideration. Laryngoscope 97:1392, 1987.
24. Breda SD, Choi IS, Persky MS, Weiss M. Embolization in the treatment of epistaxis after failure of internal maxillary artery ligation. Laryngoscope 99:809, 1989.
25. DeFillip GJ, Rubinstein M, Drake A, Koopman C. The role of angiography and embolization in the management of recurrent epistaxis. Otolaryngol Head Neck Surg 99:597, 1988.
26. Hicks JN, Vitek G. Transarterial embolization to control posterior epistaxis. Laryngoscope 99: 1027, 1989.
27. Welsh LW, Welsh JJ, Scogna JE, Gregor FA. Role of angiography in the management of refractory epistaxis. Ann Otol Rhinol Laryngol 99:69, 1990.
28. Garth RJ, Cox HJ, Thomas MR. Haemorrhage as a complication of inferior turbinectomy: A comparison of anterior and radical trimming. Clin Otolaryngol 20:236, 1995.

29. Bolger WE, Parsons DS, Potempa L. Preoperative hemostatic assessment of the adenotonsillectomy patient. Otolaryngol Head Neck Surg 103:396, 1990.

30. Mabry RL. Inferior turbinoplasty: Patient selection, technique, and long-term consequences. Otolaryngol Head Neck Surg 98:60, 1988.

31. Mabry RL. Surgery of the inferior turbinates: How much and when? Otolaryngol Head Neck Surg 92:571, 1984.

32. Barat M, Shickowitz MJ. Nasofrontal abscess following rhinoplasty. Laryngoscope 95:1523, 1985.

33. Schaefer SD, Ronis ML. Cephalexin in the treatment of acute and chronic maxillary sinusitis. South Med J 78:45, 1985.

34. Rudolph R. Pseudomonas infection in the postoperative nasal septum. Plast Reconstr Surg 70:87, 1982.

35. Thomas GG, Toohill RJ, Leham RH. Nasal actinomycosis following heterograft. Arch Otolaryngol 100:377, 1974.

36. Kamer FM, Binder WJ. Pseudomonas infection of the nose. Arch Otolaryngol 106:505, 1980.

37. Matsuba HM, Thawley SE. Nasal septal abscess: Unusual cause, complications, treatment and sequelae. Ann Plast Surg 16:161, 1986.

38. Drettner B. Pathophysiology of paranasal sinuses with clinical implications. Clin Otolaryngol 5:277, 1980.

39. Sakakura Y, Majima Y, Saida S, Ukai K, Miyoshi Y. Reversibility of reduced mucociliary clearance in chronic sinusitis. Clin Otolaryngol 10:79, 1985.

40. Herzon FS. Bacteremia and local infections with nasal packing. Arch Otolaryngol 94:317, 1970.

41. Bell RM, Pae GV, Bynoe RP, Dunham ME, Brill AH. Post-traumatic sinusitis. J Trauma 28:923, 1988.

42. Williams REO. Healthy carriage of *Staphylococcus aureus:* Its prevalence and importance. Bact Rev 27:56, 1963.

43. Slavin SA, Rees TD, Guy CL, Goldwyn RM. An investigation of bacteremia during rhinoplasty. Plast Reconstr Surg 71:196, 1983.

44. Syndnor A, Gwaltney JM, Cocchetto DM, Scheld M. Comparative evaluation of cefuroxime axetil and cefaclor for treatment of acute bacterial maxillary sinusitis. Arch Otolaryngol Head Neck Surg 115:1430, 1989.

45. Rosenvold LK. Intracranial suppuration secondary to disease of the nasal septum. Arch Otolaryngol 40:1, 1944.

46. Maniglia AJ, Goodwin J, Arnold JE, Ganz E. Intracranial abscesses secondary to nasal, sinus and orbital infection in adults and children. Arch Otolaryngol Head Neck Surg 115:1424, 1989.

47. Lewin ML, Argamaso RV, Friedman S. Localized cerebritis following an aesthetic rhinoplasty. Plast Reconstr Surg 64:720, 1979.

48. Shaw RE. Cavernous sinus thrombophlebitis: A review. Br J Surg 40:40, 1952.

49. Lacy GM, Conway H. Recovery after meningitis with convulsions and paralysis following rhinoplasty: Cause for pause. Plast Reconstr Surg 36:254, 1965.

50. Casaubon JN, Dion MA, Labrisseau A. Septic cavernous sinus thrombosis after rhinoplasty. Plast Reconstr Surg 59:119, 1977.

51. Thomas SW, Baird IM, Frazier RD. Toxic shock syndrome following submucous resection and rhinoplasty. JAMA 247:2402, 1982.

52. Hull HF, Mann JM, Sand CJ, Gregg SH, Kaufman PW. The toxic shock syndrome related to nasal packing. Arch Otolaryngol 109:624, 1983.

53. Younis RT, Gross CW, Lazar RH. Toxic shock syndrome following functional endonasal sinus surgery: A case report. Head Neck 13:247, 1991.

54. Wagner R, Toback JM. Toxic shock syndrome following septoplasty using plastic septal splints. Laryngoscope 96:609, 1986.

55. Huang IT, Podkomorska D, Murphy MN, Hoffer I. Toxic shock syndrome following septoplasty and partial turbinectomy. J Otolaryngol 15:310, 1986.

56. Breda SD, Jacobs JB, Lebowitz AS, Tierno PM. Toxic shock syndrome in nasal surgery: A physiochemical and microbiologic evaluation of Merocel and NuGauze nasal packing. Laryngoscope 97:1388, 1987.

57. Wilson JA, Von Haacke PT, McAndrew PT, Murray JAM. Toxic shock syndrome after nasal surgery. Rhinology 25:139, 1987.

58. Jacobson JA, Kasworm EM. Toxic shock syndrome after nasal surgery. Arch Otolaryngol Head Neck Surg 112:329, 1986.

59. Barbour SD, Shales DM, Guertin SR. Toxic-shock syndrome associated with nasal packing: Analogy to tampon associated illness. Pediatrics 73:163, 1984.

60. Eschelmann LT, Schleunig AJ, Brummett RE. Prophylactic antibiotics on otolaryngologic surgery: A double blind study. Trans Am Acad Ophthalmol Otolaryngol 75:387, 1971.

61. Weimert TA, Yoder MG. Antibiotics and nasal surgery. Laryngoscope 90:667, 1980.

62. Larrabee WF. Prophylactic antibiotics in nasal surgery. Arch Otolaryngol Head Neck Surg 116: 1125, 1990.

63. Stevens CN, Stevens MH. Quantitative effects of nasal surgery on olfaction. Am J Otolaryngol 6:264, 1985.

64. Goldwyn RM, Shore S. The effects of submucous resection and rhinoplasty on the sense of smell. Plast Reconstr Surg 41:428, 1968.

65. Champion R. Anosmia associated with corrective rhinoplasty. Br J Plast Surg 19:182, 1966.

66. Kimmelman CP. The risk to olfaction from nasal surgery. Laryngoscope 104:981, 1994.

67. Parkes ML, Griffiths CO. Arterial-venous aneurysm after rhinoplastic surgery. Arch Otolaryngol 86:91, 1967.

68. Guyuron B, Licota A. Arteriovenous malformation following rhinoplasty. Plast Reconstr Surg 77:474, 1986.

69. Sykes JM, Toriumi D, Kerth JD. A devitalized tooth as a complication of septorhinoplasty. Arch Otolaryngol Head Neck Surg 113:765, 1987.

70. Flannagan JC. Epiphora following rhinoplasty. Ann Ophthalmol 10:1239, 1978.

71. Hunts JH, Patrinley JR, Stal S. Orbital hemorrhage during rhinoplasty. Ann Plast Surg 37:618, 1996.

72. Flowers RS, Anderson R. Injury to the lacrimal apparatus during rhinoplasty. Plast Reconstr Surg 42:577, 1968.

73. Lavine DM, Lehman JA, Jackson T. Is the lacrimal apparatus injured following cosmetic rhinoplasty? Arch Otolaryngol 105:719, 1979.

74. Thomas JR, Grinner N. The relationship of lateral osteotomies in rhinoplasty to the lacrimal drainage system. Otolaryngol Head Neck Surg 94:362, 1986.

75. Cheny ML, Blair PA. Blindness as a complication of rhinoplasty. Arch Otolaryngol Head Neck Surg 113:768, 1987.

76. Marshall DR, Slattery PG. Intracranial complications of rhinoplasty. Br J Plast Surg 36:342, 1983.

77. Chandler JR. Traumatic cerebrospinal fluid leakage. Otolaryngol Clin North Am 16:623, 1983.

78. Hallock GG, Trier WC. Cerebrospinal fluid rhinorrhea following rhinoplasty. Plast Reconstr Surg 71:109, 1983.

79. McCabe BF. The osteomucoperiosteal flap on repair of cerebrospinal fluid rhinorrhea. Laryngoscope 86:537, 1976.

80. Montgomery WW. Cerebrospinal rhinorrhea. Otolaryngol Clin North Am 6:757, 1973.

81. Hirsch O. Successful closure of cerebrospinal fluid rhinorrhea by endonasal surgery. Arch Otolaryngol 56:1, 1952.

82. Mattox DE, Kennedy DW. Endoscopic management of cerebrospinal fluid leaks and cephaloceles. Laryngoscope 100:857, 1990.

83. Nabawi P, Maffee M, Phillips J, Capek V. The success rate of metrizamide CT cisternography in the evaluation of cerebrospinal fluid rhinorrhea. Comput Radiol 6:343, 1982.

84. Cooper PW, Kassel EE. Computer tomography and cerebrospinal fluid leak. J Otolaryngol 11: 319, 1982.

85. Ommaya AK. Spinal fluid fistulae. Clin Neurosurg 27:363, 1976.

86. Charles D, Snell D. CSF rhinorrhea. Laryngoscope 89:822, 1979.

87. Calcaterra TC. Extracranial surgical repair of CSF rhinorrhea. Ann Otol Rhinol Laryngol 80: 108, 1980.

88. Papay FA, Maggiano H, Dominguez S, Hassenbusch SJ, Levine HL, Leventu P. Rigid endoscopic repair of paranasal cerebrospinal fluid fistulas. Laryngoscope 99:1195, 1989.
89. Yessenaw RS, McCabe BF. The osteo-mucoperiosteal flap in repair of cerebrospinal fluid rhinorrhea: A 20-year experience. Otolaryngol Head Neck Surg 101:555, 1989.
90. DeJong RH. Toxic effects of local anesthetics. JAMA 239:1166, 1978.
91. Covino BG. Systemic toxicity of local anesthetic agents. Anesth Analg 57:387, 1978.
92. Wiley EN. Cocaine mud. JAMA 238:1813, 1977.
93. Fairbanks DNF. Cocaine: Friend or foe. Otolaryngol Head Neck Surg 100:638, 1989.
94. Ash M, Wiedemann HP, James KB. Cardiac complication from use of cocaine and phenylephrine in nasal septoplasty. Arch Otolaryngol Head Neck Surg 121:681, 1995.
95. Hay GG. Psychiatric aspects of cosmetic nasal operations. Br J Psychiatry 116:85, 1970.
96. Gifford S. Cosmetic surgery and personality change: A review of some clinical observations. In Goldwyn RM, ed. The Unfavorable Result in Plastic Surgery. Boston: Little, Brown, 1984, pp 21-43.
97. Spillman D. Medico-legaler Beitrag zum Thema Fremdkörper Aspiration: Aspiration von Nasen Tamponadem mit Todesfolge. Laryngol Rhinol Otol 60:56, 1981.

60

Porous Hydroxyapatite Granules to Eliminate the Hourglass Deformity in Advancement Genioplasty

P. Craig Hobar, M.D. ▪ James F. Paul, D.D.S., M.D. ▪ H. Steve Byrd, M.D.

*A*dvancement genioplasty through a horizontal osteotomy of the mandible consistently produces good results in patients with retrogenia or microgenia. However, a disruption of the smooth contour of the inferior border of the mandible at the site of the osteotomy may detract from the overall improvement. The advancement may produce a noticeable depression at the osteotomy site, commonly referred to as the "hourglass deformity."

Although the goals of genioplasty may be met in a patient, an hourglass deformity at the junction of the osteotomy and mandible posteriorly may diminish the aesthetic result.

Extending the osteotomy posteriorly minimizes this deformity but places the osteotomy dangerously close to the course of the inferior alveolar nerve and may lead to an unfavorable osteotomy split. Our method of choice to avoid the hourglass deformity and maintain a smooth inferior mandibular border is to augment the area with porous hydroxyapatite granules.

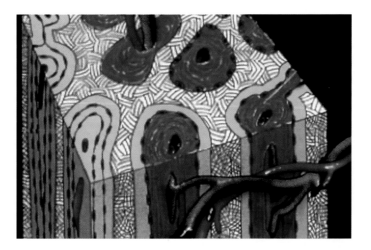

Porous hydroxyapatite granules are extremely biocompatible and allow fibrovascular ingrowth, providing both stabilization and resistance to infection. Resorption does not occur to a clinically significant degree.

TECHNIQUE

Porous hydroxyapatite granules (Pro Osteon 200; Interpore Cross International, Irvine, Calif.) are available in 0.8 ml syringes or 2 or 5 ml vials. The granules are emptied into a sterile container and mixed with a fresh sample of the patient's blood, which is usually drawn by the anesthesiologist or nurse at the time of mixing. Approximately 0.9 ml of blood is mixed with every 1 ml of hydroxyapatite granules.

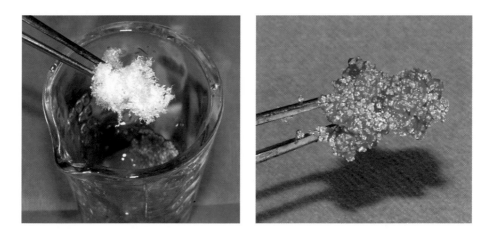

Microfibrillar collagen (Avitene) is then added (usually 300 to 400 mg per 5 ml of granules) and mixed until the desired consistency is achieved. The end point is reached when the granules adhere to one another. The mixture is easy to manipulate.

A mixture of porous hydroxyapatite, the patient's blood, and microfibrillar collagen is used to fill the concave region at the posterior junction of the osteotomy and the mandible.

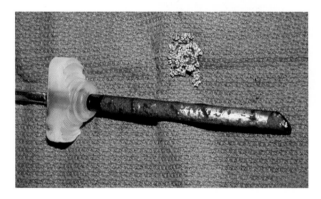

The mixture is then packed into specially coated glass syringes (Interpore 200). The syringes should only be used once or twice because the internal walls become scratched by the granules, making ejection of the material difficult.

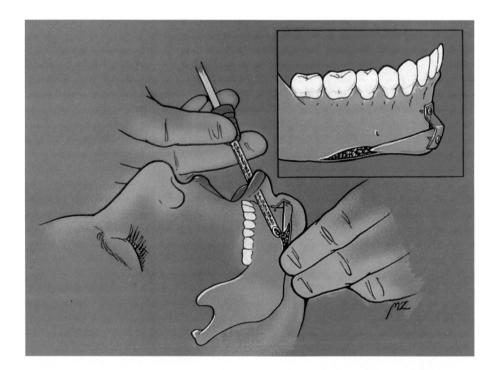

The discontinuity at the inferior mandibular border resulting from the osteotomy is palpated, and the concavity is effaced with the porous hydroxyapatite mixture. The mixture is injected subperiosteally into the concave junction. Enough of the mixture is used to fill the concavity and produce a smooth contour of the inferior border of the mandible. The mixture is molded with firm external manipulation. Approximately 1 ml is used per side.

CASE ANALYSIS

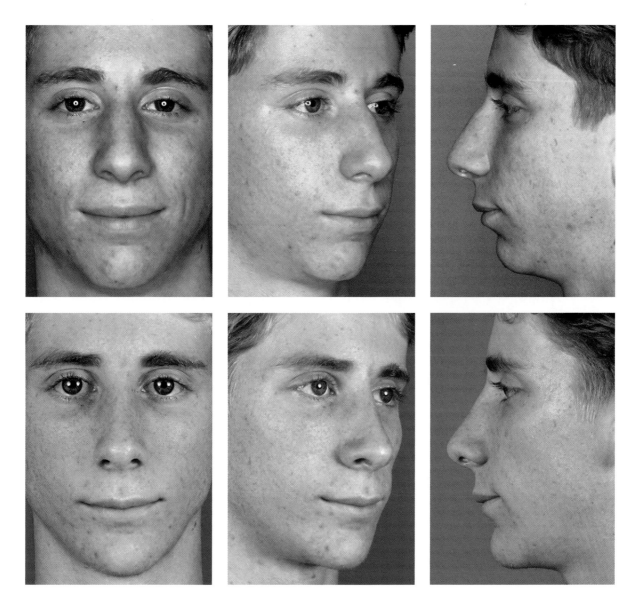

This 19-year-old man requested rhinoplasty and correction of his weak chin. Analysis revealed an underprojected chin with a slight deficiency of vertical dimension. The nasal length was relatively excessive. A refining rhinoplasty with 2 mm of shortening was performed in conjunction with a sliding genioplasty. The genioplasty consisted of a 10 mm advancement and a 3 mm increase in vertical dimension. Porous hydroxyapatite granules were used to fill in the osteotomy site.

61

Coding of Reconstructive and Cosmetic Rhinoplasty Procedures

Raymond V. Janevicius, M.D.

*A*lthough CPT coding for nasal procedures is relatively straightforward, problems may arise on two fronts: What constitutes a global code for these procedures? And how does one distinguish between reconstructive and cosmetic rhinoplasty? No distinction is made between open rhinoplasty procedures and endonasal procedures. These are considered "approaches" and the CPT Code Book does not differentiate between the two.

Primary Procedures

A tip rhinoplasty, whether for trauma or for purely cosmetic reasons, is coded 30400 if no other nasal procedure is performed (i.e., osteotomy, septal surgery). The code is global and includes all components of a tip procedure, including cephalic trim or other cartilage excisions, cartilage suturing, and scoring techniques. If, however, a distant graft (e.g., conchal cartilage) is used, it is appropriate to code separately for the graft (21235).

Code 30400 includes surgery on *both* alar cartilages since it reads "nasal tip." One does not code separately for surgery on each alar cartilage.

If surgery is performed on the bony pyramid in addition to the tip rhinoplasty, then code 30410 is used alone. Thus a rhinoplasty that includes a cephalic trim, dorsal reduction, and osteotomies is coded 30410. One does not code separately for the tip work because this is included in the global code, 30410.

Commonly Used CPT Codes for Nasal Surgery

30400	*Rhinoplasty, primary;* lateral and alar cartilages and/or tip
30410	*Rhinoplasty, primary;* bony pyramid, lateral and alar cartilages and/or tip
30420	*Rhinoplasty, primary;* bony pyramid, lateral and alar cartilages, and/or tip, including major septal repair
30430	*Rhinoplasty, secondary;* minor revision (nasal tip)
30435	*Rhinoplasty, secondary;* intermediate revision (bony work with osteotomies)
30450	*Rhinoplasty, secondary;* major revision (nasal tip and osteotomies)
30460	*Cleft lip rhinoplasty,* including columellar lengthening; tip only
30462	*Cleft lip rhinoplasty,* including columellar lengthening; tip, septum, and osteotomies
30520	*Septoplasty or submucous resection,* with or without cartilage scoring, contouring, or replacement with graft
20912	*Septal cartilage graft* (septal donor site)
21210	*Bone graft* to nose (includes obtaining graft)
21230	*Rib cartilage graft* to nose (includes obtaining graft)
21235	*Ear cartilage graft* to nose (includes obtaining graft)

A septorhinoplasty is coded 30420. This code is also global and includes septoplasty/submucous resection, bony pyramid surgery, and tip surgery. One should not unbundle these procedures (e.g., by using both 30420 and 30410) because 30420 includes all the component procedures.

When a septoplasty or submucous resection is performed alone (not in conjunction with tip or bony dorsum surgery), the code 30520 should be used. This code is global and includes all components of septal surgery (resection, scoring, suturing, etc.).

Cosmetic Vs. Reconstructive Procedures

Rhinoplasty CPT codes do not distinguish between cosmetic and reconstructive procedures. Code 30410, for example, describes cosmetic reduction of a dorsal hump with osteotomies. Code 30410 also describes dorsal straightening after trauma that requires osteotomies. ICD-9 codes indicate the *reasons* why procedures are performed. For a purely cosmetic procedure use code V50.1. For a posttraumatic procedure use ICD-9 codes 738.0 (acquired nasal deformity), 733.81 (malunion of nasal fracture), or 905.0 (late effect of nasal fracture).

Commonly Used ICD-9 Codes for Nasal Surgery

470	Deviated nasal septum
478.1	Nasal airway obstruction
733.81	Malunion nasal/septal fracture
738.0	Acquired nasal deformity
754.0	Congenital nasal/septal deformity
905.0	Late effect of fracture of skull or facial bones
V50.1	Plastic surgery for unacceptable cosmetic appearance

When performing a procedure that is part cosmetic and part reconstructive, however, one needs to itemize which procedure is done and for what reason (this is not unbundling). The reasons for each procedure are indicated with appropriate ICD-9 codes.

A septoplasty is performed for breathing obstruction secondary to a post-traumatic nasal septal deviation in a young woman. She requests that you narrow her nasal tip "while you are there." Since a portion of this procedure is cosmetic, it is coded as follows:

CPT	Procedure	ICD-9
30520	Septoplasty	470
		478.1
		905.0
30400-51	Tip rhinoplasty	V50.1

Cosmetic procedures cannot be submitted to third-party payers for re-imbursement.

Secondary Procedures

Secondary rhinoplasty codes are also global. A "minor" revision (nasal tip) is coded 30430. An "intermediate" revision (bony work with osteotomies) is coded 30435. When a "major" revision (tip and osteotomies) is performed, use the code 30450.

If septal surgery is performed during these secondary procedures, it should be coded *separately* (30520-51). Unlike the 30420 code (primary septorhino-plasty), *none of the secondary rhinoplasty codes includes septal procedures.* This inconsistency in the CPT Code Book need not be a source of confusion if one understands what is included in each global code.

As with primary rhinoplasty, the specific reasons for performing the procedures are indicated by using the proper ICD-9 codes.

Other Codes

The nasal fracture codes (21325-21355) are not used for septorhinoplasty procedures, although one may be treating the sequelae of trauma. The nasal fracture codes are used to describe reductions of acute fractures. When osteotomies or septal surgery is performed on *healed fractures,* use septorhinoplasty codes.

CPT code 30620 should not be used for septorhinoplasty procedures. This code describes "septal dermoplasty," a procedure for telangiectatic nasal bleeding in which the septal mucosa is removed and replaced with a skin graft. Unfortunately the text for this code used to read "reconstruction, functional, internal nose" and has caused some confusion because of the use of the term "reconstruction." Septal procedures should be coded 30420 or 30520.

Coding Example

A patient on whom a cosmetic rhinoplasty was performed several years ago is involved in an accident and fractures his nose. He is seen several weeks later after he develops breathing difficulty. Examination reveals that the nasal dorsum is deviated to the left. The septum is deviated into the left nasal cavity, and air entry is diminished on the left side. A septorhinoplasty is performed to correct the deformity and relieve breathing difficulty. No tip work is necessary.

Diagnoses

738.0	Acquired nasal deformity (1)
905.0	Late effect of fracture of nasal bones (2)
470	Deviated nasal septum (3)
478.1	Airway obstruction (4)

Procedures

30435	Rhinoplasty, secondary (osteotomies) (1,2)
30520-51	Septoplasty (3,4)

Since a previous rhinoplasty had been performed, the secondary rhinoplasty code is used. Because none of the secondary rhinoplasty codes includes septal surgery, the septoplasty is coded separately.

PART NINE

Personal Approaches

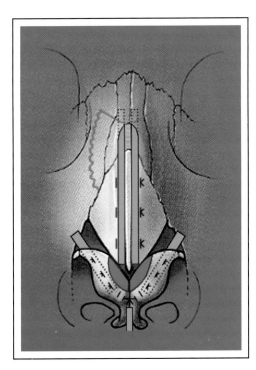

Gunter's Approach

Jack P. Gunter, M.D.

*R*hinoplasty has been a passion for me since I first began my career. It is the most difficult cosmetic surgery procedure to perform with consistently predictable and reproducible results. I have found accurate diagnosis to be the critical cornerstone on which all subsequent planning and execution rely. I have also found I do better technically with increased surgical exposure. Consequently, the external approach has become central to my technique.

After making an accurate diagnosis the surgeon must be able to determine the etiology of the deformity before establishing the goals of surgery and devising an operative plan. Assuming the correct goals and operative plan are established, it should be relatively straightforward to reconstruct a framework that will produce the desired aesthetic result if the surgeon understands the anatomy of the osseocartilaginous framework and its effect on the external appearance of the nose, obtains adequate exposure for operating, and has the equipment and materials needed. The unknown variable, however, is postoperative healing. At the current time we cannot adequately stabilize the osseocartilaginous framework to resist displacement and/or distortion by swelling and scar tissue contraction, but good planning and precise execution help minimize these unpredictable postoperative changes.

To obtain consistently good results, the surgeon performing rhinoplasty must be well versed in nasal anatomy and an expert in facial and nasal analysis. Expertise gained by watching others operate and performing rhinoplasty procedures on a regular basis is invaluable. Good record keeping is essential for tracking the surgeon's progress; the surgeon must keep accurate operative notes (I prefer pictorial) that can be studied when the patient returns to learn which techniques are most successful and reliable and take standardized pre- and postoperative photographs to evaluate the aesthetic results. Finally, once proficiency is obtained, teaching rhinoplasty techniques to colleagues helps further refine skills. Publishing and presenting papers at meetings have forced me to reexamine my thinking and ultimately have served to educate me as much as the audience it was intended for, if not more.

PATIENT CONSULTATION

The patient's initial call to the office is critical to establishing good patient rapport and ultimately obtaining a successful rhinoplasty result. The patient's questions should be answered in a friendly, yet professional manner that is informative and conveys an eagerness to help. This should be followed by sending the patient pertinent but brief information about the office, staff, surgeon, operative procedure in question, and what to expect at the first consultation.

At consultation, after being greeted by a friendly, helpful front office staff member, the patient is seen by a nurse who obtains the patient's personal and health history. I prefer for the nurse to leave before I see the patient so that we can talk privately. After a brief introduction and small talk to put the patient at ease I review the pertinent information to be certain I understand the patient's problem as well as his or her expectations to determine if they are realistic. The examination includes a complete facial and nasal analysis (see Chapter 4) and an endonasal examination using a nasal speculum, adequate lighting (preferably a headlight), and vasoconstriction, if indicated.

Having made a diagnosis and determined the etiology of the patient's deformity, I talk to the patient about the goals of surgery. Since I am not facile in computer imaging, I trace on cephalometric paper taped over standardized photographs what I think the goals of the surgery should be. The patient should always be advised that the images produced are used to establish goals only and do not guarantee results. I tell the patient that the results will be close to those drawn but probably will not be exactly the same. If the patient seems unrealistic about what can be achieved, I prefer not to operate rather than deal with an unhappy patient after surgery.

The patient then talks to the patient coordinator about scheduling the procedure, cost of surgery, and payment. The patient coordinator must be familiar with all aspects of the surgery so she can answer the patient's questions knowledgeably. She should be very positive about the procedure and make the patient feel comfortable about scheduling the surgery. When surgery is scheduled, a nominal fee is required to ensure the patient is committed to proceed. Although I do not use them, some offices make follow-up phone calls and send letters to patients after the consultation, which is probably a good idea when one is first starting.

Each surgeon must develop a protocol for patient consultation that he or she is comfortable with, but the importance of the initial phone call, the consultation itself, and the evaluation and preoperative management of the patient cannot be overemphasized.

BASIC PRINCIPLES

The following principles have helped me in developing my personal technique.

1. *Obtain adequate exposure.* To obtain adequate exposure it is generally necessary for me to use an open approach. This allows me to visualize the deformity undistorted by traction, permits me to use both hands while operating under binocular vision, and gives me more options for using different surgical maneuvers. The disadvantages of the open approach are (1) the transcolumellar scar, although it is seldom a problem if sutured correctly, (2) the increased operating time to reconstruct the osseocartilaginous framework before closing and to close the columella incision properly, (3) more postoperative edema than with the endonasal approach, which also takes longer to subside, and (4) a more difficult correction if an unsightly columellar scar occurs.

2. *Resect minimal amounts of tissue.* Overresection of cartilage results in a weakness that is more easily distorted by scar tissue contraction. To those who ask, "What is the minimal width to leave a lateral crural rim strip?" my standard answer is, "It should be kept as wide as possible without compromising the aesthetic result." It is important to remember that underresection is usually easier to correct than overresection.

3. *Maintain a balance between the osseocartilaginous framework and the skin sleeve.* An aesthetically sculpted nose is obtained by fitting skin tightly over a well-constructed osseocartilaginous framework. Since skin will only shrink so much, if the framework is too small, the skin will not fit tightly around it and will have little sculpting effect. Too much of an imbalance will result in a deformity. The adage "You can make a No. 3 size nose out of a No. 4 nose, but you can't make a No. 2" is based on this principle.

4. *Use original tissues for reconstruction.* No other cartilage in the body can simulate the delicate cartilages of the nasal tip. When the original cartilages can be used to shape the tip framework, I can think of very little justification for using cartilage from other areas other than to help stabilize or shore up the original cartilages.

5. *Avoid "visible" grafts if possible.* Visible grafts are grafts that touch the underneath surface of the skin and contribute to the shape in that area. Examples are tip grafts (onlay, umbrella, shield shape, etc.) and dorsal onlay grafts. Examples of nonvisible grafts are dorsal spreader grafts, alar

spreader grafts, lateral crural strut grafts, and most columellar struts. With age the nasal skin gets thinner, and the visible grafts sometimes show through the skin, presenting an unnatural appearance. However, at times they may be the only choice available, and the surgeon should be well versed in their use.

6. *Secure all grafts in place.* I have always found it difficult to fashion an undermined pocket the exact size and shape to hold a graft in the desired position. I find it much easier to suture them in place, which is facilitated with the open approach. An example is dorsal spreader grafts. When I placed them in pockets dissected using the endonasal approach, the pockets were either too large, allowing them to fall below the level of the dorsal septum, or too small, forcing the dorsal edge higher than the septum and resulting in a dorsal ridge. With the open approach they can be sutured directly to the septum at exactly the correct level without concern that they will become displaced.

7. *Stabilize the osseocartilaginous framework as much as possible.* Stabilization of the reconstructed framework protects against displacement and distortion caused by edema and scar tissue contraction. This is especially necessary when the open approach has been used. The open approach usually involves more extensive dissection than the endonasal approach and disrupts more of the supporting elements of the nose.

8. *Don't quit until the nose looks as good as possible.* I tell all my patients I've never performed a perfect rhinoplasty. There is always some imperfection when healing is complete. Therefore I never guarantee a perfect result, but I do tell them I will not leave the operating room until their nose looks as good as I can make it. Your best chance of getting an excellent result is on the first try. Since a revision is usually more difficult, the surgeon should not leave the operating room until he or she is satisfied the nasal shape is as good as possible.

9. *Shape the nose with the dressing.* I believe the dressing is important since it is possible to shape the nose to some extent with the dressing. For example, when lengthening a short nose without using grafts (see Chapter 30), the dressing should be placed with the nose in the lengthened position. If the dressing is placed so it rotates the nose upward, it will more than likely stay rotated, but it certainly will not heal in the lengthened position. I try to shape the nose with the dressing to make it look as good as possible. This does not guarantee that it will look good when it heals, but I assure you that if the nose does not look good when the patient leaves the operating room, it will not look better later.

OPERATIVE TECHNIQUE
Anesthesia

Both general endotracheal and IV sedation anesthesia for rhinoplasty have pros and cons. Certainly for short procedures, when very little bleeding is anticipated, IV sedation may be preferable. However, I have had some problems with blood pooling in the hypopharynx in patients under IV sedation. An unprotected airway in a patient with a decreased cough reflex poses serious problems. For this reason I prefer general endotracheal anesthesia. I always place a nasogastric tube during the operation and suction any blood that enters the stomach in an effort to reduce postoperative nausea and vomiting. The patient receives perioperative antibiotics only starting 30 minutes prior to the incision. No postoperative antibiotics are given.

Before prepping the patient I swab the interior of the nose with oxymetazoline and inject the external nose and septum with 10 ml or less of a mixture of 50 ml of 0.5% lidocaine and 0.5 ml of 1:1000 epinephrine. Strips of 1-inch NuGauze approximately 18 inches in length soaked in oxymetazoline are used for packing the nose. The face and nose are then prepped with one-half strength povidone-iodine solution, and the patient is draped in a sterile manner.

Incisions

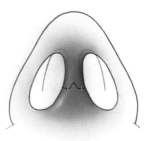

The transcolumellar incision is marked just anterior to the flare of the feet of the medial crura. The design of the incision is not critical as long as it is a broken line and made perpendicular to the skin surface. The one I find easiest to close and am presently using is the inverted notched incision. After the incision is marked, two superficial crosscuts are made on each side of the notch to facilitate precise closure at the end of the operation.

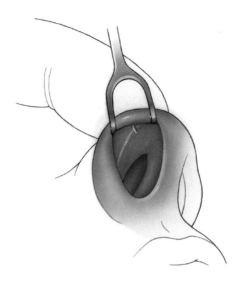

The marginal incision site is visualized by placing a 12 mm double-pronged skin hook inside the alar rim with the medial hook at the vestibular apex. The caudal margin of the lateral crus is identified by putting mild tension on the skin hook and pushing the ala into the vestibule with the fourth finger. This brings the caudal margin into prominence. The edge can usually be seen under the vestibular skin or identified by feeling the step-off with the back end of the knife handle. Another superficial crosscut is made across the incision site midway between the hooks, again to facilitate accurate closure.

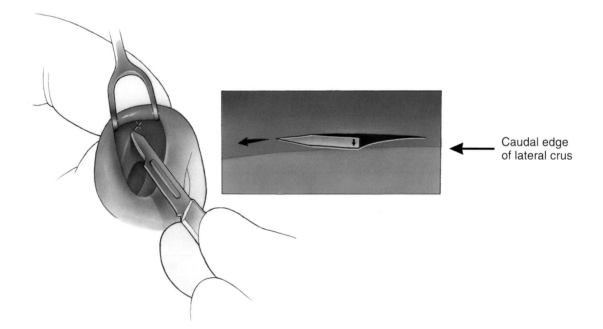

Caudal edge
of lateral crus

With the skin hook still in place the marginal incision is begun just lateral to the apex and extends laterally along the caudal margin of the lateral crus. To avoid cutting into the cartilage, the back edge of the No. 15 blade is pushed against the caudal edge of the cartilage with the cutting edge rotated slightly away from the caudal margin. While feeling its back edge against the cartilage the knife is slid along the caudal margin. The incision extends to within 1.5 cm of the piriform aperture rim.

Attention is then directed back to the starting point lateral to the apex, where the incision is continued medially along the caudal margin just inside the roll of the columella to slightly past the level of the transcolumellar incision. The most difficult part of the incision is in the area of the apex. Sometimes it is difficult to gain adequate exposure in this area with the double-pronged skin hook, and some surgeons prefer to make the incision along the columella first and then connect the medial and lateral incisions across the vestibule with small scissors.

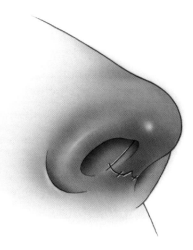

The transcolumellar incision is made last with a No. 15 blade, keeping the blade perpendicular to the skin surface and taking care to avoid cutting the caudal margins of the medial crura. It meets the marginal incision laterally and continues superficially past it for 2 to 3 mm. This extension past the junction with the transcolumellar incision forms a crossmark for orientation during closure. A No. 11 blade is used for cutting the notch.

Undermining

Undermining over the lateral crura, columella, and upper lateral cartilages is performed with small, sharp, pointed scissors, leaving little or no soft tissue on the perichondrium. It extends 2 mm past the osseocartilaginous cartilage junction onto the nasal bones, where the points of the scissors are used to scratch through the periosteum. A periosteal elevator is used to elevate the periosteum. Since periosteum does not stretch, it is impossible to elevate it as a continuous sheet. Although it will tear, the subperiosteal plane is still desired for elevation.

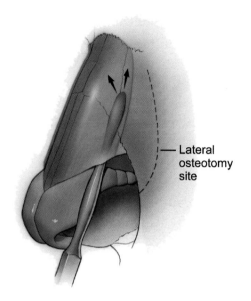

Over the bony dorsum undermining extends laterally only as far as needed for exposure. Since it is never raised as far as the lateral osteotomy site, there will be some periosteum left attached to the bone for stability anterior to the lateral osteotomy site. Undermining over the lateral crura and upper lateral cartilages goes only as far as needed for exposure.

I undermine the soft tissue off the medial surfaces of the medial crura so that I can better visualize the crura and more precisely place sutures through the crura. Undermining continues through the soft tissue of the membranous septum to access the caudal septum. If a columellar strut is to be used, a pocket is undermined between the feet of the medial crura toward the nasal spine. It stops short of the nasal spine to leave a soft tissue pad at the base of the pocket between the strut and the spine so that the end of the strut will not flip back and forth over the spine during upper lip movements.

With the caudal end of the septum now exposed work can begin on the septum. However, it is delayed until the dorsum has been reduced as needed: if septal cartilage is resected, the remaining dorsal septum must be at least 8 to 10 mm in width to maintain support. If the septoplasty is performed first leaving a dorsal width of 8 to 10 mm, lowering of the dorsal septum if indicated cannot be accomplished without some risk.

Dorsal Surgery

If dorsal reduction is indicated, it is the surgeon's preference whether to reduce the bony or the cartilaginous dorsum first. I usually treat the bony dorsum first using either a rasp or a guarded air-driven drill to reduce and/or smooth the bony dorsum. Before the bony dorsum is lowered to its correct height, some reduction of the cartilaginous dorsum is performed to compare the two to make certain the dorsum is not being overcorrected. The amount of reduction will depend on the final tip projection. Therefore the surgeon must determine what the final tip projection will be before doing the final dorsal reduction.

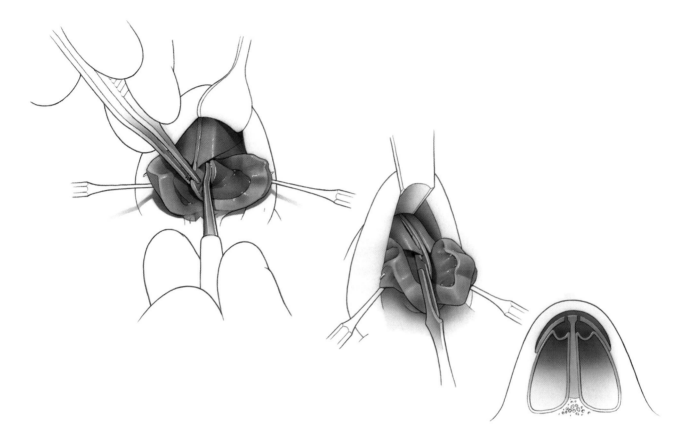

Reduction of the cartilaginous dorsum is begun by elevating the mucosa off both sides of the dorsal septum with a small elevator, leaving submucosal tunnels 5 to 6 mm in depth. This elevation is carried onto the medial under-surface of the upper lateral cartilages. A No. 15 blade is used to separate the upper lateral cartilages from the dorsal septum by incising through their junctions bilaterally. The dorsal septum is then lowered incrementally, checking it periodically to avoid overresection. The upper lateral cartilages are lowered along with the dorsal septum but kept slightly higher because they will lose some of their projection when the skin redrapes over these flaccid cartilages. When the bony dorsum and the dorsal septum are close to the correct height, they are left to be finished after the osteotomies are performed since the nasal bones can lose projection after osteotomies if they are unstable or move posteriorly when infractured. Although some surgeons perform the osteotomies at this point, I defer this to the end of the procedure. Osteotomies are the most traumatic part of the operation, and if done early, they can cause swelling that may hinder intraoperative evaluation.

Septal Surgery

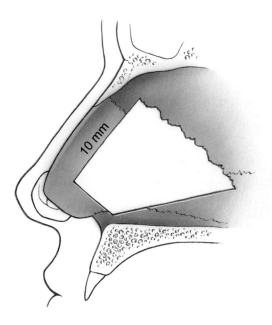

After the dorsum is reduced, any necessary septal surgery is performed to procure cartilage grafts or straighten a deviated septum, making certain that the cartilaginous support of the nose is not lost. This is done by maintaining an intact L-shaped strut of dorsal and caudal septum for support of the lower two thirds of the nose. The width of the L-shaped strut will vary, but 10 mm is a good rule of thumb.

The nasal packing is removed and elevation of the mucoperichondrium started at the caudal septum on the side to which the septum is deviated. If only the septum is to be harvested for grafting, the dissection is started on the side that the surgeon finds easiest. Small, sharp, pointed scissors are used to scratch through the perichondrium until a bluish hue appears through the cartilage, signaling penetration of the perichondrium. The mucosa with its intact perichondrium is then elevated off and around the area to be resected. If the deviation is extensive or a large piece of cartilage is needed for reconstruction, the mucoperichondrium is elevated off the entire septum, maxillary crest, and anterior two thirds of the vomer and perpendicular plate.

The most difficult part of the elevation is in the area of the maxillary crest anteriorly where the mucoperiosteum of the crest fuses with the mucoperichondrium of the septum. The lining in this area is tightly adhered to the osseocartilaginous junction. It is easiest to elevate this area by starting at the septal–maxillary crest junction posteriorly where the mucoperichondrium and mucoperiosteum are less adherent and continue the elevation as far anteriorly as possible.

With the mucoperichondrium now elevated to the septal–maxillary crest osseocartilaginous junction anteriorly, an incision *(A)* is made through cartilage only parallel to the caudal end of the septum, starting inferiorly at the junction of the cartilage with the maxillary crest 10 mm posterior to the caudal margin. It is extended to within 10 mm of the dorsum. An incision *(B)* is made from the anterior end of the caudal incision paralleling the dorsal septum to the junction of the perpendicular plate of the ethmoid, leaving a 10 mm dorsal width. Through these incisions the mucoperichondrium is elevated off the opposite side in the area to be resected. A Mayo or double-action scissors is then used to extend the dorsal incision through the perpendicular plate of the ethmoid. The septal border abutting the maxillary crest posterior to the incision is then elevated off the maxillary crest *(C)*. If the maxillary crest is deviated and resection is indicated, an angled elevator is used to elevate over the ridge down to the floor of the nose to expose the area for resection.

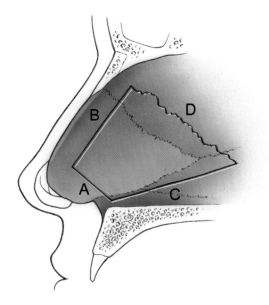

With the incisions made on the caudal and dorsal septum and the inferior septum elevated off the maxillary crest, the area to be resected is freed on three sides. The fourth side *(D)* is freed by using an angular elevator to break through the thin perpendicular plate of the ethmoid from the posterior-superior end of the dorsal incision to the posterior end of the freed inferior septal/vomer border. This completely frees the area to be excised, which is composed of both cartilage and the perpendicular plate of the ethmoid. The perpendicular plate of the ethmoid is excised to make certain as much cartilage as possible has been resected. Since the junction of the cartilage with the perpendicular plate of the ethmoid is irregular, it is difficult to separate the two without leaving some of the cartilage attached to the perpendicular plate. Also pieces of the thin, pliable perpendicular plate can be used as small onlay grafts, and thicker pieces can be burred smooth and drill holes placed to be used as struts to help straighten any curvature of a deviated cartilaginous dorsum or a C-shaped caudal segment.

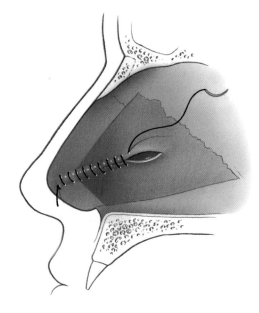

If the mucosa is accidentally perforated during the elevation or resection, it presents no problem if there is no opposing perforation. If there are opposing perforations in any area of the anterior one half of the mucoperichondrium, at least one side needs to be closed. This can be done readily by passing a suture (4-0 or 5-0 chromic suture on a small curved needle) through the muco-perichondrium anteriorly where it is easy to tie, leaving a tag on the free end. A simple running stitch is continued posteriorly to the perforation and closes the perforation, continuing past the posterior end and then running back anteriorly where it is tied to the tag of suture left at the original knot anteriorly.

It is usually impossible to get this large piece of cartilage out of the nose through a transfixion incision, and separation of the upper lateral cartilages from the septum is usually required for removal. Any straight pieces of cartilage or perpendicular plate of the ethmoid that are left after cutting the grafts or any portions of deviated cartilage that can be cut so they are straight should be placed back in the area of resection and stabilized with sutures to avoid overlapping so they can be used if any revisional surgery is necessary.

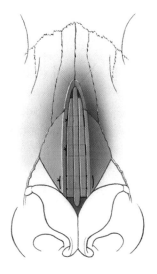

Dorsal spreader grafts, which are used in almost all cases of significant hump removal, especially if short nasal bones are present, to prevent upper lateral cartilage collapse are placed after finishing the septal surgery. In addition to preventing upper lateral cartilage collapse, they may be used to widen the dorsum or straighten a curved dorsal septum. They are placed at the same level as the dorsal septum and can extend up to the osseocartilaginous junction to prevent upper lateral cartilage collapse or extend further superiorly to help control the width of the bony dorsum after osteotomy. If the dorsal septal strut is curved, it can be straightened by making partial-thickness cuts the entire width of the strut perpendicular to the dorsal septum on the concave side. This will make this area of the septum more flaccid so it can be straightened and suture stabilized by using the spreader grafts to "sandwich" the septum between them. Spreader grafts can also be extended caudally past the septal angle to aid in lengthening the nose (see Chapter 30) or to aid in increasing tip projection (see Chapter 11).

Nasal Tip Surgery

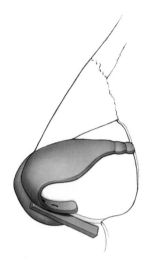

A piece of the septal cartilage is used for a columellar strut in almost all patients undergoing open rhinoplasty. The strut is useful for increasing or maintaining tip projection but mainly to stabilize the medial crura to serve as a foundation for shaping the tip. It also helps to maintain the width of the columella, which can be lost if the medial crura are sutured directly together. The strut is placed in the previously made pocket between the medial crura.

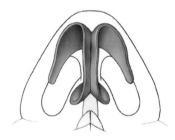

When suturing the strut to the medial crura it should be kept in mind that the normal relationship of the medial crura is that the cephalic edges abut and the caudal edges that give the columella its width are separated.

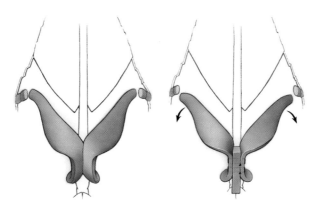

If the medial crura are sutured directly to the columellar strut, they become parallel to each other. The strut will help maintain columellar width, but a downward torque will be placed on the lateral crura. This is especially true the closer the sutures get to the level of the medial walls of the domes. Sometimes the torque is desirable, but if the cartilages are flaccid, very little torque may be produced, of which the surgeon should be aware.

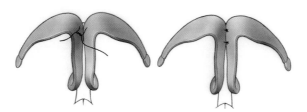

To try to avoid torque, one or two sutures are placed just inside the cephalic margins of the medial wall of the domes at an equal distance from the tip-defining points and tied before placing the columellar strut. This will maintain the abutment of the cephalic margins and counteract the tendency for them to flare when the strut is sutured in place.

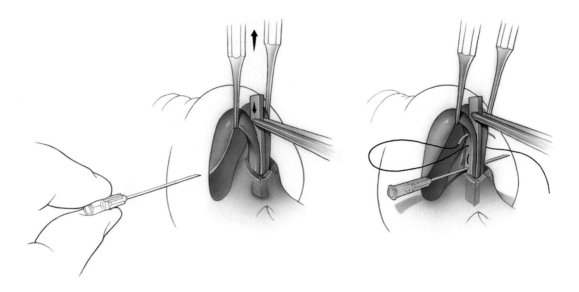

When attempting to increase tip projection with a columellar strut a double-pronged skin hook should be placed in the underneath surface of the domes at the apices of the nostrils and pulled away from the nasal spine. The strut is placed in the undermined pocket between the medial crura and forced toward the spine. A 25-gauge needle is then passed through the medial crura and the strut, which is sandwiched between them to maintain the tension while the strut is sutured in place. This will increase tip projection very little but will stabilize the cartilages so the lateral crura can be advanced medially with horizontal mattress sutures to increase projection of the domes. This method is only capable of providing 2 mm of tip projection at most.

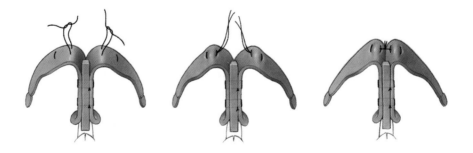

Techniques that will give more tip projection are advancing the medial crura on extended spreader grafts and using tip grafts. I find the most reliable way of increasing tip projection is to use an autologous rib cartilage graft with an internal Kirschner wire extended 10 mm from the base placed in a drill hole in the maxilla (see Chapter 11). However, this method is used almost exclusively in secondary rhinoplasty.

Another reason a columellar strut is used is to control the degree of the columellar-lobular angle. The angle can be increased or decreased by the way it is sutured to the strut. If the medial crura are strong and stiff, it may be necessary to partially incise the crura at the angle before suturing them to the strut, but if they are weak and flaccid, partial incision may not be necessary.

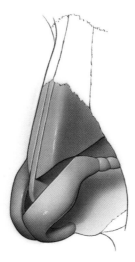

Attention is now directed to the lateral crura. The shape and size will determine if any cartilage needs to be resected. In most cases, especially if a reduction in tip fullness is desired, the scroll area of the cephalic margin will be resected, again keeping as much cartilage as possible without compromising the aesthetic result. In general, lateral crura with minimal bowing oriented so there is no alar retraction are desired. The domes should be angular enough to form subtle tip-defining points with the desired distance between them. How angular and how much distance will depend on the thickness of the skin.

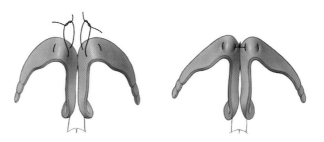

The angulation of the domes and the distance between the tip-defining points can be controlled with transdomal horizontal mattress sutures. If the lateral crura are distorted or malpositioned, they will have to be corrected by methods described in Chapters 23 and 40.

Osteotomies

Before the tip is stabilized completely, any indicated osteotomies are performed so that final trimming of the dorsum can be accomplished. Medial osteotomies are performed only if the bony dorsum is excessively wide, the nasal bones are deviated, or the bony dorsum is excessively narrow and needs to be widened with spreader grafts.

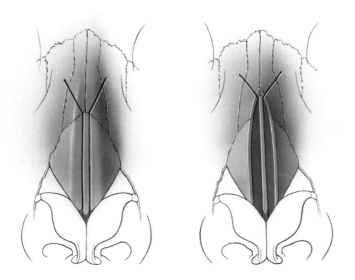

Medial osteotomies are performed with a 7 mm osteotome starting at the inferior junction of the nasal bones with the dorsal septum and angled toward the medial canthus, trying to avoid the thick bone at the root of the nose. The angle of the osteotomies will depend on whether a hump has been removed and, if so, how much. The more hump removed, the closer to the root the osteotomies will begin, which will require a greater angle to stay away from the root. If no hump has been removed, the junction of the inferior edge of the nasal bone with the septum will be further away from the root and will require less angle. The leading edge of the osteotome must be very sharp to get the osteotome started in the right direction. If a hump has been removed and there is an open roof, the inside edge of the nasal bone will curve inward as it is followed superiorly. A dull osteotome has a tendency to follow the inward curve and will end in the thick bone of the root. The further it travels into the root, the thicker the bone is and the more difficult it is to outfracture. Medial osteotomies should end no higher than the level of the medial canthus.

I prefer performing lateral osteotomies internally. Although I do not object to percutaneous osteotomies, they do not give me the control that internal osteotomies do. The osteotomies are performed by making an opening with Iris scissors through the vestibular skin anterior to the end of the inferior turbinate. The scissors are inserted down to the periosteum lateral to the piriform aperture rim and spread just enough to accommodate a curved osteotome with a small guard on the lateral edge. The edge of the piriform aperture is felt with the blade of the osteotome. By pressing the guard against the lateral surface and palpating it with the index finger of the free hand, the blade is "walked" to the desired starting position on the rim. This is usually at the level of the attachment of the anterior end of the inferior turbinate. This is slightly more anterior-superior than the most posterior point of the piriform aperture edge.

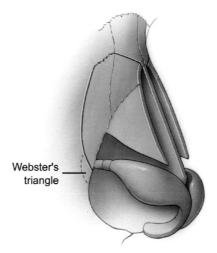

Webster's triangle

Theoretically, if the osteotomy is started low (at the most posterior point of the piriform aperture), infracture could move the anterior end of the inferior turbinate medially and compromise the airway in that area. Starting the osteotomy more superiorly on the rim avoids this but dictates that the osteotome should be angled toward the maxilla at the start to allow the osteotome to get to the nasal cheek junction, where it continues superiorly. As it moves superiorly it curves toward the nasal root. It stops at the level of the medial canthus, where it should be a few millimeters from the lateral end of the medial osteotomy. Gentle digital pressure is applied to create a greenstick infracture. Under ordinary circumstances a greenstick fracture is preferred because a complete fracture is unstable and more difficult to control.

If a medial osteotomy was not performed, the infracture is accomplished by rotating the guard of the osteotome toward the dorsum while gently moving the free end of the osteotome medially. This will result in a greenstick fracture from the superior end of the osteotomy site through the weakest line of the nasal bone. With the osteotomies completed and the tip projection set the bony dorsum, upper lateral cartilages, and septum are refined as indicated to the correct height. The ends of the upper lateral cartilages are sutured back in place to the septum for stabilization. The final tip shape is completed and the skin redraped so that the surgeon can take a final look.

Splints, Closure, and Dressings

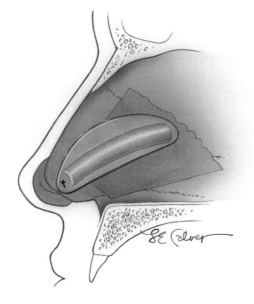

Before closure is begun, a soft plastic splint with an airway on the sides is placed into each nostril. Although the airways may get clogged with blood and mucus, the advantage of this type of splint is that the inferior turbinates press against the splint airways to sandwich the septum between the flat side of the splints, thereby immobilizing the septum in the midline. A 3-0 through-

and-through monofilament suture is placed through the anterior end of the splints and caudal septum to hold them in place; however, this is usually delayed until after closure of the incisions so one last look can be taken before the anterior ends of the splints are brought forward into the vestibule, which causes increased fullness of the alae.

Aligning the crosscuts and suturing the wound with a single layer of 6-0 monofilament nylon suture closes the transcolumellar incision. Magnifying loops may be used for more accurate closure. The marginal incision is closed with 4-0 or 5-0 chromic catgut after aligning the crosscuts. Occasionally a marginal suture may cause some slight notching or distortion of the alar rim. It should always be removed and replaced to avoid a permanent irregularity of the rim. Alar base resections, if indicated, are performed after the closure is complete and before the splints are sutured in place.

The nose and face are cleansed with a wet sponge. Alcohol and a layer of Mastisol are applied to the nasal skin and adjacent cheek skin. Steri-Strips are then taped to the nose to help mold the nose to the best aesthetic shape possible. A padded, sticky aluminum cast is symmetrically bent over a tapered ½- or ¾-inch rod, placed over the nasal bones, and gently squeezed to mold the nasal bones in position. The caudal end of the cast should not reach the supratip area. If it does, squeezing of the cast causes the caudal end to rise, pulling the supratip skin off the framework and creating a dead space in the supratip area. This will fill with blood or serum and can cause an undesirable fullness in that area. Pledgets of Gelfoam impregnated with an antibiotic ointment are placed in each nasal vestibule to pack any redundant vestibular skin back into place. A 1-inch strip of paper tape 2½ inches long is placed on each cheek so the tape of the moustache dressing can be stuck to the cheek tapes instead of the skin. This keeps the skin from becoming irritated and macerated when the moustache dressings are changed.

The nasogastric tube is suctioned and the patient is awakened and taken to the recovery room. The patient is allowed to go home later that day. The patient returns to the office 6 to 7 days later, at which time the splints, cast, and sutures are removed in that order. The patient is routinely seen at 2-week, 4-month, 1-year, and 2-year intervals thereafter.

CASE ANALYSES

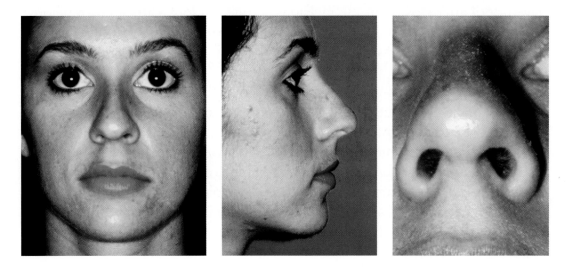

This 22-year-old woman complained of difficulty in breathing through the left side of her nose and desired cosmetic improvement of her nasal appearance. Her main concerns were her "large nose" with a small nasal hump and fullness of the tip. On the frontal view a very narrow nasal dorsum and borderline bony base width were noted. The tip was wide and lacked definition. The alar base width was within normal limits. On the profile view the nasofrontal angle was in good position, but there was increased projection of the tip off the facial plane, resulting in a fullness of the columellar-labial angle and slight tension of the upper lip. The basal view showed increased fullness of the nasal tip. Internally the septum was deviated to the left, partially blocking the airway on that side.

The goals of surgery were to widen the nasal dorsum, narrow and sculpt the nasal tip, remove the nasal hump to develop a straight nasal bridge with a slight supratip break, and set the nose closer to the facial plane, thereby relieving some of the fullness in the columellar-labial angle and tension on the upper lip.

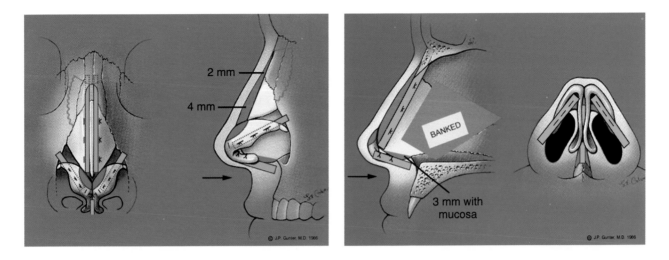

With the patient under general endotracheal anesthesia the nose was injected with 1% lidocaine with 1:100,000 epinephrine and hyaluronidase. The internal nose was packed with gauze soaked with oxymetazoline. Bilateral marginal incisions were connected to a stair-step transcolumellar incision, and the soft tissue was elevated off the osseocartilaginous framework. The nasal bones were lowered approximately 2 mm with a rasp. Bilateral submucosal tunnels were developed at the dorsal septum/upper lateral cartilage junction, and the upper lateral cartilages were separated from the dorsal septum with a No. 15 blade. The cartilaginous septum was lowered approximately 4 mm with angled scissors, and the upper lateral cartilages were trimmed minimally. Medial osteotomies and outfracturing were performed to aid in widening the nasal dorsum.

An extended complete transfixion incision was made to free the attachments of the columella to the caudal septum. The caudal margin of the septum with its mucoperichondrium was removed to reduce the fullness at the columellar-labial angle. The mucoperichondrium was elevated off the left side of the nasal septum. The septal deformity was corrected by partial resection, and the resected cartilage was carved into dorsal spreader grafts that were placed bilaterally and sutured with 5-0 Vicryl to widen the dorsum. A columellar strut was placed in a pocket undermined between the medial crura and sutured with 5-0 Vicryl for stabilization.

The cephalic margins of the lateral crura were trimmed, and the vestibular skin was elevated off the underneath surface of the lateral crura to the attachment at the caudal margins. Strips of septal cartilage (3 × 25 mm) were placed on the underneath surface of the lateral crura and sutured with 5-0 Vicryl to straighten the crura. Transdomal horizontal mattress sutures were placed to narrow the domes and move them closer together. The remaining septal cartilage was placed back in the septal pocket. The incisions were closed with 4-0 chromic catgut sutures and interrupted 6-0 black nylon to the transcolumellar incision. Septal splints that had been placed before closure were sutured with through-and-through 3-0 black nylon, and an external dressing using Steri-Strips and an aluminum cast were placed.

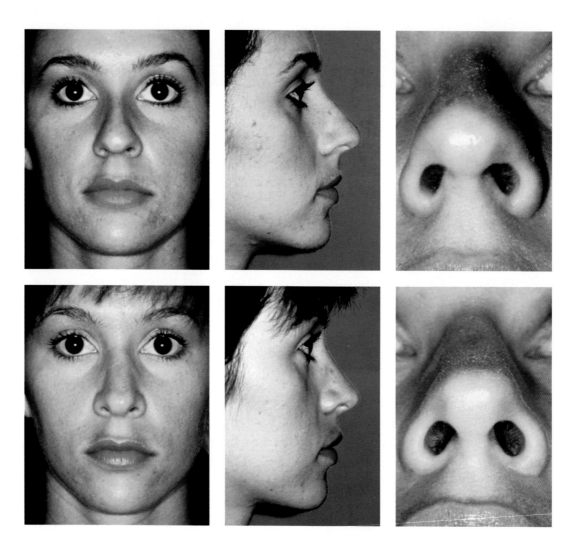

One year postoperatively the patient exhibits widening of the dorsum with more sculpting and decreased width of the nasal tip on the frontal view. On the profile view the nose sets back closer to the facial plane, and the fullness of the columellar-labial angle has been improved. On the basal view the tip is more symmetric, although the distance between the tip-defining points could be narrower.

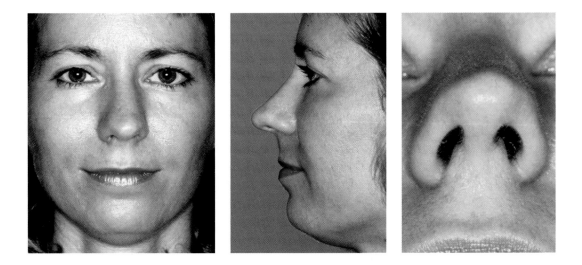

This 38-year-old woman had nasal airway obstruction, greater on the right than the left. Her allergist had her on a regimen of prednisone and steroid nasal sprays. In addition to improved breathing, she requested cosmetic improvement of her nose. On the frontal view the tip and dorsum leaned to the left. The bony base appeared wide, as did the supratip area. Alar base width was borderline. On the lateral view the nasofrontal angle was in good position with a straight dorsum and a slight supratip break but with increased projection of the nasal tip. There was very little nostril show on the profile view with increased fullness of the columellar-labial angle. The chin appeared weak in the anterior as well as the vertical direction. The basal view revealed a wide nasal tip that leaned to the left with some asymmetry of the nostrils. The internal examination demonstrated mild hypertrophy of the turbinates with deviation of the septum that was causing significant airway obstruction.

The surgical goals were to straighten the dorsum and tip, narrow the bony base, and decrease tip projection. In addition, the tip needed to be reshaped. Improvement of the nasal airway was a major goal. A mentoplasty would be performed to advance the chin and increase the vertical height.

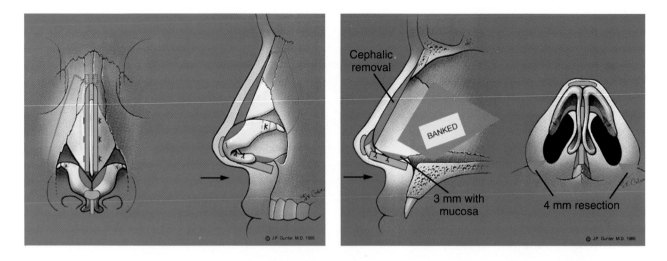

The patient's face was prepped and draped in a sterile manner after administration of a general endotracheal anesthetic. A mentoplasty was performed prior to the rhinoplasty. An extended arm Silastic implant that overlapped the inferior mandibular border was used. The nose was injected with 1% lidocaine with 1:100,000 epinephrine and hyaluronidase. The internal nose was packed with gauze soaked with oxymetazoline. An extended complete transfixion incision was made to release supporting elements of the caudal septum to the tip to aid in decreasing tip projection. Bilateral marginal incisions were connected to a stair-step transcolumellar incision and the soft tissue elevated off the osseocartilaginous framework.

The dorsum was rasped, submucosal tunnels were made, and the upper lateral cartilages were separated from the septum. The septum and upper lateral cartilages were lowered with angled scissors. The mucoperichondrium was elevated off the left side of the nasal septum, and the nasal septum deformity was corrected by partial resection and a swinging door–type flap. Part of the resected septal cartilage was used for spreader grafts, which were placed along the sides of the dorsal septum and sutured with 5-0 Vicryl to help straighten the dorsal septum. Lateral osteotomies were performed to shift the nasal bones to the midline. The upper lateral cartilages were sutured to the spreader grafts and septum at the septal angle for stabilization.

The cephalic margins of the lateral crura were trimmed. Laterally, the vestibular skin was undermined off the underneath surface of the lateral crura near their junction with the accessory cartilages. The cartilages were transected in this area, overlapped 3 mm, and sutured with through-and-through 5-0 Vicryl to reduce projection of the lateral crura. Part of the caudal septum along with the mucosa was removed to decrease fullness in the nasolabial angle. A columellar strut was placed between the medial crura and sutured with 5-0 Vicryl to help stabilize the tip. Transdomal horizontal mattress sutures of 5-0 clear nylon were placed in the dome areas bilaterally to increase the angulation of the domes and move them closer together. A resected cephalic margin from one of the lateral crura was used as an onlay graft over the domes to soften the angulation of the domes.

The internal incisions were closed with 4-0 chromic catgut sutures, and the transcolumellar incision with interrupted 6-0 black nylon. At this point it was evident that decreased tip projection had caused flaring of the nasal alae, and bilateral alar base resections were performed, resecting approximately 4 mm of skin at the widest portion. These wounds were sutured with 6-0 nylon sutures. Septal splints that had been placed before closure were sutured with through-and-through 3-0 black nylon. An external dressing using Steri-Strips and an aluminum cast were placed.

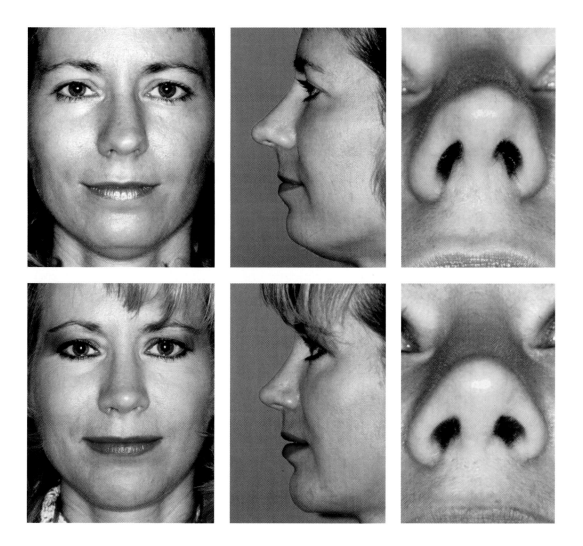

One year postoperatively the frontal view shows the dorsum and tip in the midline. The fullness and asymmetry of the tip and supratip areas have been corrected, and there is good width of the alar bases. On the profile view there is a slightly concave dorsum with decreased tip projection and a small supratip break. The basal view shows a triangular tip with improved nostril symmetry. The mentoplasty improved the nasal/jaw relationship.

63

Sheen's Approach*

Jack H. Sheen, M.D.

*O*ver the past 35 years aesthetic rhinoplasty has evolved from a generic, reductive operation to a highly individualized, problem-specific operation that often combines augmentation with reduction. My experience has been marked by the following conceptual and technical milestones that have contributed to an ongoing exploration and advancement of nasal surgery: (1) vestibular stenosis: diagnosis of a surgical consequence; (2) etiology and treatment of supratip deformity: the dynamic relationship of soft tissue contour to skeleton; (3) etiology and treatment of the tip with inadequate projection: tip graft design; (4) practical aesthetics of balance: the augmentation-reduction approach to rhinoplasty; (5) support of the middle vault: functional and aesthetic effects; (6) malposition of the lateral crura: recognition and management; and (7) the significance of the middle crura: clinical and aesthetic considerations. This chapter recounts my experience with rhinoplasty over the past 30 years and traces my personal evolution in rhinoplasty by defining significant milestones along the way.

My rhinoplasty odyssey began in 1972 when I nervously presented my first paper on secondary rhinoplasty. I was already brazen and unconventional in my approach to nasal surgery. Soon after, Tom Baker, who has been in the audience, courageously offered me, unknown and unproven, a place on the Baker-Gordon symposium faculty in 1973, giving me a forum in which I could demonstrate surgery and express my ideas. Also on that faculty were my formidable colleagues, Tord Skoog and Fernando Ortiz-Monasterio. With lasting gratitude to Tom Baker and Howard Gordon, I considered myself launched.

*Reprinted with minor modifications from Sheen JH. Rhinoplasty: Personal evolution and milestones. Plast Reconstr Surg 105:1820, 2000.

VESTIBULAR STENOSIS: DIAGNOSIS OF A SURGICAL CONSEQUENCE

By the mid-1970s I was examining hundreds of secondary rhinoplasty patients each year. I observed that an estimated 80% had some loss of vestibular volume with mild to severe impairment of the nasal airway.[1] Clearly, something was wrong with our surgical technique. I might add that something also was wrong with our postoperative follow-up. When I shared my observation with colleagues, most shrugged, saying they never saw it. The fact is that it was not expected practice to look. It surprised me at the time that many plastic surgeons did not critically examine the inside of the nose postoperatively; many did not even have adequate light and a nasal speculum in their examination room.

When analyzing the problem I focused on what was then a routine step in rhinoplasty: trimming the caudal edge of the upper lateral cartilage with right-angle scissors.[2-8]

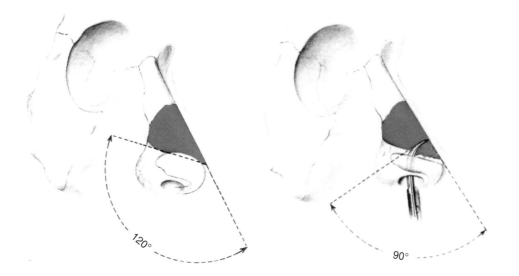

The caudal edge of the upper lateral cartilage is approximately 120 degrees from the dorsal plane *(A)*. Because the upper lateral cartilage is triangular, a straight cut along the caudal end results in a mucosal deficit, inevitably leading to scarring and stenosis *(B)*.[9]

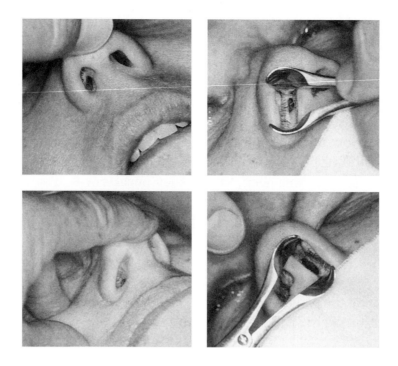

Note the severe vestibular stenosis resulting in airway impairment following routine aesthetic rhinoplasty.

The changes that resulted were, first, discarding the right-angle scissors and, second, performing a submucous dissection of the cartilage, which preserved mucosa except for the rare case in which exceedingly redundant mucosa is conservatively trimmed. This left an intact mucosa, functioning internal valves, and a normal airway. Today less than 15% of secondary rhinoplasty patients I see have any loss of vestibular volume; of those, only a few have severe vestibular stenosis.

ETIOLOGY AND TREATMENT OF SUPRATIP DEFORMITY: THE DYNAMIC RELATIONSHIP OF SOFT TISSUE CONTOUR TO SKELETON

Thirty years ago supratip deformity was commonly seen in rhinoplasty patients. The prevailing opinion was that supratip deformity was most often caused by inadequate resection of the dorsum, overlapping lateral walls, or excess scar formation.[10-14] The prevailing treatments were further dorsal reduction, "thinning" dissections, and steroid injections. The prevailing outcomes were recurrent supratip deformities and multiple procedures, many resulting in increased scarring and at times irreparable defects.

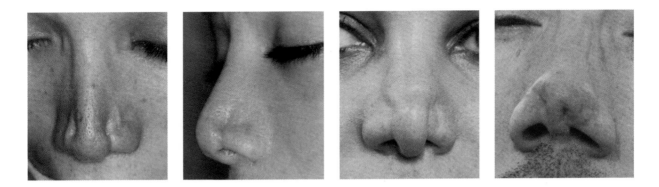

These patients had undergone tissue thinning procedures in attempts to reduce the arch of skin over the lower third of the nose.

The only thought about prevention, as suggested by Safian[15] and Deneke and Meyer,[16] was to undercut the anterior septum to allow room for granulation tissue. But I had a contrary idea about supratip deformity. I had observed that the soft tissue often could be compressed down to the septal edge.

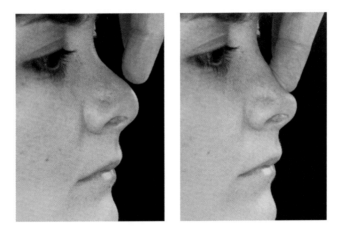

Pressing the supratip down to the anterior septum made it apparent that the supratip deformity was related to the limits of soft tissue contractility, not the height of the skeleton. No amount of lowering that septum would reduce the arch of skin overlying it. The skin had simply reached its limit of contractility. Sometimes fibrous tissue would fill in the space, making the area feel firm but never providing enough structure for a straight contour. Realizing that a soft structure needs a supportive framework to maintain shape, I hypothesized that augmentation, not reduction, was the answer.

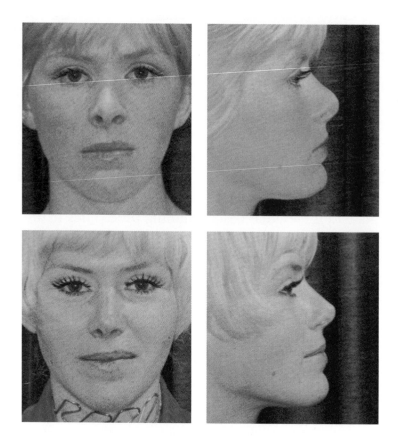

This case, presented at the 1973 Baker-Gordon Symposium, demonstrates the correction of a supratip deformity by augmentation of the dorsum and tip grafting.

In 1973 and 1974 a secondary rhinoplasty patient with a supratip deformity and a lot of time and resources was flying across the country and around the world to consult with plastic surgeons about her nose. It was Fernando Ortiz-Monasterio who recommended that she come to me for her secondary rhinoplasty. Meanwhile, Ralph Millard had heard of my unorthodox concept of supratip deformity and in 1975 invited me to his symposium in Miami to prove myself in front of an audience of 500 and a faculty of experts, including himself, Gustav Aufricht, Reid Dingman, Paul Natvig, John Lewis, and Blair Rogers. Because I knew that this patient had consulted with every surgeon on the faculty and that she was willing to have the procedure performed during the symposium, I could not possibly refuse. At surgery I showed that the anterior septum at the area of the supratip had already been lowered about 4 mm, as recommended by Dr. Safian.[17,18] I then augmented the dorsum, producing a fine, straight dorsal edge, permanently eliminating the supratip convexity.

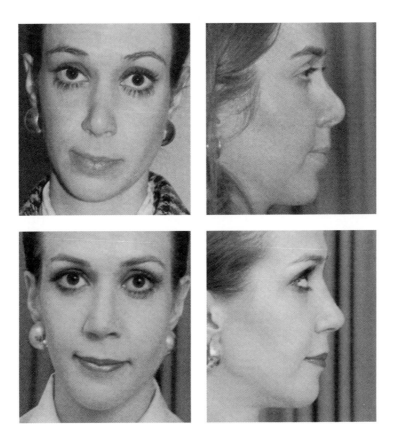

This patient, operated on at the Millard Symposium, demonstrates the effectiveness of augmentation for supratip deformity.

In 1975 I formally presented my clinical material on supratip deformity, which included a report of 100 consecutive secondary rhinoplasty patients, representing a major change in the approach to secondary rhinoplasty. Eighty-two percent of the noses were corrected by dorsal augmentation.[19]

Besides the diagnosis and treatment of supratip deformity, the other aspect of this milestone is prevention. Understanding that the size of the skeletal framework must be proportionate to the size (and character) of the overlying soft tissue, the surgeon can prevent supratip deformity by retaining adequate dorsal support.

ETIOLOGY AND TREATMENT OF THE TIP WITH INADEQUATE PROJECTION: TIP GRAFT DESIGN

A question that was frequently asked in my early days was, "Do you do the tip first or the dorsum first?" It just so happened that I usually set the height of the dorsum first, allowing for final adjustments. The reason was based on my insight into supratip deformity. I realized that the height of the dorsum must be limited by the size and character of the skin sleeve; it could be reduced only so much without deforming. After determining the limit of reduction I was faced with the challenge of achieving adequate tip projection relative to the appropriate dorsal height. I was then using only conventional tip techniques: cephalic trimming of the alar cartilage and scoring at the dome to maximize projection. For most noses this technique was successful, but not for all. I observed that there was a characteristic group of noses in which the alar cartilages were inherently inadequate to project the tip beyond an appropriate dorsal line. Predictably, these noses would have poor postoperative contours (including supratip deformity from attempts to lower the dorsum to the level of the tip). I named this problem "The Tip With Inadequate Projection" and began plotting a solution.

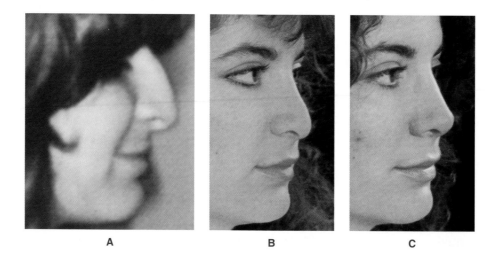

A   B   C

This patient exhibits a tip with inadequate projection *(A)*. Conservative dorsal reduction produced a supratip deformity *(B)*. Note that the tip projection remained unchanged after primary surgery. The result is shown 7 years following placement of a dorsal graft and tip graft *(C)*.

Soon came the realization that aesthetically the tip lobule itself—the area between the columellar-lobular junction and end point of the tip—was lacking in structure. The next logical step was to devise a way to support just that area. Various grafts to fill out the tip such as a small button, a tent pole, and a fleur-de-lis graft had been suggested by Millard, Gorney, Falces, and others.

As far back as 1946 Maliniac suggested small grafts of septal or conchal cartilage to fill out the tip of the cleft lip-nose.[20-22] None of these designs could provide the necessary projection to correct the tip with inadequate projection or the scarred, postsurgical nose.

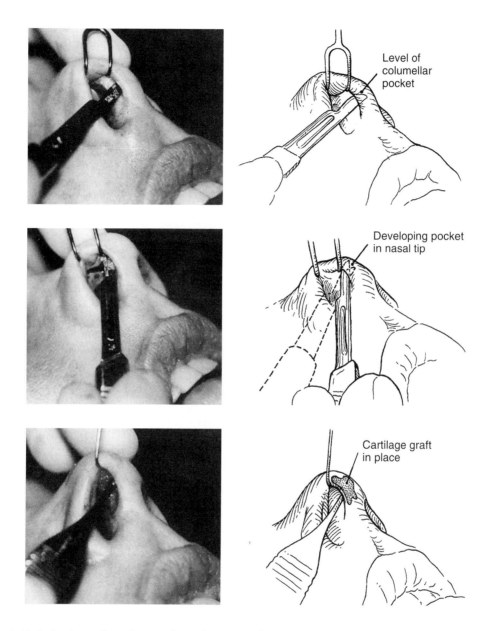

In 1968 I designed a tip graft technique that, except for the shape and number of grafts, remains unchanged.[23] An opening incision is made at the columellar-lobular junction and a pocket is developed, based at the columellar-lobular junction and extending anteriorly into the tip lobule. Using the columellar-lobular junction as a base, the graft(s) is placed under just enough tension to extend the tip to the desired position. The original graft had the configuration of a cross section of a molar; some saw it as a shield. The width of the top varied, depending on the thickness of the soft tissue. With thick tissues the graft was made narrow to improve the mechanical advantage. With thin skin the top was wider. I was now using this technique not only for deficient primary tips but also in secondary cases in which the alar cartilages had been overly resected. The use of tip grafts greatly enhanced the results in a wide variety of cases. At first the patients and I were "all smiles."

Soon there were problems. Some of the grafts became visible as the edges blanched the overlying skin. Others slipped upward or sideward, creating asymmetries and unsightly contours. To correct these mishaps, additional grafts were placed to obtain good contour and symmetry. To prevent them, I then changed my tip augmentation technique to use multiple grafts as a routine.

By the mid-1970s I had added ear cartilage to the tip graft materials (under the influence of Burt Brent) and was beginning to use crushed cartilage with excellent results. The first remarkable case using crushed cartilage involved a scarred, postsurgical nose with multiple grooves in the tip lobule. Clearly, the usual tip graft would not have corrected this problem. What I wanted was not so much to project the tip lobule but to expand it. So I crushed nine pieces of cartilage and carefully stuffed them into the tip.

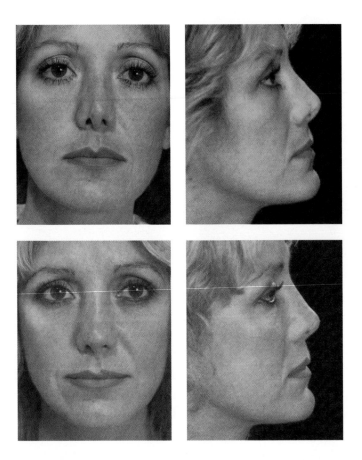

The patient is shown 4 years postoperatively.

With the success of this case crushed cartilage emerged as an extremely useful and versatile graft material. Noses with thin skin, asymmetries, visible single grafts, and flat lobules can be improved with the use of crushed cartilage grafts. With thousands of tip grafts time has proved that they are effective and they last over the long term.

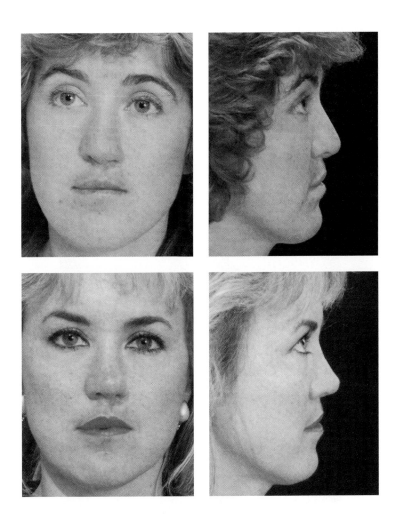

The long-term effectiveness of these grafts is exhibited in this 10-year follow-up photograph of a secondary cleft lip-nose.

The tip grafts I use today are made of septal, ear, or rib cartilage.[24] They are used either unmodified, bruised, crushed, or morselized, often in combination. A combination of solid grafts for support and projection and soft grafts for fill and contour is a versatile and effective solution to a variety of tip deficits. A buttress graft of ethmoid bone is sometimes used to stabilize the position of loose grafts within the pocket. Recently I have been using tangential sections of the ninth rib—solid, crushed, or morselized. Early results are good, but the verdict is still out.

PRACTICAL AESTHETICS OF BALANCE: THE AUGMENTATION-REDUCTION APPROACH TO RHINOPLASTY

As a milestone this is my favorite. Over time I embraced the observation that *high and low and large and small manifest each other*. Raising the root of the nose diminishes the apparent projection of the base; projecting the base diminishes the apparent height of the dorsum. Narrowing the upper vault of the nose accentuates the width of the base, and vice versa. For me, this observation represents a major conceptual shift and marks the point of departure from the standard Joseph rhinoplasty as a sequence of reductive surgical steps.

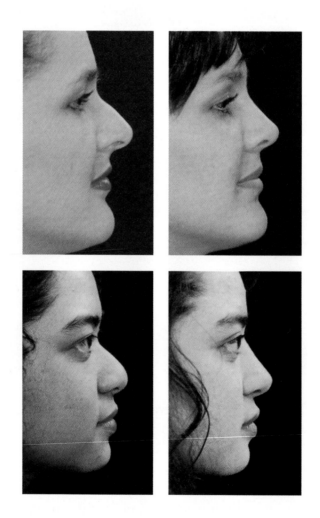

These patients can be characterized as having a low radix disproportion. They have a low root and a large nasal base, producing a "bottom heavy" nose. Minimizing the base by augmenting the root illustrates the concept of balance in rhinoplasty.

To the clinician the exciting part of this concept is the potential for practical application. If changing the nasal configuration is analyzed and planned as a matter of balance rather than reduction, then the surgeon can manipulate anatomic components to achieve aesthetic effects that otherwise would be unobtainable given the inherent limitations of an individual's tissues. Equally important is the ability to create the illusion of reduction while preserving skeletal support.[25]

Seen from this point of view, an apparent hump may be only a relative hump and therefore can be eliminated by elevating the adjacent tissue. The questions may arise, "When is a hump not a hump?" or "How do you know when a hump is a hump?" My answer is: A hump is a hump only when the rest of the nose can spare it.

Case Analysis

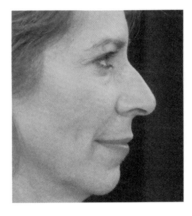

A 39-year-old woman, 5 feet 10 inches tall, had findings that may be summarized as follows:
- Low radix disproportion
- Bony arch to nasal base disproportion
- Ultraprojecting base
- Nostril-lobule disproportion
- Long nose with drooping nasal tip
- Flaring nostrils

This was a large nose on the large face of a tall patient. The patient, who wanted a smaller, more retroussé nose, was advised about tissue limitations and about the danger of sacrificing contour for size. In my experience, given the particular base-heavy structure of her nose, a conventional reductive rhinoplasty would likely result in an unattractive, surgical-appearing nose. It was explained that the nose could be made to appear more refined by improving the angles and proportions.

Twenty-five years ago I would have used the root as a point of reference in reducing this sizable hump. But 25 years ago I had not yet seen literally thousands of supratip deformities that resulted from this misjudgment. This patient had a low radix disproportion[26]; that is, the root was low relative to the base. If the dorsum were lowered to a plane in line with the radix, the dorsal skin would not be supported and a supratip deformity would likely result.

The alternative of raising the radix has three positive effects: (1) minimizing the dorsal convexity, (2) preserving skeletal structure, and (3) diminishing the apparent size of the base. In this case the nasal base itself posed challenges. The alar base was relatively wide, the nasal tip was ultraprojecting, and the nostrils were disproportionately long relative to the tip lobule. The nostril-lobule disproportion had to be addressed.[27] My plan was to increase lobular size by tip grafts and decrease the nostril size by alar resection. Projection of the nasal base would be countered by root augmentation.

The frontal contour was also a problem of balance. The bony arch was narrow, which contraindicated osteotomy and suggested augmentation to diminish the relative width of the base. Spreader grafts provide continuity of the middle vault and ensure function of the internal valves. Conservative reduction of the flaring nostrils, including lobular and vestibular sides, and preserving a medial flap for a smooth sill[28] would narrow the alar base without compromise to contour or function. Nostrils can be reduced only so much without distortion. Therefore augmentation of the upper vaults is of great benefit because it minimizes the amount of alar resection required to adequately narrow the base.

The surgical plan was as follows:
- Transfixion incision of the columella, anterior third only
- Wide skeletonization
- Rasping of the radix to prepare for graft
- Trimming of dorsum
- Development of spreader graft pockets
- Septal submucous resection to harvest graft material
- Placement of bruised cartilage grafts at the root
- Placement of spreader grafts
- Trimming of caudal edges of upper lateral cartilages
- Augmentation of lateral bony arch, bilateral
- Alar resection, lobular and vestibular excision
- Placement of tip graft

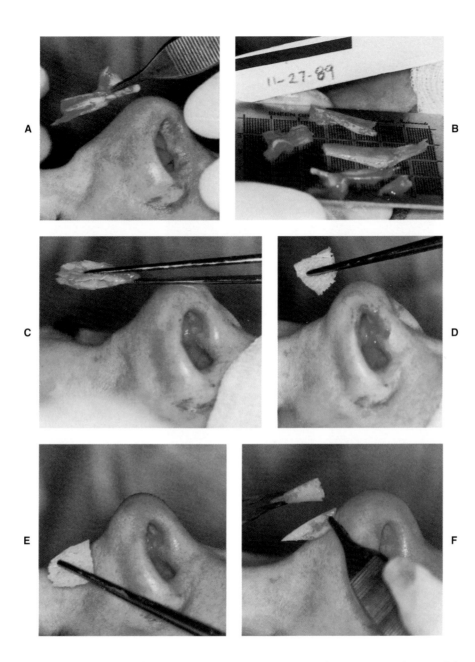

The anterior segment of the middle vault is resected *(A)*. Note the visible septal T, which effectively supports the lateral walls and spreads the apices of the internal valves *(B)*. The specimens obtained from the septum to correct airway obstruction and for use as grafts are demonstrated *(C)*. The root graft consists of segments of bruised or morselized septal cartilage layered and sutured together. Crushed cartilage grafts to be placed over each lateral wall of the bony arch are shown along with the spreader grafts before placement *(D to F)*.

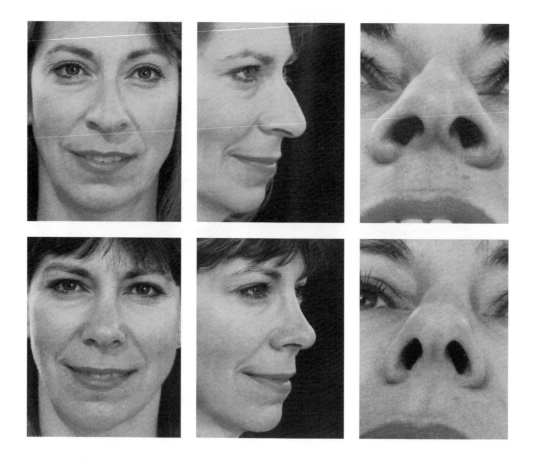

This patient, shown 14 months after surgery, exemplifies the concept of augmentation-reduction to achieve a balanced nose. She now has a balanced, retroussé nose. Increased width of the bony arch and a narrower base have improved balance. Elevation of the root diminishes the apparent size of the base. The basal view shows a narrower base in addition to a smooth sill, the result of preservation of a medial flap with the alar resection. The nose is not small, but it is correct in contour and function. A large nose, especially one with a projecting base, can be a trap. The soft tissue will not contract down to an overly reduced skeleton without sacrificing contour. With an understanding of this very real limitation, every surgeon performing rhinoplasty should be inspired by the possibilities presented by selective augmentation.

SUPPORT OF THE MIDDLE VAULT: FUNCTIONAL AND AESTHETIC EFFECTS

With the exception of Tord Skoog, who replaced the dorsal roof following reduction of the anterior septum,[29] no one in the early days of rhinoplasty attached much importance to the integrity of the middle vault. Lowering the dorsum was just another routine step in a reductive operation. In the 1950s and 1960s surgeons actually tried to produce "scooped" noses. Lipsett took pride in creating a dorsum that was "razor thin." Postsurgical noses of that era were characteristically caved in on the sides and functionally compromised.

Like everyone else, I was taught to routinely perform an osteotomy and to resect the dorsum, thinking only of reduction. Narrower, smaller, lower, shorter: those were our goals. But even as I was dutifully narrowing my patients' noses I began to observe three recurring postoperative problems: (1) narrowing of the internal valves with impaired airways; (2) visible fall-in of the middle vault, seen on the oblique view; and (3) inverted V deformity, a visible demarcation between the middle and bony vaults, apparent on the frontal view. As increasing numbers of secondary rhinoplasty patients streamed through my examining room, this observation became crystallized. I realized that our surgery was causing a discontinuity between the middle and bony vaults. I guessed, wrongly, that the upper lateral cartilages might separate from their bony attachment during rasping, thus causing them to fall in. But this idea was dispelled in the anatomy laboratory, where I discovered that a horse trainer would have difficulty pulling the cartilages away from the nasal bones. It wasn't until I met one particular primary rhinoplasty patient that the etiology and treatment of middle vault impairment began to emerge.

Short Nasal Bones

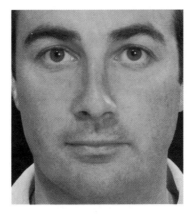

A male patient with no history of prior surgery requested that I improve his airway without changing the nasal contour. When I examined him with a nasal speculum, the septum was obviously straight and the airways were wide open. "I can't see anything wrong with the inside of your nose," I said. He gave me a quizzical look and inhaled deeply. "Well I still can't breathe," he insisted. I looked again. "Yes, now I can breathe," he said, his breath fogging the speculum. "But when you take that instrument out, I can't." Then, when examining him without the speculum, I saw that on inspiration, the internal valves collapsed against the septum. Thinking about normal anatomy, I placed a cotton applicator at the apex of the internal valve and asked the patient to breathe. With the applicator in place, he breathed well.

Now I was faced with two questions: Why were the internal valves collapsing and what could be done about it? A careful look showed a nose that was long and narrow with practically no bony arch. On palpation the nasal bones were found to be less than a centimeter long. It was clear then that the middle vault was lacking the support usually provided by a substantial bony arch. Thus began my campaign of measuring every bony arch I saw. I concluded that most nasal bones extend about half the distance between the radix and the angle of the septum. Twenty-five percent of that distance I considered to be short. I then realized the clinical significance of the length of nasal bones for rhinoplasty patients and reported my findings in 1976 at the meeting of the American Society of Plastic and Reconstructive Surgeons in Boston.[30]

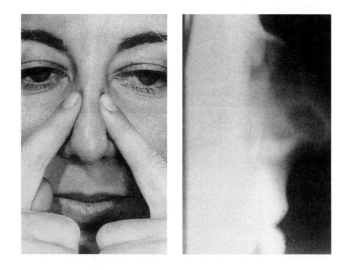

Diagnosis of short nasal bones often can be made by visual examination. Palpation verifies the boundary of the caudal bony arch. An x-ray film shows the nasal bones to be about 1 cm long.

Significantly, in the nose with short nasal bones the middle vault is not held laterally by the support of the bony arch. Medially, the primary support to the internal valves is the broad anterior edge of the septum, or the top of the septal T. When the anterior septum is resected to lower the dorsum, the walls will fall medially and airway impairment and an inverted V deformity may result. In patients with short nasal bones osteotomy is contraindicated, and something must be done to expand the internal valves.

Spreader Grafts

Returning to my milestone patient with short nasal bones, I must say that at the time I was just fishing for ideas. With the cotton applicator came the answer: A sticklike graft placed along the anterior edge of the septum would spread the apex of the internal valve (just like the applicator), moving the medial portions of the lateral walls outward. This would widen and support the patient's long middle vault and improve his airway. The graft was named for its function: spreader graft.[31-33] The technique I used for this patient remains unchanged except for the sequence. The initial incision extends through the perichondrium. The narrow pocket is developed with a Cottle perichondrial elevator, flat side against the septum, maintaining a mucosal attachment at the anterior septum. In the past I made the pockets and then reduced the dorsum. Today I reduce the dorsum and then make the pockets to ensure an anterior mucosal attachment, which prevents slippage of the graft.

With the success of spreader grafts for this patient the technique was soon extended for use in the postsurgical nose (without a dorsal graft), asymmetries of the dorsum, and selected primary patients.

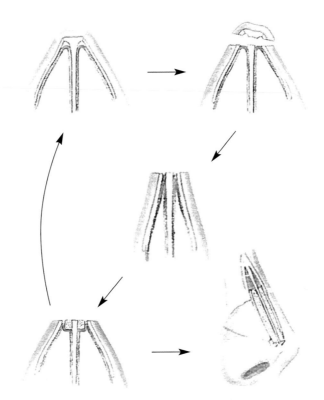

Spreader grafts replace the broad, anterior portion of the septal T that is removed with any significant dorsal hump. Therefore these grafts prevent the functional and visible sequelae of middle vault fall-in as well as restore middle vault support in the postoperative patient or in patients with short nasal bones.

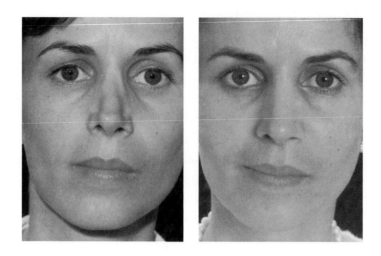

Inverted V deformity is frequently seen in patients with short nasal bones. This patient with an appropriate dorsal height is shown before and after spreader graft placement. Had she needed dorsal augmentation, spreader grafts would not have been necessary because the width of the dorsal graft would provide the necessary support.

MALPOSITION OF THE LATERAL CRURA: RECOGNITION AND MANAGEMENT

Malposition is not the best term for this anatomic feature, but I have used it since the early 1970s, so it is too late to take it back. I now realize that what I observed as a malposition of the lateral crura is not an abnormal position of the cartilage, but a somewhat common variation of normal anatomy. I had learned that the normal, expected position of the alar cartilage almost parallels the alar rim. Gray's *Anatomy of the Human Body* describes the cartilage as diverging from the alar rim at about 15 degrees.[34] So when I observed alar cartilages at a 60-degree cephalic slant, it seemed to me that they were malpositioned.[35,36]

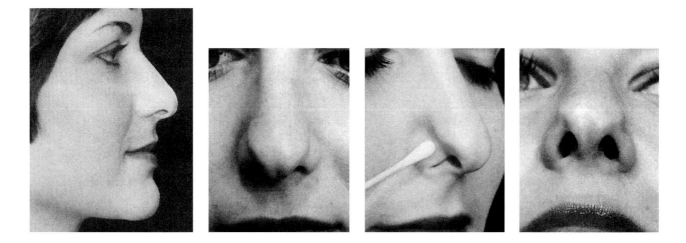

The first patient who brought my attention to the position of the alar cartilages demonstrated a dramatic picture of malposition. On the frontal view the nasal tip was ball-like and bordered by parentheses. The cephalic orientation of the latera crura was clearly visible with the characteristic parentheses, which mark the margins of the alar cartilages. Pressure on the alar rim revealed a sharp outline of the position of the lateral crus. On the basal view there was notching in the alar rims where the cartilages angled cephalad. The poorly supported alae and the square perimeter of the base are characteristic. However, the cartilages can be either broad or narrow at the tip.

I realized that the standard approach to trimming the cartilages would not be effective and might cause distortion. I then decided to dissect out the alar cartilages and rotate them downward to provide substance and support to the rims.

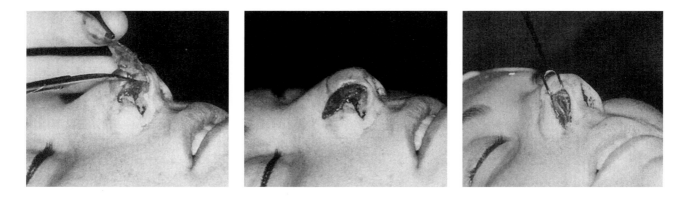

The lateral crus is dissected from the vestibular skin. The completely dissected lateral crus is demonstrated. Note the repositioned crus in the newly formed pocket, parallel to the alar rim.

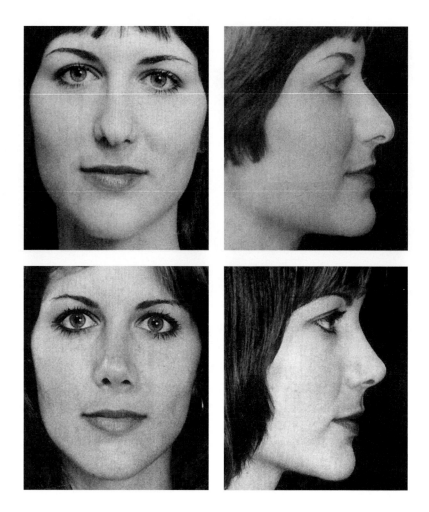

The patient is shown 14 months after surgery with good support to the alar rims, thereby eliminating the tip parentheses, and improved tip projection.

After this I began to find malposition of the alar cartilages in a variety of forms and degrees. However, the characteristic findings were consistent: lack of alar rim support and some degree of visible parentheses, which manifest the caudal edges of the cephalically positioned lateral crura. "Malpositions" were everywhere. This recognition became important as the clinical relevance and application became increasingly apparent. If a significant malposition is unrecognized preoperatively, the standard cephalic trim of the alar cartilage may result in postoperative distortions. For example, the usually safe intra-cartilaginous incision is made parallel to the alar rim, but if the cartilages are cephalically rotated, this technique may result in transection of the cartilages, often creating visible stumps or knuckles postoperatively. Secondary rhino-plasty patients with undiagnosed or untreated malpositions share identifiable defects; most notable are tip deformities and notching of the alar rims.

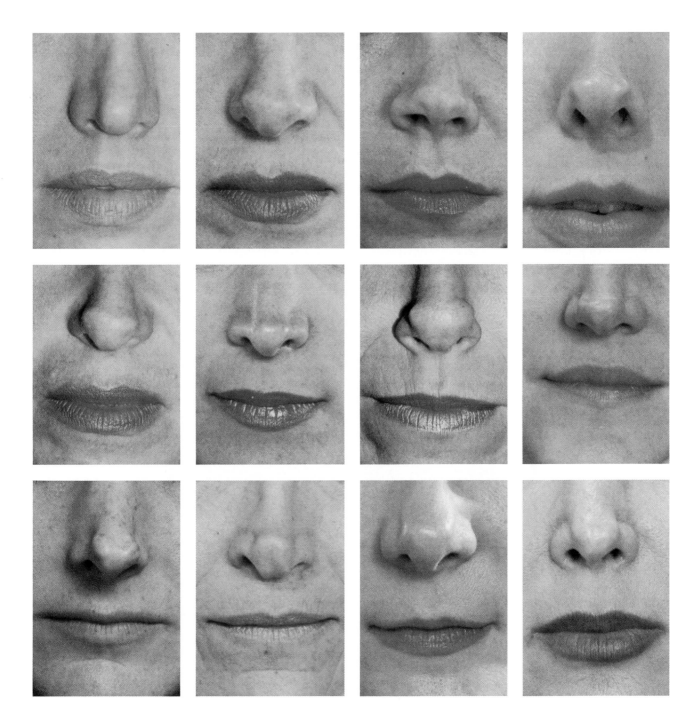

These patients all had undiagnosed malposition treated by standard tip refining techniques that resulted in tip distortions. Note that all have notched alar rims and visible stumps of the remaining lateral crura.

Now that malposition had made itself known, what was to be done? Obviously diagnosis was paramount. At first my treatment was straightforward: repositioning of the lateral crura. With experience I abandoned that technique because of the occurrence of some distortion at the apex of the nostril.

Then I experimented with the more radical technique of total resection of the lateral crura, then replacing them as free grafts along the alar rims. A third option is to leave them alone.

Whether to leave the cartilages alone depends more on the patient's desires than on any other factor. I always ask, "What do you think of your nose on the frontal view?" If the patient does not specifically mention the round tip, I then ask, "What about these grooves here, do they bother you at all?" If the patient says no, then I will plan a conservative approach—a tip graft to project and define the tip and alar rim grafts for support. The improvement is good, but subtle. For many patients this conservative result is quite satisfactory, and for the surgeon who may not be comfortable with resecting the cartilages and reconstructing the base, this is certainly the safest technique.

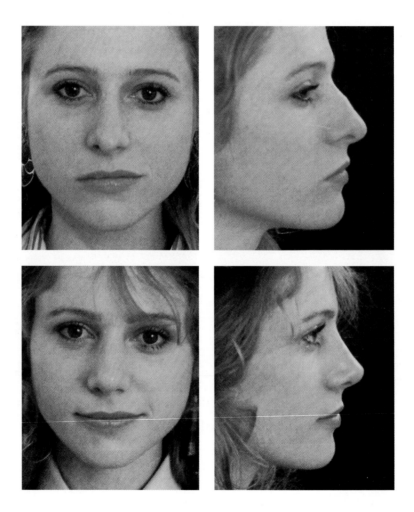

This patient had malposition of the crura, which was treated by leaving the alar cartilages untouched. A tip graft was placed, and the alar rims were supported by grafted strips of cartilage. The patient also had a root graft, spreader grafts, and a slight reduction of the dorsum.

Resection of the cartilages and replacing them in the alar rims are technically challenging. The dissection from the vestibular side is difficult. However, with experience the dissection becomes easier, faster, and less traumatic. The grafts are effectively fixed in position by 5-0 plain sutures. I do not recommend this technique to the occasional nasal surgeon. Placing fragile strips of alar cartilage in meticulously made pockets requires a familiar and respectful touch. But for me, this has been the most successful technique to support the alar rims in cases of malposition.

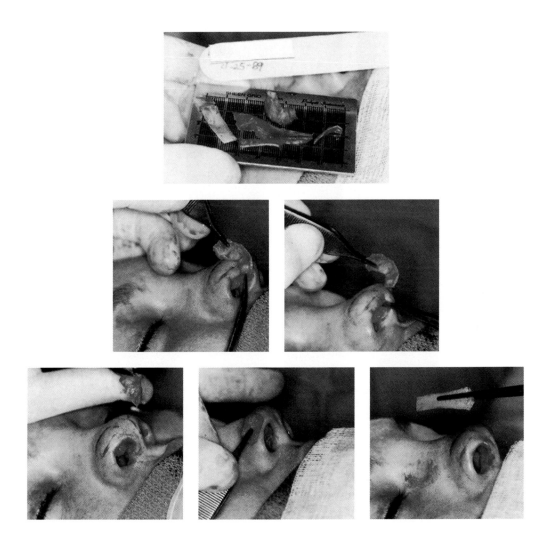

The surgical steps to correct malposition are shown. The specimen from the rhinoplasty is shown. Note the degree of bony deformity. The right lateral crus is dissected out to the medial genu. The lateral crura are completely removed and the trimmed lateral crus positioned for suturing in the alar rim. The dorsal graft of the septal cartilage is shown prior to placement.

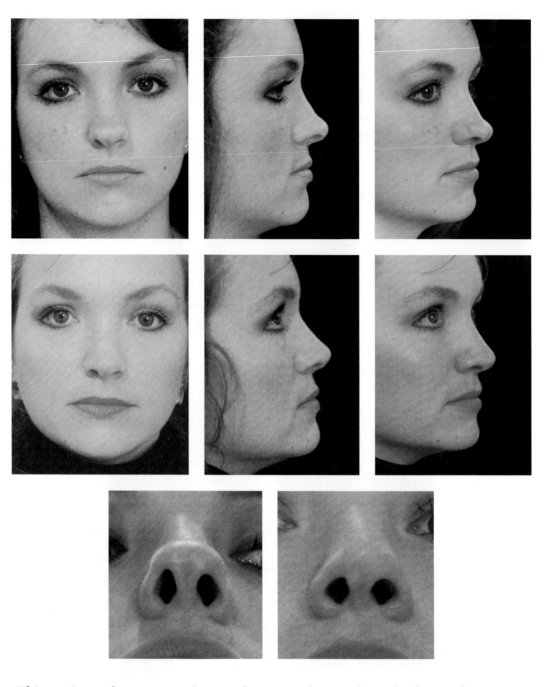

This patient whose surgical procedure was shown above had complete resection of alar cartilages lateral to the medial genu and replacement with narrow strips of cartilage to support the alar rims. She also had tip grafts and a dorsal graft.

Regardless of the method of treatment, the most important aspect of malposition is recognition. The position of the lateral crura relative to the alar rim should be assessed in every rhinoplasty patient to prevent untoward results, to modify technique as necessary, and to ensure the best aesthetic result for patients whose alar cartilages require special management.

THE SIGNIFICANCE OF THE MIDDLE CRURA: CLINICAL AND AESTHETIC CONSIDERATIONS

This milestone is an example of how one can look at something every day, for years, and never really see it. I was taught that an alar cartilage consists of two segments, the medial and lateral crus, which join at the dome or lateral genu. Medical illustrations confirmed this impression, showing a long, continuous structure bent in the middle. It never occurred to me to question the accepted anatomy. When researching it later, I found that Gray's *Anatomy*[34] mentions, almost parenthetically, a *transitional* area but gives no description, nor is it represented in any illustration. No wonder it went unnoticed. I had never heard or read any reference to it, nor seen it illustrated in presentations, let alone any mention of a possible clinical significance.

Informed by the accepted anatomy, I had been intently studying alar cartilages but was still perplexed by unanswered questions. The many variations in the surface anatomy of the tip remained a puzzle. In particular I was interested in the angulation at the columellar-lobular junction and the various facets seen in different nasal tips. From the beginning I could get some results I was proud of, such as the one I often used in my early presentations.

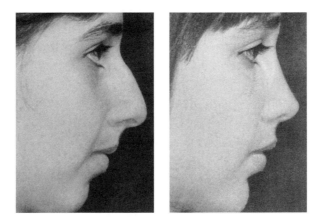

This patient, operated on in 1968, happened to have the ideal cartilages for the standard tip refining technique. Then, as I gained experience, I could not understand why the same technique failed to produce consistent results. I could not create the desired facets and angulations at will. I felt that until these features were understood, I could not adequately diagnose and control tip contours.

One day, quite unexpectedly, I saw what I had been looking at. In an anatomy laboratory I had dissected out and exposed an entire alar cartilage. At once it was obvious. Between the medial and lateral crus there was a distinct segment that extended from a medial genu to a lateral genu: a middle crus.

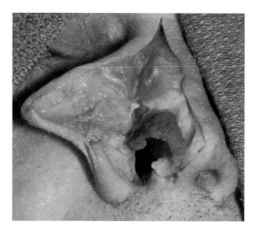

Cadaver dissection exhibits three distinct segments of the alar cartilage. The middle crus (red portion) is bounded by the medial and lateral genua.

With that observation the surface anatomy of the nasal base finally made sense. The base consisted of three definite units: the columella, the tip lobule, and the alar rims. The columellar-lobular junction indicated the medial genu, or the angulation between the medial and middle crura. This angle I defined as the *angle of rotation.* The height of the lobule reflected the length of the middle crura, and on the frontal view the tip was defined by the distance between the lateral genua. This distance was determined by the *angle of divergence,* or the relationship of the middle crura to each other. Thus for me, the middle crus was the missing link in nasal tip anatomy. With it, diagnosis and management of a variety of nasal base configurations was possible.

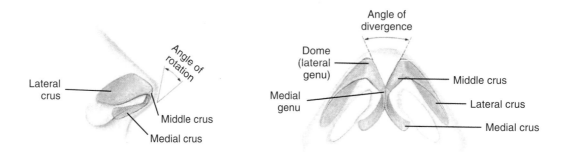

The three-segment anatomy of the alar cartilage is depicted. The angle of rotation at the medial genu defines the columellar-lobular junction; the angle of divergence determines the intercrural distance.

One frequently encountered configuration is the broad tip. Keeping the relationship between the middle crura in mind, one can see that a broad tip is the manifestation of a wide angle of divergence. Conversely, a narrow angle of divergence creates a pointed tip, lacking the attractive defining point of the lateral genu seen on the oblique view.

The length of the middle crura also determines characteristic tip contours. What I termed a "tip with inadequate projection" usually reflects short middle crura. To the extreme, a "snub" nose is the result of very short or nonexistent middle crura.

Historically, these noses have often been treated by composite grafts to lengthen the columella. With critical observation, however, it is apparent that the columella is not the primary problem. The lack of projection is usually caused by a deficient tip lobule, that is, short middle crura. The logical treatment for a deficient lobule is to place tip grafts to project and define the nasal tip, thus duplicating the role of the middle crura.

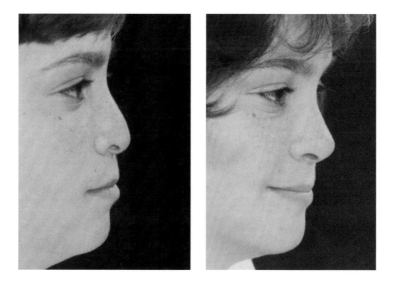

This patient has a typical "snub" nose that reflects short middle crura, resulting in inadequate projection of the nasal tip. She is shown 8 years after tip grafting.

Less common but also typical in appearance is the tip with long middle crura. Long middle crura are manifest by a tall lobule or a long infratip segment. In these cases the nasal tip appears to be square on profile. Recognition of long middle crura is necessary for a satisfactory result because techniques that address only the lateral crura will not effect the desired change. Only excision of part of the middle crura will decrease the height of the lobule.

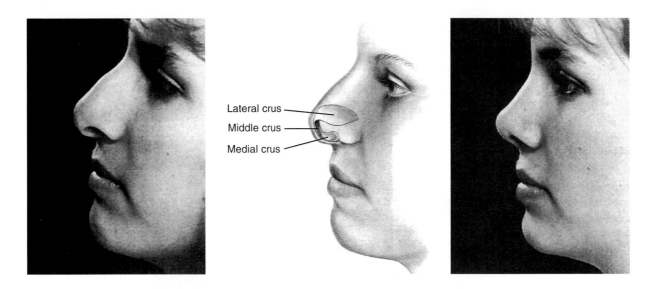

Lateral crus
Middle crus
Medial crus

This patient had a square nasal tip reflecting long middle crura with a wide angle of rotation. The graphic depicts the three-segment alar cartilage as it relates to surface contour. Note the postoperative result obtained by partial resection of the middle crura and tip grafting.

Understanding the alar cartilage as a three-part structure, with each part having a specific role in the contour of the nasal base, and understanding that the size, shape, and position of each component influences the aesthetics of the tip enable the surgeon to analyze the anatomic basis for each patient's nasal contour and to plan an operation that is appropriate and effective.

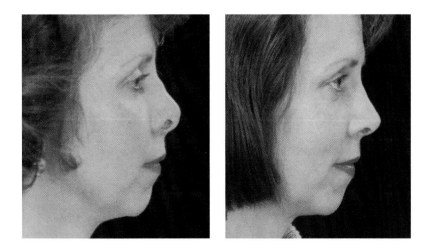

Critical analysis of the individual patient's alar cartilage—the size, shape, and position of each component—enables effective surgical management of the nasal tip, as demonstrated in this patient. She is shown following resection of the crura lateral to the medial genu and reconstruction with septal cartilage grafts to the dorsum and nasal tip. Ear cartilage was used to support the alar rims.

Finally, I would like to comment on the "endonasal" method of rhinoplasty, which, when I learned it, was the only method. All of the observations, realizations, and resulting changes have been made under the conditions of an endonasal approach and could not have been made otherwise. Some of the techniques such as placing free grafts in discrete pockets are not applicable to the "open" method, but the principles still apply. This is not the time or place for a comparison with the now popular open method, but one reflection is salient. Much of what I have learned and continue to learn from nasal surgery is dependent on seeing and touching the nose in its normal, covered state. As I operate, a dynamic takes place between me and the nasal tissues, between what I am imposing on the nasal contour and what it will accept. I would find it difficult to duplicate the subtlety of this experience working on exposed skeleton. At present I would make one exception—the case of malposition. Because of the technical difficulty of repositioning or replacing the lateral crura, it may be that the open approach enables more controllable management of malpositioned cartilages.

It is an interesting experience to reflect on the evolution of one's thinking on a particular subject over a long period of time. My subject is small, but for me, the possibilities have always been great. I like noses. I like to think about changing them and I like to think about changing the ways in which we change them to achieve ever improving and predictable results. To that end, these are my seven personal milestones to date. I'm working toward an even number.

REFERENCES

1. Sheen JH. Aesthetic Rhinoplasty, 1st ed. St. Louis: CV Mosby, 1978, p 26.
2. Converse JM. Surgical Treatment of Facial Injuries, 3rd ed. Baltimore: Williams & Wilkins, 1974, p 782.
3. Rees TD, Wood-Smith D. Cosmetic Facial Surgery. Philadelphia: WB Saunders, 1973, p 439.
4. Brown JB, McDowell F. Plastic Surgery of the Nose. St. Louis: CV Mosby, 1951, pp 118-119.
5. Lewis JR. Atlas of Aesthetic Plastic Surgery. Boston: Little, Brown, 1973, p 119.
6. Deneke HJ, Meyer R. Plastic Surgery of Head and Neck. New York: Springer-Verlag, 1967, p 102.
7. Aufricht G. Rhinoplasty and the face. Plast Reconstr Surg 43:219, 1969.
8. Joseph J. Nasenplastik und sonstige Gesichtsplastik nebst Mammaplastik. Oxford, England: Willem A Meeuws, 1931, p 141.
9. Sheen JH. Aesthetic Rhinoplasty, 1st ed. St. Louis: CV Mosby, 1978, pp 26-37.
10. Rogers BO. Rhinoplasty. In Goldwyn RM, ed. The Unfavorable Result in Plastic Surgery. Boston: Little, Brown, 1972.
11. Lewis JR. Correction of the supratip hump. In Millard DR, ed. Symposium on Corrective Rhinoplasty. St. Louis: CV Mosby, 1976, p 161.
12. Rees TD, Wood-Smith D. Cosmetic Facial Surgery. Philadelphia: WB Saunders, 1973, pp 456-460.
13. Rees TD, Krupp S, Wood-Smith D. Secondary rhinoplasty. Plast Reconstr Surg 46:332, 1970.
14. Meyer R. Secondary rhinoplasty. In Berman W, ed. Rhinoplastic Surgery. St. Louis: CV Mosby, 1989, pp 223-226.
15. Safian J. Fact and fallacy in rhinoplasty. Plast Reconstr Surg 12:24, 1953.
16. Deneke HJ, Meyer R. Corrective and Reconstructive Rhinoplasty. New York: Springer-Verlag, 1967, p 451.
17. Sheen JH. Secondary rhinoplasty surgery. In Millard DR, ed. Symposium on Corrective Rhinoplasty. St. Louis: CV Mosby, 1976, chap 16.
18. Sheen JH. Secondary Rhinoplasty Surgery (Videotape #9610). Creating the Balanced Nose. Arlington Heights, Ill.: Plastic Surgery Educational Foundation.
19. Sheen JH. A new look at supratip deformity. Ann Plast Surg 3:498, 1979.
20. Maliniac JW. Rhinoplasty and Restoration of Facial Contour. Philadelphia: FA Davis, 1946, pp 238-240.
21. Millard DR. Adjuncts in augmentation mentoplasty and corrective rhinoplasty. Plast Reconstr Surg 36:48, 1965.
22. Falces E, Gorney M. Use of ear cartilage grafts for nasal tip reconstruction. Plast Reconstr Surg 50:147, 1972.
23. Sheen JH. Achieving more nasal tip projection by the use of a small autogenous vomer or septal cartilage graft. A preliminary report. Plast Reconstr Surg 36:35, 1975.
24. Sheen JH. Tip graft: A 20-year retrospective. Plast Reconstr Surg 91:48, 1993.
25. Sheen JH. The radix as a reference in rhinoplasty. Perspect Plast Surg 1(1):33, 1987.
26. Sheen JH, Sheen AP. Aesthetic Rhinoplasty, 2nd ed. St. Louis: Quality Medical Publishing, 1998, pp 808-825 (reprint of 1987 ed.).
27. Sheen JH. Aesthetic Rhinoplasty, 1st ed. St. Louis: CV Mosby, 1978, p 81.
28. Sheen JH. Aesthetic Rhinoplasty, 1st ed. St. Louis: CV Mosby, 1978, pp 210-215.
29. Skoog T. Plastic Surgery. Philadelphia: WB Saunders, 1974, pp 233-239.
30. Sheen JH. New concepts in rhinoplasty. Presented at the Annual Meeting of the American Society of Plastic and Reconstructive Surgeons, Boston, 1976.

31. Sheen JH, Sheen AP. Aesthetic Rhinoplasty, 2nd ed. St. Louis: CV Mosby, 1987, pp 530-536.
32. Sheen JH. Spreader graft: A method of reconstructing the roof of the middle nasal vault following rhinoplasty. Plast Reconstr Surg 73:230, 1984.
33. Sheen JH. Spreader graft revisited. Perspect Plast Surg 3(1):155-163.
34. Gray H. Anatomy of the Human Body, 28th ed. Philadelphia: Lea & Febiger, 1967, p 1119.
35. Sheen JH. Aesthetic Rhinoplasty, 1st ed. St. Louis: CV Mosby, 1978, pp 432-461.
36. Sheen JH, Sheen AP. Aesthetic Rhinoplasty, 2nd ed. St. Louis: CV Mosby, 1987, pp 988-1011.
37. Sheen JH, Sheen AP. Aesthetic Rhinoplasty, 2nd ed. St. Louis: Quality Medical Publishing, 1998, pp 25-45 (reprint of 1987 ed.).
38. Sheen JH. Middle crus: The missing link in alar cartilage anatomy. Perspect Plast Surg 5(1):31, 1991.

64

Tardy's Approach

M. Eugene Tardy, Jr., M.D.

It is often said that there are many ways of achieving the same surgical end [in tip surgery]. What is not added is that there are usually differences in the price to be paid. The wise man sorts these out.

Richard Webster, M.D.

No single universal technique for refining the wide variety of nasal tip configurations exists. The rhinoplasty surgeon must possess an arsenal of different surgical approaches and techniques, applying the most appropriate as a consequence of the specific anatomy encountered.

In the course of performing and teaching conservative rhinoplasty surgery in the last three decades, a systematic graduated anatomic approach to nasal tip surgery has been developed. This system depends entirely on the anatomy encountered (and the precise diagnosis of that anatomy) and selecting the least traumatic, most predictable, and most conservative sculpturing technique in the majority of anatomic situations, reserving less predictable and more aggressive approaches for the instances in which the perceived anatomy demands more dramatic sculpturing to achieve a preconceived result.

In the vast majority of patients undergoing primary rhinoplasty it is desirable to preserve a generous intact caudal segment (complete strip) of alar cartilage, extending from the medial crural footplate attachment to the caudal septum to the lateral crural sesamoid attachment to the piriform aperture, and avoid the less predictable healing consequences of various forms of vertical dome division interrupted strips. Symmetry is thus enhanced, trauma is diminished, and predictable, controlled healing is facilitated. Setting the master surgeon apart from the novice is, in part, the ability to accurately predict and compensate for the favorable and unfavorable healing factors that continue to influence nasal appearance for many years after primary surgery.

Successful rhinoplasty is initially preceded by exacting analytic assessment of the nasal configuration, the deformity, and its relationship to the surrounding features. A realistic estimate of surgical correction, based on the possibilities and limitations imposed by the characteristics of the nasal tissues, is formulated—the preoperative "game plan." Based on his analysis the surgeon must construct an operative plan predicated on the anatomy and deformity encountered, orchestrating the operation fluidly to achieve the intended long-term stable result. Both before and during the operation the surgeon must envision the ultimate appearance. The goal of surgery is to fashion a natural nose that is in harmony with its surrounding facial features, does not draw attention to itself, and results in a happy patient and proud surgeon. Only with continued experience and study, coupled with a continual impartial analysis of one's own long-term results, can this surgical finesse be developed and refined.

Each patient's unique nasal configuration and anatomic structure require individual operative planning in surgical reconstruction. No single technique, even though mastered, can satisfactorily correct the varied anatomic patterns encountered. This fundamental principle is most critical in tip sculpturing techniques. It is essential to regard rhinoplasty as an operation planned to reconstitute and shape the anatomic features of the nose into a new, more pleasing relationship to one another as well as to the surrounding facial features without altering the physiologic function of the nose. Indeed, septal reconstruction to improve function and enhance nasal alignment is a fundamental requirement in the majority of rhinoplasties.

Rhinoplasty should be approached as an anatomic dissection of the nasal structures requiring alteration, conservatively shaping and repositioning these elements and reducing resection and sacrifice of tissue to a minimum. Far more problems and complications arise from overcorrection of nasal abnormalities than from conservative correction. Inappropriate techniques applied persistently without regard for the limitations imposed by the existing anatomy create frequent complications. One truism remains valid: "It is not what is removed in rhinoplasty that is important, but what is left behind." Furthermore, it is mandatory that the dynamic aspects of operative rhinoplasty be fully comprehended since all surgical steps in the correction of the nose are interrelated and interdependent.

TIP SCULPTURING CONCEPTS

Sculpturing techniques can be broadly classified as those that preserve a complete strip of intact caudal alar cartilage and those that interrupt that caudal segment to produce an incomplete or interrupted strip. Numerous variations in each technique exist, but the procedures to be discussed in each category retain fundamental similarities. If tip shape and attitude may be refined by preserving the majority of the alar cartilage while reorienting tip anatomy by suture techniques, risk is diminished.

The concept of a *systematic graduated anatomic approach* implies the application of the most conservative, most predictable sculpturing operations and incisional approaches to nasal tips requiring minimal or subtle changes; as the anatomic deformity encountered becomes more severe, progressively less conservative approaches are used as required. Emphasis is always placed on conservatism in managing nasal tip structures, replacing radical dissection with cartilage reorientation and repositioning whenever possible.

When considering nasal tip surgery alternatives and variations it is useful to differentiate between incisions, approaches, and techniques. This important distinction has not always been noted in the literature and teaching in the past, leading to confusion and misunderstanding about the indications for and the long-term results of individual surgical approaches and techniques.

Incisions are in reality only methods to gain access to nasal tip structures and by themselves exert no major influence on the final tip contour and appearance. If the incision chosen weakens or divides one of the important fundamental tip support mechanisms, then the dynamics of healing change and the consequent loss of tip support may create loss of tip projection.

Approaches to the tip may be conveniently divided into nondelivery and delivery open categories. Tip approaches provide exposure of the tip structures for analysis and modification. Relatively clear indications for each approach exist and will be discussed in detail. Techniques are those sculpturing and/or suturing modifications carried out on the alar cartilages that effect a minor or major shape change, projection alteration, and possibly a dynamic cephalic rotation of the tip to enhance the nasal appearance. The technique chosen preoperatively often dictates the approach to be used, a decision made as a result of precise preoperative evaluation and diagnosis of the anatomy of the alar cartilages and the ultimate result desired.

TIP SUPPORT MECHANISMS

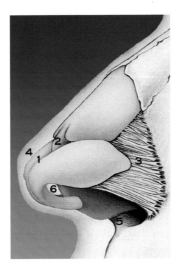

A fundamental understanding of and respect for the various major and lesser tip support mechanisms play an all-important role in executing tip incisions in tip contouring procedures. They consist of (in varying degrees of importance from patient to patient) (1) the contour, size, thickness, and strength of the alar cartilages, (2) the attachment of the medial crural footplates to the caudal septum along with the size and strength of the medial crura, and (3) the fibrous attachment of the caudal edge of the upper lateral cartilage to the cephalic edge of the alar cartilage.

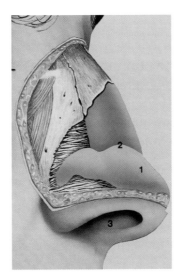

Of lesser but still vital importance to tip support can be listed (1) the nasal tip interdomal ligamentous aponeurosis, (2) the cartilaginous septal dorsum, (3) the nasal spine, (4) the strength and resilience of the medial crura, (5) the thickness of the tip skin and subcutaneous tissues, and (6) the supportive strength of the alar sidewalls.

In every surgical procedure on the nasal tip the operation will inevitably ultimately result in (1) preservation of tip projection, (2) increase in tip projection, or (3) decrease in tip projection. Anatomic situations will be regularly encountered in a diverse rhinoplasty practice in which each of these outcomes will be desirable and intended. In the majority of Caucasian rhinoplasties, however, it is critical to preserve and maintain the already existing (preoperative) tip projection while favorably altering the contour and attitude of the alar cartilages, avoiding at all costs the loss of vital tip support with the consequent potential decrease in projection ("tip ptosis"). Respect for tip support mechanisms facilitates a predictable outcome.

Incisions should be planned to preserve as many tip support mechanisms as possible. Alar sculpturing techniques should likewise respect this principle by conserving the volume and integrity of the lateral crus while maintaining an intact complete caudal strip of alar cartilage.

The rhinoplasty literature is often less than clear about the important distinction between what constitutes an incisional approach to the tip cartilages and a technique for modifying those cartilages. Eponyms attached to surgical procedures further confuse the issue for the learner and expert alike. In this chapter clear distinctions will be drawn between these concepts since their understanding is vital to achieving superior operative results.

INCISIONS

Within themselves incisions are only a method to gain access to the underlying cartilaginous and soft tissue substructures of the nose. Although specific incisions possess particular virtues, experienced surgeons can modify the cartilaginous structures of the tip through almost any incision; each surgeon, however, generally develops preferred incisional approaches with which he has gained experience and dexterity. Nonetheless, it is not the incisions themselves that are important but what is accomplished through those incisions that count in long-term favorable results. Without exception the choice of the incisions should be governed by the anatomy of the tip and its related nasal structures. Whenever possible, less invasive incisions (and dissection) are preferred since they result in greater control of the healing process.

In selecting the appropriate incision(s) for gaining access to the tip and supratip areas the surgeon should take into account whether the incision:
1. Provides reasonably unencumbered visualization and/or access to the alar cartilages
2. Preserves whenever possible the important tip support mechanisms
3. Avoids interference with other incisions contemplated in the same area
4. Lends itself well to healing without contraction or undue scarring

Alar Cartilage Incisions

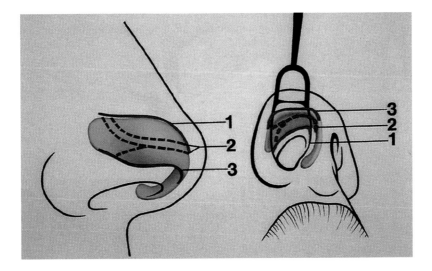

Preferred incisional approaches to gain access to the nasal tip cartilages include the intercartilaginous *(1)*, transcartilaginous *(2)*, and marginal *(3)*. Both the intercartilaginous and the transcartilaginous incisions may be used individually as the sole incisional approach to the alar cartilage, preferably when a conservative volume reduction (cephalic trim) of the medial-cephalic margins of the lateral crus and domes is desired, leaving an intact complete strip of alar cartilage. One incision thus suffices for tip modeling and dissection trauma is minimal.

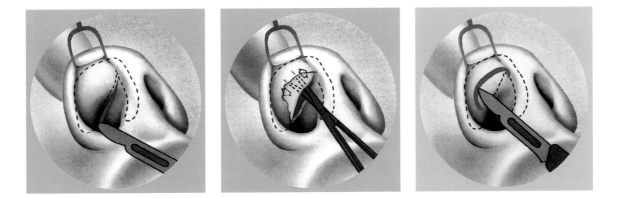

Through the intercartilaginous incision a retrograde (eversion) approach may be accomplished while the cartilage-splitting approach is carried out through the transcartilaginous incision. It is worthy of emphasis that both these incisional approaches ultimately divide and eliminate one of the vital major tip support mechanisms—the attachment between the caudal aspect of the upper lateral cartilage and the cephalic aspect of the alar cartilage.

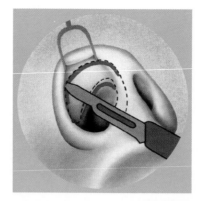

Although the marginal incision may be used alone, particularly when correcting minor tip asymmetries in revision tip surgery, it classically is combined with the intercartilaginous incision in the delivery approach to the alar cartilage, creating a bilateral chondrocutaneous flap that is delivered through the nostril for direct vision modeling and refinement. Ideally, the marginal incision is positioned 1 mm inside (cephalad to) the palpable caudal margins of the lateral crus, allowing for ultimate ease of incision closure and further protecting the soft tissue alar margin. As the marginal incision is carried medially into the area of the soft triangle and facets, care must be taken to maintain complete precision of the cut along the caudal edge of the lateral crus, dome, and upper medial crus where the incision courses perilously close to the alar and columellar margins.

Septal Incisions

Septal transfixion incisions useful in exposing the nasal tip structures are categorized as complete, partial (limited), hemi-, and high.

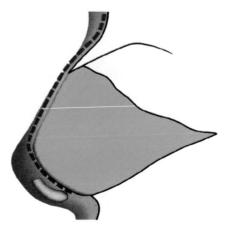

The complete transfixion incision, ordinarily a continuation of the intercartilaginous or transcartilaginous incision, separates the caudal end of the septum from the membranous septum and the medial crura therein. If truly complete (sweeping posteriorly to the nasal spine), a major tip support mechanism—the attachment of the medial crural footplates to the caudal septum—is interrupted, thus inevitably creating a major loss of tip support and possibly loss of tip projection.

When indicated, this incision favorably frees the tip completely from the more stable structural elements, provides excellent access to the nose, allows exposure to the nasal spine and depressor septi muscle, and exposes the septum for elevation of one or both mucoperichondrial flaps. Our initial approach to the overprojecting nose usually is initiated by a complete transfixion incision to effect intentional tip retroprojection.

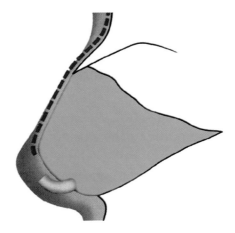

When limited access to the nasal tip and nose will suffice (as in the majority of nasal operations), a limited partial transfixion is preferable, preserving the major tip support mechanism while allowing adequate exposure. The partial incision may be carried from just beyond (caudal to) the anterior septal angle to any extent just short of the medial crural attachment to the caudal septum. When combined with the intercartilaginous or transcartilaginous incisional approach, the partial transfixion may be limited to one side only, exposing the septal angle and supratip dorsum by extending the transcartilaginous or intercartilaginous incisions medially to encounter the partial transfixion. Exposure is entirely adequate, scarring is diminished, controlled healing is facilitated, and the liabilities of the complete transfixion are negated.

The hemitransfixion incision is created unilaterally at the junction of the caudal septum and columella, particularly in procedures in which the caudal septum is deviated or requires resection modification for tip rotation or columellar adjustment.

The high septal transfixion incision is a useful alternative in septorhinoplasty incisional approaches. Tip support mechanisms are preserved and incisions in vestibular skin are minimized. Tip rotation and nasal shortening of the central component of the nose are facilitated without altering the relationships of the caudal septum to the columella and nasal tip structures. Tip support remains undisturbed by the incision.

PRINCIPLES OF ENDONASAL ALAR CARTILAGE SCULPTURING

When confronted by a nasal tip requiring aesthetic alteration the rhinoplasty surgeon must initially bring all of his diagnostic skills to bear on the accurate analysis and diagnosis of the deformity. Inspection complemented by extensive palpation of the contour, thickness, bulk, resilience, and extent of the alar cartilages with their surrounding soft tissues and bony relationships generally affords an accurate understanding of the existent anatomy (with the possible exception of revision rhinoplasty), upon which a strategic surgical plan can be devised. Surgical decisions related to incisional approaches and alar sculpturing techniques should be predicated principally on the anatomy encountered and tip dynamics contemplated; everything else is of secondary importance. The technical steps chosen in tip surgery should accomplish cartilage contouring by the most conservative manner possible, preserving or reorienting structures in preference to resection. Attempts should be made to "mimic nature" in reduction rhinoplasty, reducing volume or reorienting cartilage so that the final altered alar cartilages will retain their positive characteristics while being surgically relieved of a portion of their undesirable characteristics. Tip surgery, except in the otherwise near-perfect tip, is almost always a compromise or series of compromises in which the surgeon and patient must "pay a price" for almost any surgical alteration in the form of support sacrifice and various degrees of scarring. The control of these compromises and healing characteristics become all critical if surgical errors are to be avoided in the attempt to accomplish more than the tissue anatomic characteristics will permit. Limitations must then be recognized and respected.

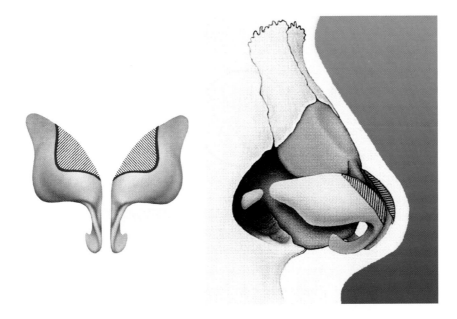

Several vital principles then are worthy of strong emphasis when considering alar cartilage contouring. These apply in the overwhelming majority of rhinoplasty operations. Almost all traditional tip "techniques" share in common the principle of volume reduction of the alar cartilage (cephalic trim), usually confined to the broad cephalic portions of the lateral crus and dome, with an occasional thinning resection of the medial crural contribution to the dome when indicated. This volume reduction may include a portion of the "scroll" formed by the upper lateral cartilage–alar cartilage relationship. Alar volume reduction creates a "dead space," which will be ultimately filled with scar tissue, undergoing contracture in a variable manner. This space may ultimately be diminished by a variable upward visor-like rotation of the alar cartilage. To reduce scar formation and cephalic contraction, all underlying vestibular skin residual from alar reduction (unless clearly redundant) should be preserved.

Preserving a complete caudal strip of intact cartilage (complete strip), extending from the medial crural footplates to the lateral cephalicmost tip of the alar crus, is desirable in the majority of rhinoplasties. Tip support and projection are enhanced, irregularities in healing are minimized, symmetry is probable, and a relative resistance to cephalic tip rotations is retained. The more alar cartilage left undisturbed consistent with adequate aesthetic tip correction the more predictable is the healing process.

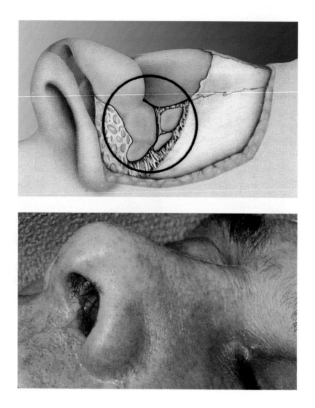

The superolateral portion of the lateral crus, attached by connective tissue to the bony piriform margin (at times with various interposed sesamoid cartilages), should be left intact and not resected. Support for the lateral nasal sidewall is thus preserved (avoiding potential inspiratory collapse), possible dimpling stigmata are avoided, and potential undesired alar cephalic retraction is unlikely.

In the vast majority of rhinoplasties the surgeon either preserves or increases existing projection of the nasal tip; much less often is reduction in tip projection required. Therefore identifying and preserving the tip-defining point of the alar cartilage dome are mandatory for optimal tip definition and projection.

In most patients in whom preservation of a complete strip of alar cartilage does not result in satisfactory definition and refinement, a shape and attitude change may be induced in the residual caudal strip with suture techniques without resorting to a vertical incisional interruption of the complete strip.

If a decision is made to interrupt the complete strip to achieve an added narrowing refinement and/or increased projection, the overlying skin canopy must ideally be of sufficient thickness to camouflage any irregularities or offsets that would otherwise become palpable and/or visible in the long-term postoperative period.

Alar Cartilage Approaches

In the final analysis contouring with volume reduction of the alar cartilages falls principally into three general categories: (1) cephalic cartilage volume reduction with preservation of an intact complete caudal cartilage strip, (2) cephalic cartilage volume reduction with caudal complete strip preservation with a shape change induced by sutures or by cartilage incision procedures, and (3) cephalic cartilage volume reduction with vertical division of the dome and/or lateral crus medially or laterally. Onlay or infratip lobule cartilage grafts may be employed with any of the above to achieve tip projection, support, camouflage, and contour.

To achieve alar cartilage contouring, one of several available approaches to the cartilages must be chosen, based on the anatomy encountered and the degree of exposure required to satisfactorily effect a pleasing contour modification. The systematic graduated anatomic system to nasal tip surgery may be classified according to approaches as follows:
1. Nondelivery approaches to the lower lateral cartilages
   a. Transcartilaginous approach
   b. Retrograde (eversion) approach
2. Delivery approaches to the lower lateral cartilages
   a. Bipedicle chondrocutaneous flap approach
3. External (open) approach

Nondelivery Approaches

Any surgical approach that requires minimal dissection disturbance of the alar cartilages generally ensures more symmetric healing and produces fewer risks of unpredictable healing. Since tip surgery constitutes a bilateral operation in which ultimate symmetry is all important, minimal disturbance to an already symmetric tip makes operative sense. Although believed by some to be technically more difficult because of reduced visualization, in reality the competent experienced surgeon finds little technical difficulty in employing nondelivery techniques. We prefer nondelivery approaches in all patients whose anatomy will permit its use.

Additional virtues include (1) a relative resistance to cephalic rotation, (2) a single incisional approach, (3) preservation of existing tip projection, and (4) a relative resistance to tip retrodisplacement and postoperative tip ptosis. The latter two factors are operable only if a complete strip technique is maintained.

Transcartilaginous (Cartilage-Splitting) Approach. In patients in whom conservative tip volume reduction (cephalic trim) is indicated and minimal tip rotation is desirable, the transcartilaginous (cartilage-splitting) incisional approach is useful and predictable. Advantages include a single incision, diminished tip edema and scarring, complete preservation of facets, and, if a complete strip is preserved, relative resistance to cephalic rotation in patients in whom tip attitude and projection are already anatomically correct. Postoperative tip ptosis or retrodisplacement is largely avoided. Properly performed in selected anatomic situations, predictable healing with preservation of symmetry and support is consistently achieved. In patients demonstrating abnormal divergence of the intermediate crura with a wide intercrural distance, the cartilage-splitting approach is insufficient for proper repair since in these patients the domes must ordinarily be exposed and sutured together for satisfactory narrowing. Thus the transcartilaginous approach is contraindicated in patients with thin skin, strong cartilages, and bifidity (the "dangerous triad").

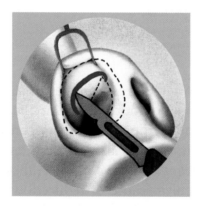

Retracting the left ala with a wide double hook, a single incision through vestibular skin only is sited and executed several millimeters cephalad to the caudal margin of the alar cartilage.

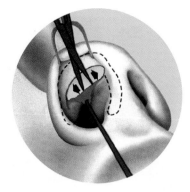

With delicate curved, sharp scissors the vestibular skin is undermined easily by pushing motions using a sharp scissors and elevated from the portion of the cephalic alar cartilage to be removed. Spreading in the subperichondrial plane already hydraulically dissected by local anesthetic facilitates atraumatic bloodless elevation. The lateralmost portion of the lateral crus remains undisturbed. The undersurface of the lateral crus and dome is now clearly uncovered for further inspection, final diagnosis, and sculpture.

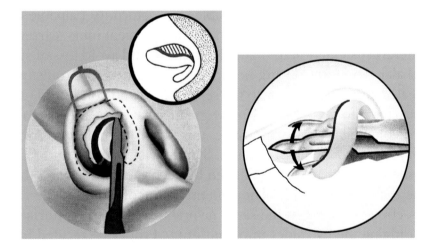

The alar cartilage is next transected at a predetermined level; dissection of the overlying soft tissues embracing the upper lateral cartilages and septum proceeds with the knife in similar fashion as when using the intercartilaginous incisional approach. The plane dissected should be just superficial to and precisely intimate to the perichondrium enveloping the upper lateral cartilages to preserve overlying soft tissues and minimize bleeding and ultimate scar formation.

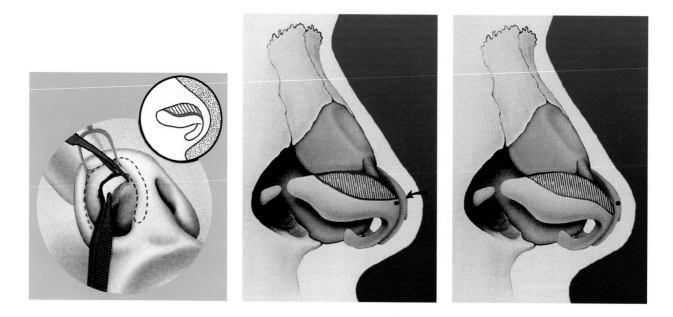

Under direct vision the predetermined amount of lower lateral cartilage is resected, preserving or reducing tip projection as desired by varying the amount of medial-cephalic alar cartilage removed from the dome areas. In patients with exquisitely thin skin the transcartilaginous incisions are ideally beveled or feathered to obviate a possible step deformity palpable or visible through skin. Caution is exercised to maintain sufficient intact cartilage at the medial-lateral crus junction to maintain strength and avoid loss of support to the lateral alar structures during healing. A separate partial transfixion incision is created at or just inferior to the septal angle and connected only to the left transcartilaginous incision. Unless greater access to the caudal septum or inferior columellar area is desirable, this initial partial transfixion allows satisfactory access to the nasal dorsum. Symmetric exposure and resection of the opposite alar cartilage are facilitated by accurately measuring the precise site of the incision bilaterally. The soft tissue uncovering on the right with knife dissection proceeds in the same favorable supraperichondrial plane as the left, bringing the two sides into continuity. Properly executed in the recommended supraperichondrial plane, décollement of the lower cartilaginous nose is accomplished with rapid sharp knife dissection and little trauma and little or no bleeding.

The new tip configuration is now assessed visually and palpably for symmetry, projection, narrowing refinement, and attitude. Further modifications of the residual intact segment or dome are possible, ranging from excision of small triangles of cartilage to shave excision of offending cartilage excesses. The objective is to render the tip more defined and delicate while preserving as much normal alar cartilage as possible, thus "mimicking nature" consistent with the volume reduction and attitude change desirable.

The transcartilaginous approach consistently generates minimal tip edema and rapid healing when carefully suture repaired, a clear virtue when precise tip definition and projection are being assessed. Since the caudal portion of the tip cartilages and alar margins remains undisturbed, predictable healing is ensured.

Retrograde (Eversion) Approach. An alternative to the transcartilaginous approach is the retrograde or eversion approach, similarly useful in patients requiring conservative tip modeling. In reality the two approaches are interchangeable.

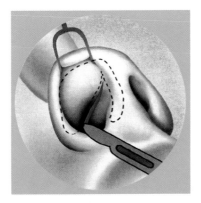

Only one incision (a bilateral intercartilaginous) is needed to access the alar cartilage; additional exposure, if desirable, can be gained by creating a vertical relaxing incision in the vestibular skin at the dome.

Indicated conservative sculpturing of the lower lateral cartilage is accomplished as desired bilaterally after retrograde undermining of the vestibular skin, again using the subperichondrial plane. The singular advantage lies in the fact that this approach eliminates any possibility of undesirable scarring or asymmetric healing in already aesthetically pleasing caudal alar cartilage margins while conservatively reducing cartilage volume and refining the nasal tip appearance. In addition, since a minimal tissue void is created, more cartilage is preserved and scar contracture is minimized. Tip rotation is therefore resisted in a similar fashion to the transcartilaginous approach if a complete strip is preserved.

Since incisions are in reality only a method to gain access to the tip-supporting structures, the transcartilaginous and retrograde approaches are essentially interchangeable; conservative volume reduction of the tip cartilages is equally possible with either approach. The key in both techniques is the preservation of equal intact complete alar segments bilaterally. Both allow the surgeon maximal control over healing; therein lies their principal virtue.

Delivery Approaches

Gross asymmetry, marked bulbosity, excessive or inadequate projection, marked bifidity, soft tissue excess requiring resection, as well as revision tip surgery are all appropriate indications for delivering the alar cartilage with its attached vestibular skin as a bipedicle chondrocutaneous alar flap. Sharp knife dissection again minimizes soft tissue trauma and scarring. Preservation of symmetry or production of symmetry in tips with unequal cartilages is theoretically enhanced by delivery of the alar cartilages for contouring under direct vision. The delivery approach facilitates suture modifications of the domal angles and interdomal region, allowing triangular refinement of broad tips.

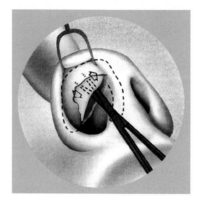

The right nostril is retracted with a wide double skin hook, and external counterpressure is applied over the cartilage with the middle finger. An intercartilaginous incision is created with a No. 15 blade just above and along the projecting rim of the upper lateral cartilage, hugging the perichondrium in the favorable tissue plane; the knife is preferred for atraumatic dissection, thus elevating the skin–soft tissue canopy precisely from the dorsal cartilaginous septum and the septal dorsum. A similar maneuver in the right nostril is accomplished; the two planes of dissection are connected by the knife in the same motion, and the incision is carried immediately anterior to and around the anterior septal angle to terminate in a partial transfixion incision. Complete transfixion incisions involving the entire length of the columella are reserved for those anatomic deformities in which (1) the caudal septum is severely deviated from the midline, (2) access to the nasal spine and depressor septi muscle is desirable, (3) tip retrodisplacement is desired, and (4) tip rotation and shortening are necessary. Complete transfixion incisions are normally disadvantageous in that they interrupt a particularly vital support to the tip of the nose—the intimate wraparound relationship of the feet of the medial crura to the caudal quadrangular cartilage.

Elevation of the soft tissues and periosteum over the nasal bones can be accomplished at this time but is ordinarily deferred until tip modeling is complete.

Each nostril is then again retracted in turn, and a curved marginal incision is created in the vestibular skin 1 to 2 mm cephalad to the caudal margin of the lower lateral cartilage. The incision extends medially past the dome area and courses variably downward along the caudal edge of the intermediate crus, depending on the exposure required.

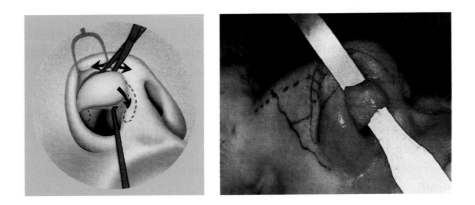

With knife dissection of the favorable soft tissue plane immediately superficial to the lateral crus and dome completed, the high point of the dome is engaged with a sharp hook and the cartilage is gently subluxated from the nostril as a bipedicle chondrocutaneous alar flap with a thin, curved elevator or closed scissors. Considerable soft tissue can be included in the delivered segment if desirable in bulky noses. Otherwise, in keeping with the dictum of conservative surgery, only the chondrocutaneous alar flap is delivered, preserving the overlying skin and subcutaneous tissues. Exposing the cartilages in this manner (intercartilaginous and marginal incisions) allows clear visualization of their anatomy and precise symmetric remodeling. Various geometric excisions or attenuating excisions may now be created near the dome area, combined with generally conservative excision of a portion of the medial-cephalic margin of the lateral crus. A simple volume reduction may be desirable, creating a cartilage of smaller dimensions with natural architecture. To adequately reduce the cartilage volume and avoid the healing development of "horns" or "notches," it will be necessary in selected patients to reduce a portion of the cephalic extent of the medial crus as well as the lateral crus or to suture the domes together in the midline with 4-0 PDS transdomal sutures.

The cartilages are now replaced in their normal anatomic beds, inspected for symmetry and adequate reduction of shape and attitude, and the marginal incisions sutured if the modified tip appearance is satisfactory. The vestibular skin is religiously preserved throughout. Every attempt is made to preserve a sufficiently generous intact caudal marginal segment of the cartilage (the complete strip) to ensure sufficient tip support and symmetry. This is of considerable importance; failure to observe its surgical significance will lead to a larger number of tip cartilage asymmetries and irregularities. Only in certain anatomic variants (wide, trapezoidal boxy tips, asymmetric tips with abnormal projection, markedly overprojected tips, certain revision surgeries) is this rule violated by cutting totally across and resecting a portion of the otherwise intact caudal segment (interrupted strip techniques). The vestibular skin is preserved throughout unless clearly redundant. Excessively thick residual cartilage segments may be further refined and reduced in their anterior-posterior dimension by careful shave excision and thinning.

Several dynamic changes will now have been effected that are critical to the surgeon's comprehension of the refinements of rhinoplasty. Freeing of the cartilages from their soft tissue fibrous attachments combined with selective cephalic segment (and partial dome) reduction or attenuation creates a narrowing refinement and a slight cephalic rotation of the nasal tip in relation to the remaining features of the nose. A new more favorable tip-supratip profile relationship is now established. The dead space resulting from lateral crus volume reduction will heal with scar, contracting during healing and tending to accentuate tip rotation (to a variable degree) while reestablishing the tip support mechanism originally provided by the fibrous tissue attachment of the upper lateral cartilage to the alar cartilage.

External Approach

In 1934 Rethi first described an approach to nasal surgery incorporating an incision across the columellar-labial junction, transecting the columella, and lifting the nasal tip to gain access to the nasal skeleton. Because of the somewhat radical nature of this approach compared to the effectiveness of traditional endonasal rhinoplasty, the Rethi approach found usefulness only in patients with unusual anatomic variants.

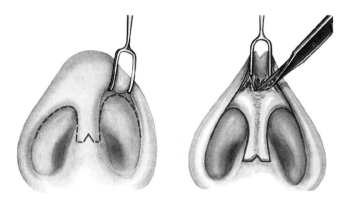

Sercer, in 1957, revived and modified the open approach by limiting the transcolumellar incision to the skin only, joining it with bilateral lateral paracolumellar incisions that were brought into continuity with bilateral marginal incisions. The entire skin of the columella above the incision was then dissected free from the adherent alar cartilages and nasal skeleton, fully revealing the anatomy of the tip structures. Padovan, Sercer's talented and thoughtful student, deserves profound credit for refining and popularizing the approach since 1966. Goodman found virtue in this so-called decortication rhinoplasty and promoted its use in North America.

In the past two decades external or open rhinoplasty has established its usefulness in the surgical correction of a variety of nasal anatomic deformities. Those surgeons who trumpet its use in every rhinoplasty operation are perhaps indiscriminate, whereas those who never employ this approach fail to add another useful tool to their surgical armamentarium.

The proper and appropriate use of the open approach clearly lies between these two extremes and, like all other rhinoplasty approaches, should be selected based entirely on the nasal anatomy encountered. It is vital to appreciate that this surgical maneuver is not in truth a technique but rather simply an alternative approach to gain access to the nasal skeleton. Not surprisingly, open rhinoplasty possesses clear virtues and liabilities, which must be balanced in each patient against the likely or intended end result.

It is further clear that certain specific nasal anatomic variants lend themselves to greater ease of correction through the open approach; I prefer this operative approach when the tip anatomy is severely distorted as well as for certain revision rhinoplasties.

Techniques

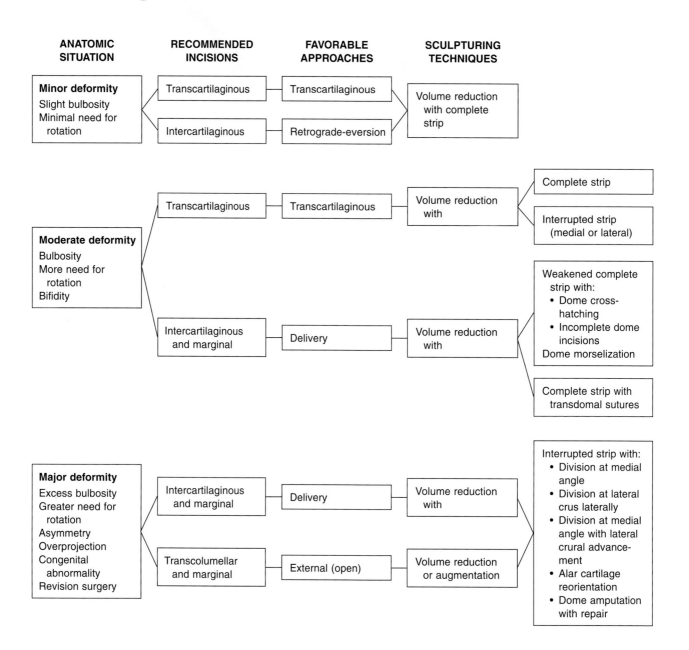

The majority of surgical techniques useful in remodeling the alar cartilages are outlined for the sake of organization. Almost all procedures devised and employed with regularity when indicated will fall within this framework of categorization, which is presented simply to organize the thought process involved and alternatives available in tip surgery as well as to introduce the concept of a graduated anatomic approach to nasal tip sculpturing maneuvers. Since tip surgery is undoubtedly the most difficult part of rhinoplasty, any system that helps to guide the planning process prior to and during surgery can conceivably be useful to the surgeon and ultimately beneficial to the patient.

The concept of a systematic graduated anatomic approach to nasal tip sculpture incorporates the application of the most conservative, most predictable, and least hazardous sculpturing techniques on nasal tips requiring subtle changes in volume, contour, and shape; as the anatomic deformity encountered becomes more abnormal, progressively less conservative approaches are used as required. This concept then requires knowledge on the part of the experienced surgeon of a variety of tip sculpturing procedures with their virtues as well as liabilities. His ability to naturally reduce, reorient, and/or reshape the alar tip structures becomes a product of sound conservative planning and facile technical execution of those plans at the time of surgery, running as few risks as possible and accepting as few compromises as possible to achieve a natural result. Two major categories of procedures encompass the vast majority of useful tip modeling operations.

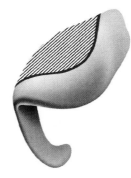

After variable reduction in volume of the cephalic (and often medial) aspect of the lateral crura, a concept uniformly employed in almost all tip operations, a generous complete strip of intact alar cartilage from the medial crura footplates to the lateral-cephalic edge of the lateral crus remains. If for valid predetermined reasons this intact cartilaginous strip is surgically divided anywhere along its extent, an incomplete or interrupted strip is created, which embodies significantly different dynamic principles and healing characteristics than when an undisturbed complete strip remains. Each of these anatomic circumstances possesses virtues and indications for use as well as liabilities and contraindications.

Within these two broad categories various principles have been applied to the shape alteration and attenuation of the complete or incomplete strip to enhance the tip appearance and refine the aesthetic result. Consideration will now be given to the anatomic indications for one or a combination of these surgical maneuvers, introducing more technically aggressive cartilage changes as the anatomic problem encountered becomes more severe.

Cephalic Volume Reduction

To add definition, shape, and attitude change to the nasal tip, a variable reduction of the volume of the cephalic margin of the lateral crus is a common maneuver in most tip operations. When the dome is broad and convex, carrying the incision into the intermediate crus will accomplish a further "thinning resection," allowing additional narrowing and definition (and potentially a slight reduction in tip projection). In tips in which a prominent "scroll" relationship exists between the upper lateral cartilage and the alar cartilage excision of the scroll, at least medially where it is usually more prominent, it is necessary to enhance tip refinement and narrowing. If the alar cartilage is heavy and thick, revealed in broad relief through very thin skin, the edge of the cut made for volume reduction should be ideally beveled to avoid an abrupt step deformity that might appear unnaturally visible on surface inspection.

Complete Strip Operations. Cephalic volume reduction, common to almost all tip techniques, may be accomplished through either the delivery approaches (bipedicle chondrocutaneous alar flap or open) or nondelivery approaches (transcartilaginous or retrograde). Every attempt should be made to preserve as much continuous caudal complete strip remnant as possible, ordinarily leaving at least a 6 to 7 mm strip remnant. In the majority of complete strip operations I prefer to preserve at least 75% of the original cartilage volume. It is always preferable to avoid creating significant subcutaneous tissue and cartilage deficits.

Seldom is it necessary to resect any of the underlying vestibular skin unless in the reduction of a large nose an excess of skin becomes apparent (as in the plunging tip undergoing considerable cephalic rotation). Vestibular skin preservation prevents large tissue voids and raw surfaces and functions as an external but intimate supporting splint or sling for the residual complete strip. If the transcartilaginous single incision approach to the tip and nasal dorsum is employed, the continuity of the vestibular skin and mucoperichondrium underlying the alar cartilage is totally undisturbed, thus protecting the nasal valve area completely.

Reduction of a significant section of the cephalic cartilaginous margin produces a wide void between the otherwise intimate relationship of the upper lateral cartilage to the alar cartilage, a tissue defect ordinarily partially filled as the complete strip and tip are rotated cephalically on the two major pivot points of the alar cartilage. Complete strip techniques tend to resist significant upward rotation, however, and are therefore ideal when significant rotation and shortening of the nose are undesirable.

Anatomic variations in the alar cartilages (and therefore topographic tip anatomy) are regularly encountered in which volume reduction alone is insufficient to accomplish a desirable narrowing refinement, attitude change, or projection alteration to the tip. Depending on the anatomy encountered, progressively systematic maneuvers are then considered to accomplish the desired end result, limiting these maneuvers to the most conservative and predictable unless forced by abnormal anatomy to employ the more aggressive (and consequently less controllable) procedures. They range from minimal surgical weakening of the complete strip to reduce convexity and "break the spring" to interruption of the complete strip by vertical division, either medially or laterally. If, however, triangular refinement of the wide tip can be achieved with transdomal suturing, this technique takes priority.

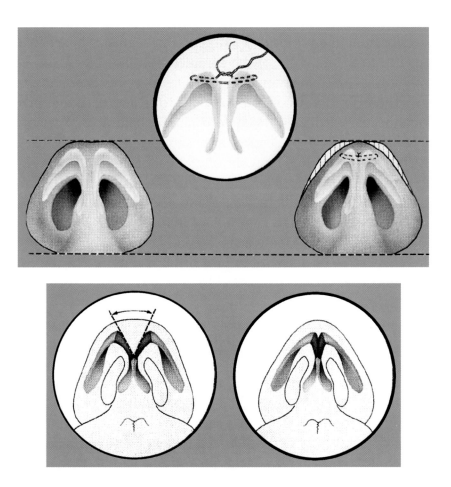

Transdomal suture narrowing is a highly effective alternative maneuver that complements complete strip techniques. A considerable narrowing refinement is possible without interrupting the complete strip integrity, thus ensuring maximal control over healing. Sutures (4-0 PDS is preferred) may be placed to appose the upper intermediate crura (interdomal suture), or the suture may be placed in horizontal mattress fashion through the intermediate and lateral crural contributions to the dome, burying the suture between domes to avoid potential eventual exposure or extrusion (transdomal suture).

Indications include alar cartilages that diverge abnormally, resulting in bifidity. Soft tissue, if abundant, should be removed between the domes. Accuracy in suture placement is critical to avoid asymmetries, but this conservative approach has much to recommend it in the patient with a wide broad tip, thin skin, and weak supporting alar skin sidewalls. Transdomal sutures thus reorient the attitude of imperfect alar cartilage, preserve or improve satisfactory tip support, and may, when deemed appropriate, be positioned to add 2 to 3 mm of stable projection to the tip by recruiting a slight amount of the lateral dome medially. Since 1970 the use of transdomal suture techniques has generated natural, stable, and predictable tip improvements. They are ideal when bifidity and wide domal angles coexist.

Incomplete Interrupted Strip Operations. Profound changes in the shape, attitude, and contour of the alar cartilages (and therefore nasal tip) generally require a calculated alteration in tip support mechanisms, particularly that support related to the integrity of the complete alar cartilage strip. Vertically dividing the complete strip at one or more sites along its lateral crural extent weakens this contribution to tip support, introduces a rotational pivot point from which the alar cartilage is likely to rotate cephalically, invariably results in some reduction in tip projection and support, and totally "breaks the spring" of the horseshoe-like crescent of alar cartilage to effect a significant change in the nasal tip width. These more aggressive procedures are reserved for anatomic situations in which thicker skin and subcutaneous tissue at the tip will be likely to cushion and camouflage minor cartilage offsets or irregularities in healing, when the dome is thick and markedly convex, and in those tips where an increase or decrease in projection is required to improve nasal tip proportions.

Although dramatic changes are possible with interrupted strip techniques, a higher price is extracted in the form of diminishing surgical control over ultimate healing. Lateral division of the complete strip anywhere lateral to the dome totally breaks the spring of the intact cartilage segment, transfers the pivot point to a new location, results in a predictable cephalic tip rotation, and may very well lead to a slight decrease in nasal tip projection. The latter problem may thus have to be compensated for by other means such as suturing the "rim strip" to the caudal edge of the residual lateral remnant of the lateral crus and supporting the medial crura and tip with a cartilaginous strut.

Medial division of the complete strip near the dome allows a medial rotation of the lateral alar wall, thereby further narrowing the tip. Undermining the vestibular skin for 2 to 4 mm medial and lateral to the interrupting incision will allow the medial crura to lie more medial (they may be sutured together in the midline, "stealing" a portion of the lateral crura to increase tip projection), and the lateral crura to advance slightly medialward as well. All edges should be carefully rounded off or blunted since no sharp angles or points occur naturally in the vast majority of normal alar cartilages.

Multiple vertical interrupting cuts may be made through the complete strip to effect medial rotation of the lateral alar walls and tip narrowing. The vestibular skin is not undermined and must remain as an intact sling or support for the multiply divided cartilage remnant. Excessive tip width is converted to a more narrow state as healing contracture pulls medially. Greater risks for asymmetric healing exist with interrupted strip techniques.

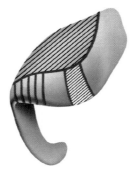

In certain cases in which overprojection of the nasal tip is the consequence of an overdeveloped alar cartilage, medial and lateral division combined with a resection of a calculated lateral segment will effect a lateral rotation of the dome and lateral crus, decreasing the excess projection while maintaining an attenuated tip that retains a moderate degree of strength and integrity. The divided lateral segments may be stabilized and secured by suture apposition with fine 6-0 PDS.

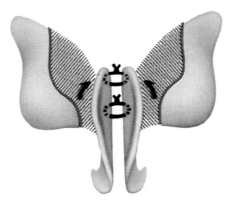

If additional projection by rotating a calculated segment of lateral crus into the medial crus is desired—an uncommonly employed technique—it can be carried out while leaving the vestibular skin intact. Suture apposition of the medial cartilage segments is necessary. The new projecting edges should be blunted by rounding for the same reason stated above (sanding the cut edges with the common Bovie cautery scratch pad is helpful). This approach is reserved for the occasional patient with extremely thick skin, abundant soft tissue, and a wide tip lacking adequate projection.

Commonly tip projection is restored or enhanced by one of the procedures discussed later in the section on adjunctive projection procedures. It is worthy of reemphasis that the interrupted strip techniques are less predictable in their healing and therefore constitute less conservative procedures than complete strip approaches, which are preferred whenever the anatomy will allow.

Dissection and Repositioning

Rarely but significantly, an anatomic situation will be encountered in which the mildly asymmetric or maloriented alar cartilages may assume a new, more desirable shape by simply dissecting the dome and lateral crura free from their soft tissue investments and repositioning them in more normal anatomic beds, creating little or no sculpturing effect. On occasion the lateral crus may lie abnormally low throughout its length along the nostril margin; dissecting it out and transposing the entire lateral crus to a site slightly more cephalad to the nostril rim will effect a more pleasant appearance while conserving alar cartilage tissue. Freeing the alar cartilage from its surrounding soft tissues may indeed allow small but definite knuckles and twists, congenital or traumatic in origin, to straighten out and assume a more natural shape.

An occasional anatomic variant is encountered in which the lateral crura of one or both of the alar cartilages is inwardly concave (instead of an outward convexity) to an extreme, imparting a pinched appearance with an unpleasant asymmetric contour to the tip.

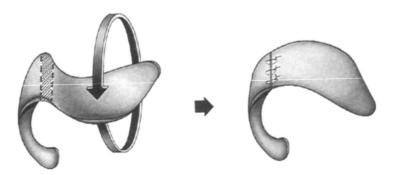

It is possible to significantly improve this condition and restore the appearance to near normal by dissecting the lateral crus completely free from its investing soft tissues, turning it over so that the convexity is now facing outward, and fixing it in place with sutures at the dome area. Exquisitely thin skin is a rule in these patients; therefore no cartilage irregularities or offsets should be created that would become apparent during healing in months to come. Conservative volume reduction of the transposed lateral crural segment may be acceptable if further tip refinement is necessary. Care should be taken to create as little dissection as possible in the surrounding perialar tissues, developing as precise a pocket for the "implant" as possible.

PRINCIPLES OF NASAL TIP PROJECTION

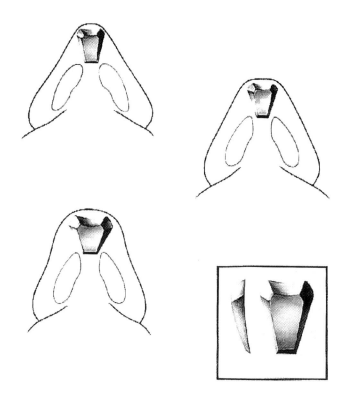

In the course of tip rhinoplasty there is frequently a need to enhance projection of the nasal tip tissues. Asymmetries, projection deficits, contour irregularities, and the frequent demands of revision rhinoplasty all call for implants of varying sizes and shapes. These may consist of stiffening and supportive implants to the columella or alae, tip grafts for refining definition, and projection and cartilage "fillers" for effacing depressions.

Only three tissues are deemed suitable for implanting into the mobile tip commonly subject to trauma—autologous cartilage, fascia, and perichondrium. Without exception allografts are contraindicated in the nasal tip. Particularly since implants are ordinarily placed quite superficially beneath the nasal skin, it is imperative that they be somewhat stiff but not inflexible, that they be well tolerated, and that they may be easily harvested, fabricated, and contoured.

Autologous cartilage and fascia are preferred when nasal tip implants are required. Cartilage harvested from the nasal septum or the external auricle, which represents a marvelous regional storehouse of spare parts for nasal structural reconstitution, persists over the long term after appropriate autografting. Fascia is derived from the supra-auricular temporalis fascia; layering and lamination can increase its bulk for contouring, effacement, and smoothing of irregularities. Postauricular perichondrium serves well for crushing cartilage grafts. On occasion mature scar derived from tissue excess elsewhere in the nose serves well for tip contouring in revision rhinoplasty.

In every rhinoplasty operation, without fail, projection of the nasal tip is either increased, preserved, or diminished. Preservation of the existing projection is the desirable surgical goal if, as is true in the majority of rhinoplasty patients, preoperative projection of the tip is satisfactory. A smaller number of patients will require an increase in the projection of the tip relative to the intended new profile line. A variety of reliable operative methods exist for creating or augmenting tip projection; these techniques will be reviewed in the following discussion. Finally, in a limited number of patients, tip projection will be decreased, either in the intentional reduction of the overprojecting tip or as a consequence of postoperative "tip ptosis" secondary to the excessive sacrifice of tip support mechanisms, a preventable but still common surgical misadventure.

Enhancement of Tip Projection

Fundamental to the techniques for increasing tip projection is the nearly unalterable principle of preserving the original tip support and projection. Further enhancement of tip projection, if desirable, can then be achieved by less adventuresome and risky augmentation techniques (usually autologous cartilage grafts).

Nasal tips that deviate markedly from the accepted range of anatomic norms (an aesthetic judgment of the surgeon) generally demand a more aggressive approach to tip sculpture and realignment. More extensive dissection is usually necessary, critical tip supports are often sacrificed, and projection enhancement techniques assume a more major role to reinforce or reconstruct tip supports and improve projection potential of the new tip.

Indications and mechanisms to enhance projection follow, with an accompanying rationale for the use of each.

Preservation of Existing Projection and Major Tip Supports

Conservative volume reduction of the alar cartilage with preservation of the tip-defining points is a valuable principle here. If the tip support provided by the medial crural footplate attachment to the caudal septum has been interrupted by a complete transfixion incision, permanent suture reattachment is vital to reestablish this important support; in most rhinoplasties no indication exists for detaching the medial crural footplates. Proper taping and splinting of the tip to close the tissue void created at the interface between the upper and lower lateral cartilage will aid in reconstructing this major tip support with favorable scar tissue development.

Improvement of Columellar Support and Thrust

The ultimate projection of the nasal tip may be improved by establishing a supportive platform and upward thrust to the columella. Autologous cartilage graft struts, positioned below and/or between the intermediate and medial crura, are effective in establishing permanent projection. "Plumping" grafts of cartilage fragments introduced into the lower columella through a low lateral columellar incision are quite useful for columellar support in conjunction with effacement of and filling out the acute columellar-labial angle. Cartilage struts should be shaped with a gentle curve to match the anatomy of the curved columella, at times aiding in the creation of a distinct desirable "double break," but should never extend to the apex of the tip skin, lest a visible "tent-pole" appearance develop.

If the medial crural footplates diverge in a widely splayed fashion, further tip support may be gained by resecting intercrural soft tissue and suturing the lower medial crura together, converting a degree of horizontal width to vertical height.

Projection With Cartilage Tip Grafts

In the past two decades greater emphasis has been placed on the value of adding contour and height (and therefore projection) to the nasal tip; pleasant definition of the tip anatomy can be achieved with carefully sculptured and judiciously positioned autologous cartilage grafts from the nasal septum or the external ear; my preference is the thicker nasal septal cartilage.

Since these grafts lie immediately subcutaneously, intimately subjacent to the skin, great care must be taken in their positioning. Exacting "pocket preparation" therefore becomes a basic prerequisite for their use, fashioning a pocket into which the graft will fit as precisely as a hand into a glove. Bilateral marginal incisions, limited to the region of the domes, allow excellent access for securing grafts into precise pockets at the infratip lobule. If desired, suture fixation of the tip graft may be accomplished through an endonasal approach by temporarily skewering the graft(s) with two No. 30 needles followed by fine suture fixation to the intermediate crura.

Carved in triangular, trapezoid, or shieldlike fashion, tip grafts may accentuate favorable tip-defining points and highlights, camouflage infratip lobule asymmetries, and lengthen the infratip lobule and can succeed in creating a more normal appearance to tips with congenital or postsurgical inadequacies. My 25-year experience with the stability and fate of tip cartilage grafts is highly satisfactory. In patients with extremely thin skin it is preferable to use other means of tip projection and contouring.

Cephalic Rotation of the Tip

An actual increase in projection or a significant illusion of increased projection may be produced by techniques designed to result in cephalic rotation of the nasal tip structures. Projection is enhanced by reorienting the attitude of tip structures in a more cephalic direction and stabilizing this reorientation. However, not all tip techniques that result in tip rotation (interrupted strip techniques) automatically create added projection, and in fact the division of the intact complete strip of alar cartilage not uncommonly produces a loss of actual tip projection, both initially and during the healing process.

Illusory Enhancement of Tip Projection

The perceptual illusion of enhanced tip projection may be created in the humped nose by simply reversing the preoperative relationship between the tip and supratip area. Incremental reduction of the cartilaginous dorsum produces a redefinition of the tip-supratip relationship, thus allowing the tip to project 2 to 3 mm forward of the supratip dorsum and ideally lead the remainder of the osseocartilaginous profile when bony hump realignment is accomplished. Satisfactory anatomic tip projection must exist prior to profile realignment to invoke this illusory principle; likewise, all tip support mechanisms must be preserved without fail since even a minute "settling" of the tip may rob it of pleasing projection and definition.

Reorientation of Attitude of Alar Cartilages

In certain patients with broad tips increased vertical height for tip projection may be recruited from the excess transverse or horizontal dimension of the alar cartilage. The classic Goldman tip technique achieves added projection from an elongation of the medial crura by rotating borrowed cartilage from the lateral crus into the medial crus, maintaining this relationship by suture apposition (see p. 1133). This interrupted strip technique can, however, lead to overprojection and collapse of the lateral alar sidewalls in improperly selected patients unless the minor tip support mechanisms (tip skin, soft tissue, alar sidewalls) are sufficiently strong and thick to compensate for the support lost by vertically interrupting the dome areas. In addition, this approach may create a distinct "surgical look" in poorly selected patients, a price too high to be paid for projection enhancement. Consequently, this technique is reserved for those few patients who demonstrate markedly inadequate lobular length, inadequate tip projection, and thick skin and supporting soft tissues and those in whom more conservative tip projection techniques are judged to be inadequate. With the favorable results obtained by cartilage tip grafts combined with complete strip techniques, little need exists in our practice for employing this more radical tip technique that permanently interrupts the residual alar cartilage segment.

In patients with well-developed broad alar cartilages, thin skin and subcutaneous tissues, and wide domal angles, the conversion of horizontal tip width to vertical tip height is more favorably carried out by positioning one or more transdomal mattress sutures through the complete strips developed after bilateral volume reduction of the alar cartilage (see p. 1131). Sutures of 4-0 clear nylon or PDS are used to permanently alter the shape, attitude, and relative projection of the dome (and therefore the tip-defining points), ensuring that the knot comes to rest between the domes, buried as deeply as possible from the tip surface epithelium. The rigid anatomic criteria listed above must be met to ensure a pleasing aesthetic outcome from this transdomal suture technique.

Reduction of Tip Projection

Conditions arise in every active rhinoplasty practice in which the abnormal anatomy demands a calculated and intentional reduction in nasal tip projection (the overprojected nose). After careful analysis of which components of the tip and lobule are responsible for the abnormal projection, an operative plan can be formulated to bring these nasal components into harmony with the rest of the nose and face. Not uncommonly this tip projection reduction can be gained by incrementally sacrificing the major tip supports that ordinarily are religiously preserved during most rhinoplasty procedures. Projection reduction is partially accomplished by a total transfixion incision to interrupt the medial crural footplate–caudal septal attachment support, a generous volume reduction of the cephalic portions of the alar cartilages, and if appropriate, vertical interruption of the residual complete strip to ensure further intentional loss of tip support. Suture reconstitution of the interrupted residual strip follows to restore continuity.

Overabundant tip projection as the consequence of a large nasal spine may suggest reduction (but never removal) of the bony nasal spine and associated overly large caudal cartilaginous septal parts.

PRINCIPLES OF TIP ROTATION

In many patients undergoing rhinoplasty cephalic rotation of the nasal tip complex (alar cartilages, columella, nasal base) assumes major importance in the surgical event, whereas in other individuals the prevention of upward rotation is vital. Although no procedure in aesthetic rhinoplasty may be considered absolute, certain well-defined and reliable principles may be invoked by the thoughtful surgeon to essentially calibrate the degree of tip rotation (or absence thereof). The dynamics of healing play a critical role in tip rotation principles; it is the control of these postoperative healing changes that distinguishes this technique from less elegant procedures. In the past overrotation of the nasal tip created an unhealthy stigma of rhinoplasty, so much so that patients routinely admonish surgeons to avoid "turning up the nose." Unless a major downward inclination of the nasal tip exists, most individuals recognize and prefer the aesthetic advantages of the stronger nose possessed of sufficient length to impart character and suitable proportions to the face, thus avoiding the "operated" look.

The planned degree of tip rotation is dependent on a variety of factors, which often include the:
1. Length of the nose
2. Length of the face
3. Length of the upper lip
4. Facial balance and proportions
5. Patient's aesthetic desires
6. Surgeon's aesthetic judgment

An important distinction must be drawn between tip rotation and tip projection. Although certain tip rotation techniques may result in desirable increases in tip projection, the converse is not true. Tip rotation and projection are in fact complementary to each other, and their proper achievement in individual patients is constantly interrelated. A classic example of this inter-dependent relationship is illustrated by the almost inevitable loss of tip pro-jection when interrupted strip techniques are chosen to enhance cephalic rota-tion; steps must be planned to restore adequate long-term tip projection by one of the several methods recommended.

Finally, distinction must be drawn between true tip rotation and the illusion of tip rotation achieved by contouring cartilage grafts placed in the infratip lobule, columella, and nasolabial angle. Favorable modifications in the tip-lip complex profile area with autologous implants may obviate entirely the need for any actual tip rotation, thus preserving a longer and at times a more desir-able nasal appearance. Reduction of the nasal profile, particularly the supra-tip cartilaginous pyramid, may also impart the illusion of rotation and a shortened nose, but at the expense of a strong and narrow dorsum.

Nasal tip rotation results fundamentally from planned surgical modifications of the alar cartilages, but increments of rotation may also be realized from additional adjunctive procedures on nasal structures adjacent to the alar car-tilages that exert a favorable influence on calibrated tip rotation methods. Shortening of the caudal septum, excision of the caudal aspect of overly long upper lateral cartilages, excision of excess columellar vestibular skin, and sep-tal shortening with a high transfixion incision are regularly employed to en-hance the effects of a planned degree of tip rotation.

Primary Principles and Dynamics of Tip Rotation

Since tip rotation is only one of the many potential objectives desirable in rhinoplasty, decisions regarding rotation must be interrelated with planning for tip volume reduction, alar cartilage thinning or reduction, and modifica-tions in the attitude and angulation of the alar cartilages.

The fundamental principles involved in tip rotation will be considered in general terms and as an overall function of the sculpture/modification of the alar cartilages. The techniques and healing dynamics described are therefore not absolute, but are reliably predictable. The overwhelming majority of tip rotation techniques may be incorporated in an organizational scheme that in-corporates three procedures preserving a complete, intact strip of alar carti-lages and three additional procedures involving interrupted strip techniques. Unique anatomic situations regularly are encountered that require modifi-cations of this scheme to achieve a more refined result, but the fundamen-tal principles elaborated remain a constant. In addition, the thickness and strength of the alar cartilages along with the character of their enveloping soft tissue and skin will dictate to a degree which techniques may be safely and predictably employed in each anatomic situation.

Complete strip techniques are always preferable tip procedures when the nasal anatomy will permit and the goals of the surgical procedure may be met without resorting to the less predictable interrupted strip procedures. Preserving a complete, uninterrupted segment of alar cartilage remnant contributes to a more stable and better supported nasal tip that tends to resist cephalic rotation during healing. In addition, tip projection is ordinarily better preserved with complete strip techniques, and asymmetric healing is less likely as long as equal alar cartilage surgery is carried out bilaterally. By maintaining the attachments of the medial and lateral crura intact the cephalic linear scar contracture to be anticipated from the skeletal tissue void resulting from the volume reduction of the alar cartilage is successfully resisted, and minimal or controlled tip rotation results.

Interrupted strip techniques combined with volume reduction of overly large alar cartilages tend to result in a more substantial degree of cephalic tip rotation. Once the complete strip of residual alar cartilage is divided (interrupted), a relative instability of the nasal tip results, upon which the forces of upward scar contraction create a variable degree of cephalic rotation, underscoring the principle that during scar contracture tissues are generally moved from areas of instability (in this case the unstable nasal tip cartilages) toward areas of stability (the bony-cartilaginous nasal pyramid).

Complete Strip Techniques

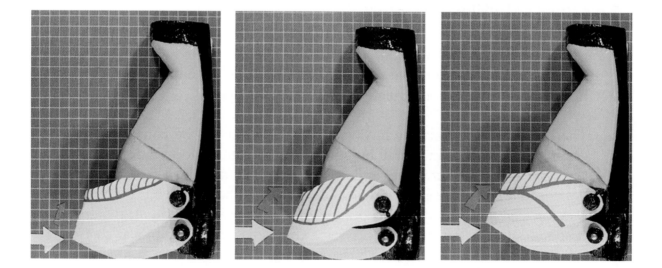

Volume reduction of the alar cartilage results in a tissue deficit of minimal, moderate, or maximal proportions, depending on the degree of cartilage removal indicated or desirable. Essentially no cephalic tip rotation results from minimal volume reduction alone, whereas the greater tissue void resulting from moderate to maximal volume reduction tends to create progressively greater degrees of minimal tip rotation. Indeed, preservation of the complete strip is regularly indicated and preferred to resist the forces of upward rotation when the preoperative nasal length is to be maintained. Complete strip techniques find further favor with surgeons wishing to preserve the normal anatomy of the nasal tip and avoid the possibilities of alar retraction, notching, and collapse, complications far more likely when interrupted strips are employed inappropriately. Substantial planned tip rotation when complete strip techniques are employed therefore depends on the addition of adjunctive procedures to achieve cephalic elevation of the tip complex.

Interrupted Strip Techniques

When the integrity and spring of the alar cartilage is broken, cephalic rotation is fostered by virtue of upward scar contracture forces acting inexorably on alar cartilage segments that are now more flail and less well supported. These techniques are particularly useful when the attitude of the alar cartilages is one of a profound downward inclination, imparting a depressed or snarl-like appearance to the nose. Caution must be constantly exercised in the use of interrupted strips in patients with thin skin and/or more delicate cartilages since the absence of good tip supporting structures sets the stage for loss of projection, alar collapse, notching, pinching, and asymmetry.

Lateral Interrupted Techniques. In anatomic situations where cephalic rotation is desirable and the anatomy of the bridge between the medial and lateral crus (the "dome") is aesthetically pleasing, lateral interruption of the residual complete strip possesses virtues. Avoiding interruption of the strip medially fosters symmetric healing and reduces the likelihood of uneven tip-defining points becoming evident months after surgery. The lateral interruption approach allows the reduced alar cartilage to be pulled moderately upward by scar tissue during healing, but because the dividing cut is sited more laterally and therefore more deeply in the soft tissues of the tip, notching, pinching, and other asymmetries are essentially prevented. By incising only through the cartilage and preserving intact the medial perichondrium and vestibular skin bridge, less projection is lost than with other interrupted strip techniques. If modification of the dome is necessary, transdomal suture techniques to narrow, refine, and even slightly project the tip may be favorably combined with lateral interruption.

Medial Interrupted Techniques. Many different methods of interruption of the residual complete strip at or near the dome have been described; each will predictably lead to some degree of cephalic rotation, and the complete strip is converted to two or more segments of flail cartilage. Planned rotation with this approach is reserved for patients with thicker skin and supporting structures to minimize undesirable consequences of asymmetric healing and even overrotation. Elevation of the medial nostril margin is more common with medial strip interruption, an onerous stigma of nasal surgery.

This method of tip refinement is useful in more extreme anatomic situations to normalize tip projection when either significant overprojection or undesirable lack of projection is encountered. In the former situation excess alar cartilage is resected and the dome architecture reestablished with fine permanent sutures, whereas in the latter instance tip height may be enhanced by elongating the length of the medial crura with techniques that borrow cartilage from the lateral crus in a "leaf-of-book" manner.

It is worthy of reemphasis that medial interrupted techniques almost always result in a moderate to major loss of tip projection, requiring adjunctive procedures to restore or augment tip projection to avoid tip ptosis.

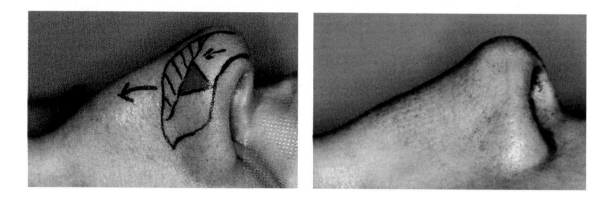

Lateral Interrupted Techniques With Suture Rotation. An ideal method for significant tip rotation would combine lateral strip interruption to preserve the integrity of the strip medially with a calibrated triangular excision of cartilage laterally and stabilization with suture fixation. The degree of rotation realized here is controllable by the surgeon, essentially eliminates most of the undesirable sequelae of interrupted strip techniques, and changes in a predictable and permanent way the attitude of the alar cartilages. The suture fixation helps to diminish loss of tip support inherent in most interrupted strip techniques. In individuals with thin or moderately thin skin with more delicate cartilages, this method is highly predictable and desirable.

As with rotation concepts discussed above with complete strip techniques, the same adjunctive techniques for enhancing tip rotation may be useful to combine with interrupted strip techniques. Overrotation, however, must be religiously avoided since the restoration of this undesirable postoperative situation to a normal appearance is often difficult or impossible.

Adjunctive Techniques

Profound tip rotation changes rely on the alar cartilage modifying techniques described above. Predictable rotation may be enhanced or may be accomplished independently by modifying nasal anatomic components (other than the alar cartilages). Indeed, when complete strip techniques are indicated, rotation depends primarily on these adjunctive methods, individually or combined. Contouring the infratip lobule, columella, and nasolabial angle with cartilage grafts significantly enhances the surgeon's ability to transform an unbalanced nose into the illusion of better length.

Major Adjuncts

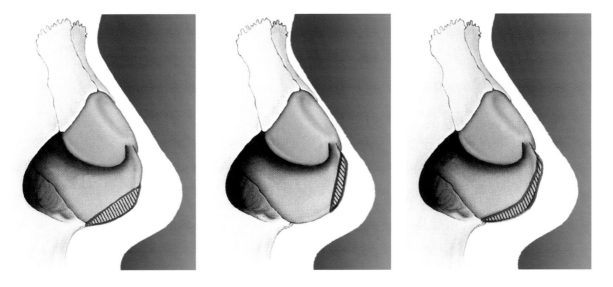

Caudal Septal Shortening. Modification of the caudal septum by resection of geometric triangles based upward will shorten the middle segment of the nose and provide room for the infratip lobule, in particular, to be lifted upward during healing. Ideally, the medial crural footplates should be left attached to the inferior caudal septum during this modification to maintain this all-important major tip support mechanism intact. Caudal septum resection is particularly useful if the septum is judged to be overlong or overdeveloped, a common circumstance in certain types of overprojected noses. A decided limit exists to the degree of rotation possible by caudal septal reduction, however, since overaggressive sacrifice of the caudal septum can result in an almost opposite effect, dropping or ptosis of the nasal tip.

If during this maneuver the medial crural footplates are detached from the caudal septum to repair a caudal subluxation or similar abnormality, they should be resutured into position to reestablish this important tip support. Excess vestibular skin or mucosa apparent after septal shortening is best excised to avoid redundancy.

Upper Lateral Cartilage Shortening. Once tip rotation is completed by whatever primary means has been selected, the caudal and medial ends of the upper lateral cartilages should be directly inspected for redundancy and excessive length. Commonly in long noses the caudal margins project inappropriately into the nasal airway after tip rotation, requiring shortening of the offending inferior margin. Redundant "scrolls" of the upper lateral interfere with the space needed to adequately effect upward tip rotation and may limit desirable tip definition procedures. Conservative excision corrects these problems.

High Septal Transfixion With Septal Shortening. When the anatomy of the tip, infratip lobule, and related structures is ideal and the surgeon wishes to maintain its preoperative condition without alteration, predictable tip rotation results from the vertical excision of a calibrated triangle of septal cartilage (and associated mucoperichondrium) that is removed through a high transfixion incision. Suture repair effects a rotational shortening of the nose while preserving the medial crural and membranous columellar attachments to the caudal septum.

Reduction of Convex Caudal Medial Crura. When the caudal aspect of the medial and intermediate crura is overly convex, a "hanging" appearance to the infratip lobule and columella imparts an unaesthetic appearance to the nasal profile as well as the frontal appearance of the tip. An apparently overlong nose results. In this anatomic variant the medial crura are ordinarily overdeveloped in their vertical dimension as well as appearing overly convex, spoiling the pleasing desirable double-break contour of the columella. Delivery and reduction contouring of the caudal margins of the medial and intermediate crura through lateral paracolumellar incisions restores proper profile and frontal configuration without sacrificing tip support, thereby resulting in a desirable lifting rotation of the infratip lobule portion of the nasal tip.

Minor Adjuncts

Complete transfixion incision frees the nasal tip from the cartilaginous pyramid and assists the upward rotation influences resulting from major rotation maneuvers described previously.

Wide skin sleeve undermining creates a broader expanse of subcutaneous scar tissue formation, thereby enhancing the degree of cephalic rotation resulting from healing scar contracture. In the vast majority of rhinoplasty procedures only sufficient skin should be elevated to gain access to the nasal hump.

Excision of excessive vestibular skin aids in proper splinting of the nasal structures in a new, more cephalic position after major upward rotation techniques have been carried out. Accurate edge-to-edge suture apposition of the trimmed vestibular skin on either side of a partial or complete transfixion incision acts much like an "internal splint" in stabilizing the tip during healing in its new upward attitude. Failure to eliminate redundant skin may result in partial nostril airway obstruction as well as reduction in the degree of tip rotation.

Proper tip taping affords appropriate external splinting to stabilize the newly rotated tip. Paper tape compression of the entire tip and infratip lobule is preferred.

Division of the depressor septi muscle, which imparts a hypermobility to the nasal tip, eliminates a strong mechanism acting against the techniques employed to create planned tip rotation. Failure to recognize this potential destroyer of cephalic rotation reduces the effectiveness of the major techniques for rotation.

Illusory Rotation Concepts

Much of sophisticated rhinoplasty surgery involves the use of illusion to result in improved balance and proportion. If the nasal length (from nasion to the tip-defining points) is in good proportion and further cephalic tip rotation is likely to result in an overly short nose, illusions of rotation result from contouring changes created at the columellar-tip junction or by further lowering of the supratip cartilaginous profile. Cartilaginous grafts placed in the columella, nasolabial angle, and even the infratip lobule region soften and open a more acute nasolabial junction and improve the appearance of the nose as well as the upper lip. Although the nose maintains its preoperative length, improved facial proportions and angle manipulation by cartilage grafting impart a more favorable appearance to the midface by resulting in the illusion of tip rotation and nasal shortening.

Autologous cartilage grafts harvested from the septum or external ear, implanted through lateral paracolumellar incisions, may be contoured to impart a double-break appearance to the columellar configuration, augment the lower one half of the columella, or "plump" the recessed or acute nasolabial to a more favorable obtuse alignment. Plumping grafts should be generously placed to maintain long-term improvement. Firm cartilage struts stabilized between the medial crura, carved in a slightly curved manner, assist predictably in contouring the columella while providing stabilization to tip support and projection.

Reduction of the cartilaginous profile to a level below that of the tip-defining points results uniformly in the illusion of nasal shortening and cephalic rotation, even though no true rotation has occurred. If projection of the nasal tip is sufficient to allow this supratip lowering without resulting in a nose too small for the surrounding features, this illusory effort will allow the surgeon to avoid unwanted shortening by true tip rotation procedures in noses of ideal preoperative length.

SUMMARY: DECISION MAKING IN SURGICAL APPROACHES TO THE NASAL TIP

Surgical approaches to the nasal tip should then be based on the existing nasal tip anatomy and the intended change in the attitude, shape, and permanent support of structures of the nasal tip. No single approach will uniformly suffice for the countless varieties of anatomic variants encountered. Thus surgical approach options must be available and chosen to provide adequate and complete access and exposure to the structures and nasal components to be modified and to result in the least traumatic exposure of the tip elements to diminish scarring and the potential for eccentric healing. The paired alar cartilages essentially create a bilateral system in which predictable and symmetric healing becomes critical to natural pleasing results. Atraumatic approaches and techniques that result in more favorable control of the healing process are clearly beneficial and preferable.

Two broad categories of nasal tip approaches exist: nondelivery and delivery approaches. Nondelivery approaches consist of the cartilage-splitting (transcartilaginous) approach and its closely related procedure, the retrograde approach. Nondelivery approaches create little trauma (and minimal intraoperative edema), leave undisturbed the caudal portion of the alar cartilages and their investing soft tissue attachments, and heal more rapidly with less swelling in the early postoperative period. Critical millimeter by millimeter judgments regarding tip-supratip relationships are thus more easily determined with those tissue-sparing approaches, and the potential complication of asymmetric healing is rendered less likely.

Delivery approaches consist of exposure and delivery of the alar cartilages as chondrocutaneous flaps via intercartilaginous and marginal incisions and the open (external) approach through transcolumellar, paracolumellar, and marginal incisions. Delivery approaches provide increased access to and exposure of the tip structures at the expense of more tissue dissection and temporary anatomic alterations. More intraoperative as well as postoperative edema and swelling inevitably result with less rapid healing. Over the long term (several years) there probably is little difference in the ultimate healing result of any approach. Whenever more extensive tissue dissection is employed in rhinoplasty, however, more potential exists for eccentric or asymmetric healing that can render an otherwise well-performed procedure less than ideal.

Given these known anatomic facts and principles, the surgeon generally can intelligently select an individual approach to the nasal tip most favorable to each patient. When subtle changes are planned in already symmetric tips, it makes clear sense to employ atraumatic nondelivery approaches. In patients with more severe deformities and departures from normal anatomy, delivery approaches possess the virtues of greater exposure for accurate analysis and more extensive repair. A further advantage of the open approach consists of its retention of preexisting preoperative tip support since intercartilaginous and transfixion incisions are not required in most cases.

DECISION MAKING IN TIP SURGERY

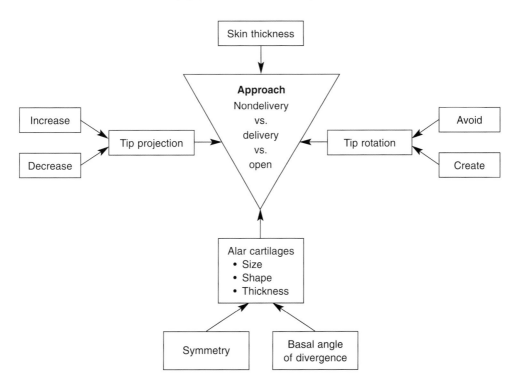

Additional important anatomic factors weigh heavily on the decision for tip approach selection. Each will influence the choice of the most favorably and anatomically judicious approach to effect tip sculpturing and refinement.

BIBLIOGRAPHY

1. Constantian MB. A model for planning rhinoplasty. Plast Reconstr Surg 79:472, 1987.
2. Daniel RK. The nasal tip: Anatomy and aesthetics. Plast Reconstr Surg 89:216, 1992.
3. Gunter JP. Tip rhinoplasty: A personal approach. Facial Plast Surg 4:263, 1987.
4. Sheen JH, Sheen AP. Aesthetic Rhinoplasty, 2nd ed. St. Louis: Quality Medical Publishing, 1998 (reprint of 1987 ed.).
5. Tardy ME. Rhinoplasty: The art and the science. Philadelphia: WB Saunders, 1997.
6. Tardy ME. Aesthetic rhinoplasty. In Bailey et al, eds. Head and Neck Surgery: Otolaryngology. Philadelphia: JB Lippincott, 1993.
7. Tardy ME, Brown RJ. Surgical Anatomy of the Nose. New York: Raven Press, 1990.
8. Tardy ME, Schwartz M. The evolution of the rhinoplasty outcome. In Daniel RK, ed. Rhinoplasty. New York: Little, Brown, 1993.
9. Tardy ME, Patt BS, Walter MA. Transdomal suture refinement of the nasal tip: Long-term outcomes. Facial Plast Surg 9:275, 1993.
10. Toriumi DM, Tardy ME. Cartilage suturing techniques for correction of nasal tip deformities. Operative Tech Otolaryngol Head Neck Surg 6:265, 1995.
11. Toriumi DM. Vascular anatomy of the nose and the external rhinoplasty approach. Arch Otolaryngol Head Neck Surg 122:24, 1996.

65

Rohrich's Approach

Rod J. Rohrich, M.D.

*R*hinoplasty is one of the most difficult and challenging operations in cosmetic surgery. The difference between a good and poor result often is measured in millimeters, leaving little room for error. The initial procedure is critical since tissues are virginal and undistorted by surgical intervention. That is why precise nasal analysis and careful preoperative planning are so crucial to a well-executed procedure. For me, excellence in rhinoplasty is an ongoing learning process based on critical analysis of my long-term results and continuing feedback from my colleagues. The goal is to consistently produce reliable, long-lasting, natural results that meet functional and aesthetic expectations. The open rhinoplasty approach has enabled me to achieve that standard. I have been a proponent of the open rhinoplasty technique for the past 15 years because it provides unparalleled exposure for accurate anatomic diagnosis and systematic technical execution.

Open Rhinoplasty Approach Rationale

Distinct Advantages
Binocular visualization
Evaluation of complete deformity
  without distortion
Precise diagnosis and correction of
  deformities
Allows use of both hands
More options with original tissues and
  cartilage grafts
Direct control of bleeding with
  electrocautery
Suture stabilization of grafts (invisible
  and visible)

Potential Disadvantages
External nasal incision
  (transcolumellar scar)
Prolonged operative time
Protracted nasal tip edema
Columellar incision separation
Delayed wound healing

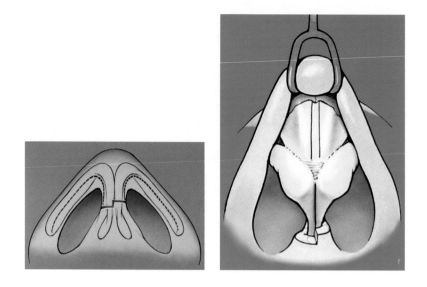

The full and undistorted exposure of the nasal framework afforded by the external approach has allowed me to obtain excellent aesthetic and functional results in patients with primary nasal deformities. It permits a binocular view of the framework so that it can be reliably and consistently modified. The major objection to the open rhinoplasty approach is the transcolumellar scar, but my patients have not found it to be objectionable. In my experience other potential disadvantages commonly cited, such as wound separation, prolonged operative time, prolonged tip edema, and delayed secondary healing, have not presented a problem.

THE CONSULTATION

Success in rhinoplasty is dependent on more than excellent technique. Good communication is crucial for understanding patient expectations and defining realistic goals. The emotional stability of the patient greatly influences the doctor/patient relationship. The initial interview serves to determine if a patient is a candidate for rhinoplasty, both physically and psychologically. At this time I encourage my patients to explain their concerns and define their expectations so that I can assess if they can realistically be achieved. Patients are asked to list specific complaints concerning nasal appearance and function and to rank problems in order of importance. It is helpful to ask the patient, "If you had only one problem that could be corrected, what would it be?" This "one thing" is then recorded verbatim in the patient's notes. It is important to learn to differentiate between healthy and unhealthy motivations for seeking rhinoplasty. Poor results are often a reflection of emotional dissatisfaction rather than technical failure. Therefore, when faced with a patient who focuses on a minor or imperceptible problem or one who is unhappy or angry with a previous surgeon, it is often wise not to proceed with surgery.

Specific nasal problems such as asymmetry, tip deformity, supratip deformity, dorsum irregularity, and septal perforation are pointed out to the patient and discussed. The patient needs to understand the proposed surgical plan and the potential sequelae. Complications are fully outlined and disclosed before obtaining an informed consent for rhinoplasty and any other indicated procedures such as rib or ear graft harvesting (see Chapter 5). Photographs demonstrate problems that will persist postoperatively or are inevitable consequences of the procedure, such as notches, grooves, and irregularities. Facial disproportions are pointed out to the patient with an explanation that facial asymmetry will not be corrected by the surgery. I personally explain to all patients what is involved in postoperative care and provide specific preoperative and postoperative instruction sheets at the time of the initial consultation. I telephone my rhinoplasty patients the evening after their surgery and see them 5 to 7 days later in the office. Patients are then examined 3 and 6 weeks and 3, 6, and 12 months after surgery and annually thereafter.

Meticulous documentation of the nasal history and anatomic findings is essential. A comprehensive nasal history helps to determine whether a patient is medically and physically able to undergo rhinoplasty. A systematic anatomic examination is also key. The surface anatomy of the nose directly reflects the underlying framework and is carefully evaluated; nasal skin thickness and texture have an effect on the rhinoplasty outcome. The soft tissue envelope is inspected to evaluate its overall condition, and the thickness of the nasal tip skin is assessed. The internal nasal examination confirms the presence of any existing functional deformity.

Systematic Nasal Analysis

Nasofrontal angle position	Alae
Bony pyramid	Width
Upper lateral cartilages	Collapse
Supratip area	Retraction
Nasal tip	Alar-columellar relationship
Projection	Columellar-labial angle
Rotation	Nasal examination
Symmetry	Internal nasal valves
Position of tip-defining points	Septum
	Turbinates

Additional documentation is provided by standardized photographic views taken preoperatively that can be compared to the postoperative views. Analysis of the patient's nasal/facial photographs is essential to rhinoplasty planning as well as for "before" and "after" documentation for medicolegal purposes. A thorough understanding of an individual patient's nasal/facial proportions is absolutely prerequisite to successful rhinoplasty. Facial proportions must always be considered since the nose is a prominent component of the overall facial characteristics. These photographs help identify non-ideal nasal/facial anatomic lines and landmarks. Then computer images are made to compare these photographic lines and landmarks with the ideal that the surgical plan is designed to achieve. An operative plan is then outlined on the rhinoplasty worksheet (see Chapter 4) and taken to the operating room with the patient's photographs and computer images.

Computer imaging has been a useful adjunct to my rhinoplasty practice for the past 8 years. It is especially helpful for the difficult secondary rhinoplasty patient. It allows me to simulate the nasal changes seen after rhinoplasty and enables the patient to visualize the projected surgical results prior to surgery. It also serves to give the patient an active role in determining what aesthetic goal is ideal and what surgical results are possible. For me, it is another means of building a bond with the patient and enhancing communication. It also helps me identify potential "red flag" patients. If the patient is unhappy with the imaging projections or requests something that is not possible or not aesthetically pleasing or proportional, I do not operate!

OPERATIVE TECHNIQUE
Anesthesia and Preoperative Management

Head placement is essential to maximize comfort and control. Since I am left-handed the patient's head is placed on the left side of the operating room table and slightly over the head of the operating room bed to hyperextend the neck and therefore minimize any excessive neck flexion for the surgeon as well as the patient.

I prefer to use general anesthesia. Following induction of general anesthesia with endotracheal intubation I use a solution of 10 ml of 1% lidocaine with 1:100,000 epinephrine to infiltrate the soft tissue envelope as well as the intranasal mucosa (Table 65-1). Injection begins posteriorly in the nasal septal mucosa at a submucoperichondrial plane, proceeding in a posterior to anterior fashion, and includes the mucosa along the entire vertical height of the septum. Next the soft tissue envelope is infiltrated. Care is taken to infiltrate evenly.

Overview of Operative Technique Sequence

Anesthesia
Incisions (transcolumellar)
Skin elevation/dissection of lower lateral cartilage/upper lateral cartilage
Intraoperative diagnosis
Assess tip projection
    Component dorsal reduction/augmentation
    Septal and/or turbinate surgery (if indicated)
Cephalic trim of lower lateral cartilage (when indicated)
    Establish final tip projection (suture technique)
Final inspection/irrigation
Osteotomies
Wound closure
    Depressor septi muscle transposition (if indicated)
Alar base surgery
    Splints and dressing

Table 65-1. Location/Volume Distribution of 1% Lidocaine With 1:100,000 epinephrine

Location	Amount (ml)
Vestibules/aperture	2
Dorsum	1
Lateral walls	2
Tip/columella	2
Distal septum	2
Inferior turbinates	1
	10

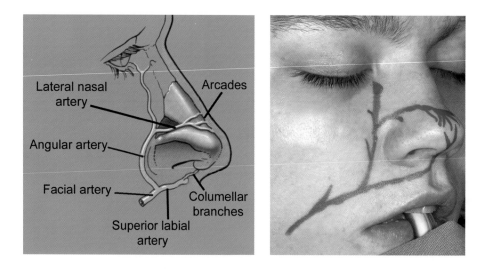

Particular attention is paid to highly vascular anatomic subunits, including the midcolumella, lateral nasal walls and dorsum, nasal tip, alar base, and intranasally along the caudal margin of the lower lateral cartilages. The anterior head of the inferior turbinate is injected if an inferior turbinoplasty is anticipated.

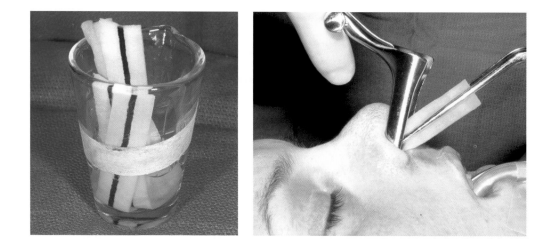

After the local anesthetic infiltration is completed, oxymetazoline-soaked cottonoid pledgets are placed into the nose. One drop of methylene blue is placed into the solution to visually differentiate it from the local anesthetic. Three pledgets are placed on each side along the middle turbinate, inferomedial septum, and superior nasal vault. Vasoconstriction of these areas will provide maximal intranasal visual exposure. Since the inferomedial septum houses the sphenopalatine vessels, vasoconstriction is especially important in this area. I prefer oxymetazoline as a vasoconstrictive agent to cocaine.

Equivalent mucosal shrinkage is achieved without the use of a controlled substance. Engorgement of the nasal mucosa or a significant septal spur obscures visualization of the intranasal vault. The pledgets should be placed prior to local anesthetic infiltration.

I place a similar throat pack into the oropharynx to minimize intragastric bleeding, which contributes to postoperative nausea and vomiting. In addition, it prevents blood from collecting at the endolarynx, which can cause laryngeal irritation with coughing or laryngospasm. The stomach is suctioned using an endogastric tube prior to extubation.

Stair-Step Transcolumellar Incision and Approach

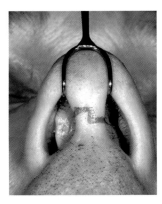

An incision is made at the narrowest part of the columella, generally near its midportion. This is done superficially to prevent injury to the underlying medial crura. A broken-line incision (I prefer a stair-step incision) is used to camouflage the scar, to provide landmarks for accurate closure, and to prevent linear scar contracture.

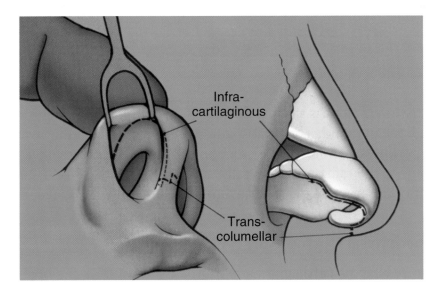

The incision is continued intranasally via an infracartilaginous incision, which approximates the caudal border of the medial crura. This incision is continued toward the apex of the middle crus. A separate incision is begun laterally in the vestibule along the caudal margin of the lateral crus of the lower lateral cartilage.

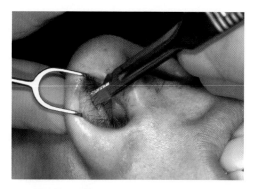

The caudal margin of the lateral crus is demonstrated by everting the ala using digital pressure externally against a double-pronged skin hook placed within the alar rim. The inferior border is visibly evident using this maneuver or can be palpated using the back of the scalpel handle. The incision is extended in a lateral to medial direction, staying along the caudal cartilage margin. The two incisions are connected at the middle crus region.

Skin Envelope Dissection

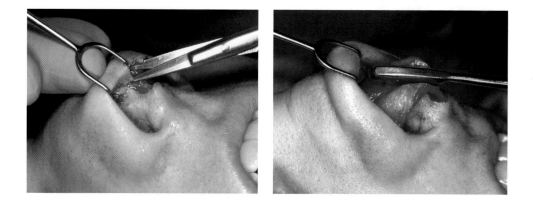

The soft tissue envelope is sharply elevated in a submusculoaponeurotic plane up to the bony pyramid. The periosteum is sharply incised and elevated with a Joseph periosteal elevator and dissection continued superiorly in a subperiosteal plane to the radix area. Laterally, subperiosteal dissection is limited to the extent necessary to allow for bony hump reduction if indicated.

Component Nasal Dorsum Surgery

I prefer to reduce the cartilaginous septum after separating the upper lateral cartilage and before performing the bony dorsum reduction. The cartilaginous dorsum is reduced initially as a separate component by lowering the septum and upper lateral cartilages in an extramucosal manner. It is important to maintain as much periosteal attachment of the bony sidewall as possible since it provides significant external support for the nasal pyramid following osteotomy.

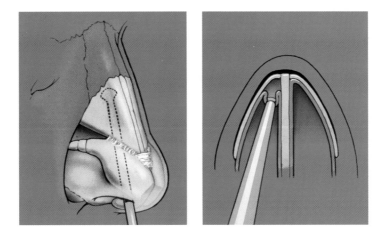

An extramucosal approach is ensured by initially creating submucosal tunnels via the dorsal septal approach and proceeding beneath the osseocartilaginous roof prior to modification of the bony dorsum. This minimizes late scarring with subsequent internal nasal valve dysfunction in addition to providing a closed space for safe placement of spreader or dorsal grafts.

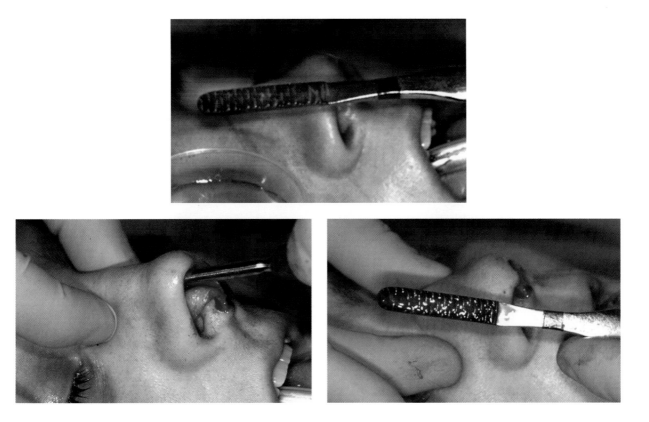

Dorsal bony humps are managed according to their size. In general, reduction of small-to-medium dorsal humps (<5 mm) is managed by simple rasping. Rasping should be performed using short strokes with the nondominant index finger and thumb for maximal control. Rasping is done at an oblique angle to prevent mechanical avulsion of the upper lateral cartilage. I prefer to use a sharp down-biting Forman diamond rasp. The superior edge of the upper lateral cartilage that projects under the nasal bone may require trimming to avoid lateral fullness following rasping.

Large dorsal bony humps (>5 mm) are expediently managed using sharp resection with a guarded osteotome. The sharp, guarded osteotome is placed at the desired level along the caudal margin of the bony pyramid and carefully driven to a predetermined point superiorly.

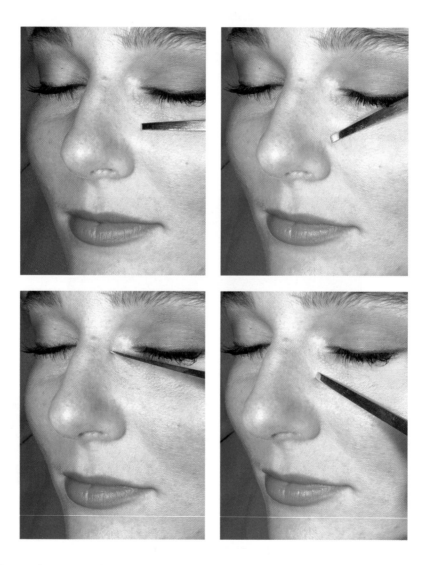

Large bony hump reductions with a significant open-roof deformity require either a dorsal onlay graft if the nasal base is normal or, more commonly, a lateral percutaneous osteotomy to close the open dorsum. The skin envelope is replaced and a three-point test performed. The newly contoured nasal dorsum is moistened to allow a finger to glide smoothly across the skin.

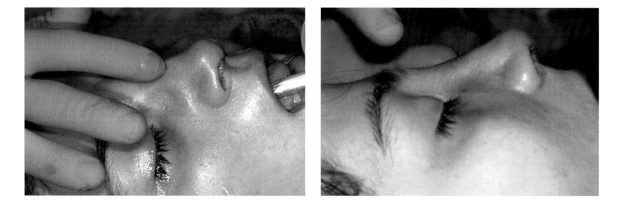

The midsagittal dorsum is palpated along its length and on either lateral side to determine if the nasal dorsum is smooth and straight.

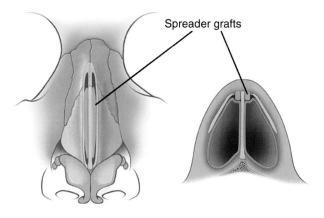

After the dorsal septum is trimmed to its desired height, if the lateral dorsal aesthetic lines are too narrow or the middle vault has an inverted V deformity, spreader grafts are indicated. The mucoperichondrium is elevated 4 to 6 mm from the dorsal septal edge bilaterally. The mucoperiosteum is also elevated from the undersurface of the nasal bones medially and from the perpendicular plate of the ethmoid. Septal cartilage grafts are preferred and are contoured to measure 25 to 30 mm in length and 3 mm in width. Spreader grafts are placed either unilaterally or bilaterally, depending on the dorsal problem.

The dorsal cephalic edges of the grafts are resected obliquely to allow them to be seated under the bony dorsum. The grafts are placed and sutured to the dorsal septum with two through-and-through horizontal mattress sutures of 5-0 PDS. If lengthening of the nose is desired, the caudal ends of the grafts are left long to extend past the septal angle. However, if lengthening is not desired, the grafts should end at the level of the septal angle. The spreader grafts can also be placed higher (visible) or lower (invisible) along the dorsal septum, depending on the clinical situation. Final dorsal trimming is carried out after the osteotomies are performed to infracture the nasal bones.

Septal Reconstruction/Cartilage Graft Harvest

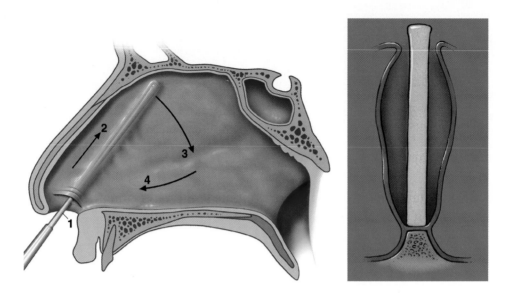

If septal cartilage harvest or septal reconstruction is indicated, the interdomal suspensory ligament is incised to expose the anterior septal angle. Starting at the anterior septal angle, a sharp No. 15 scalpel is used to incise through the perichondrium, and a Cottle elevator is placed under it. Bilateral subperichondrial superior tunnels are made with the Cottle elevator, and then the upper lateral cartilages are separated from the septum with a No. 15 blade. The perichondrium is then elevated toward the floor of the nose to the junction of the septum and the maxillary crest with the Cottle elevator. The elevation is extended posteriorly along the crest to the perpendicular plate of the ethmoid. The mucoperichondrium is elevated off the rest of the nasal septum and the perpendicular plate. This is done bilaterally using the Cottle elevator. With an angled Cottle elevator the thin perpendicular plate of the ethmoid is fractured from the posterior end of the dorsal incision down to the end of the separation of the septal cartilage from the maxillary crest.

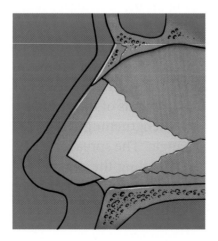

Only the amount of septal cartilage and perpendicular plate needed for the graft or that which is obstructing the nasal cavity is removed, leaving at least a 10 mm L-shaped strut for support of the lower nasal vault.

The excised cartilage is placed in a saline-moistened gauze sponge. Ideally, no mucosal tears are created, avoiding the need for repair and potential septal perforation. The opposing mucoperichondrial flaps can be reapproximated using an absorbable quilting suture (5-0 chromic or a PC-3 suture, Ethicon, Inc., Somerville, N.J.) or by placement of intranasal Doyle splints at the time of nasal closure.

Inferior Submucosal Turbinoplasty

A turbinoplasty is performed in patients with symptomatic obstructive hypertrophic inferior turbinates unresponsive to medical management (see Chapter 36). The previously placed cottonoid pledgets are removed. A pinpoint electrocautery is used to incise along the inferior margin of the turbinate down to conchal bone.

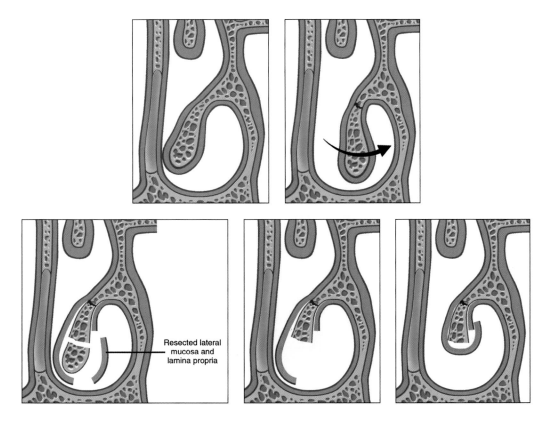

Resected lateral mucosa and lamina propria

A medial mucoperiosteal flap is elevated with a Cottle elevator to expose the desired amount of turbinate to be resected. Following sharp resection of the conchal bone the mucoperiosteal flap is laid back down, taking care to cover the cut edge of the turbinate. Failure to cover the cut edge of conchal bone may lead to postoperative crusting and/or epistaxis. No sutures are necessary for closure since the mucoperiosteal flap will self-adhere to the remaining underlying bone.

Cephalic Trim

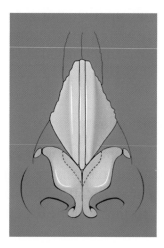

Only when the domes are bulbous or boxy, causing paradomal fullness, is a cephalic trim indicated. The cephalic portion of the middle and lateral crura of the lower lateral cartilage is modified leaving at least a 5 mm rim strip. Calipers accurately demarcate the planned incision. Excised lower lateral cartilage is used for tip or alar grafting when indicated.

Nasal Tip Suture Techniques/Grafting

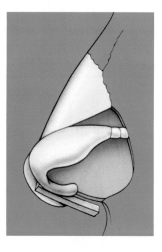

A graduated approach to nasal tip surgery involves the use of columellar struts, suture techniques, and tip grafts. An intercrural columellar strut is used either to maintain or to increase tip projection. A floating strut is usually preferred and placed between the medial crura 2 to 3 mm in front of the nasal spine. The struts are secured at the junction of the medial crura with the middle crura using a 5-0 clear PDS.

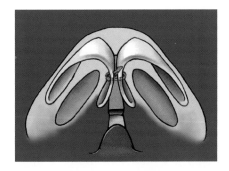

Four primary suture techniques are commonly used. Medial crural suture techniques stabilize the columellar strut between or in front of the medial crura. A columellar strut is fashioned from a septal cartilage graft to measure approximately 4 × 25 mm. With upward traction of a hook in each vestibular apex a tunnel or pocket is dissected in the soft tissue between the medial crura toward the nasal spine, leaving a soft tissue pad between the base of the pocket and the nasal spine. The columellar strut is placed in the pocket, and with the tip-defining points held at the same level under slight tension, a 25-gauge needle is placed through the feet of the medial crura and the columellar strut to stabilize the strut for suturing. A 5-0 PDS suture is used to stabilize the medial crura to the columellar strut. Two additional superior sutures are placed to stabilize and unify the tip complex. The sutures are placed so that the medial portions of the domes are sutured to the columellar strut. The strut is then trimmed to its desired shape to alter or refine the infratip lobular area.

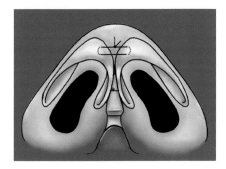

Interdomal sutures can increase infratip-columellar projection and definition or further increase tip projection. A simple 5-0 PDS suture is placed through the medial walls of the domes and tied to narrow the interdomal distance.

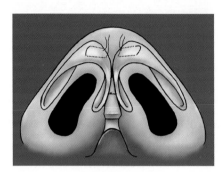

Transdomal sutures control dome asymmetry. A 5-0 PDS horizontal mattress suture is placed from the medial surface of the dome through the lateral surface, staying beneath the vestibular skin. It is passed back from lateral to medial. A double surgeon's knot is placed in the suture and tightened until the desired angulation of the dome is achieved. If narrowing of the distance between the tip-defining points is required, one end of the suture is cut short and the other left approximately 1 inch in length. The same procedure is performed on the opposite side, leaving one end of the suture long.

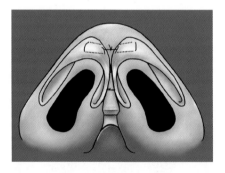

The long end is tied to the remaining suture end on the opposite side. The knot is tightened until the desired distance exists between the tip-defining points and then tied. This is a spanning suture to prevent alar notching and should be used primarily in thicker skinned patients.

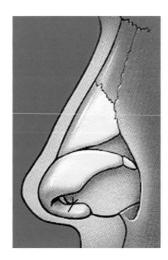

Finally, tip rotation is altered using intercrural septal sutures. This is the only instance in which a 5-0 clear nylon spanning suture is required for permanency.

Only if adequate tip projection, definition, or symmetry cannot be obtained using the above procedures are visible tip grafts used. They are used infrequently in primary rhinoplasty since visible grafts over the long term can reabsorb and become asymmetric and sharply angulated, necessitating revision in up to 30% of cases.

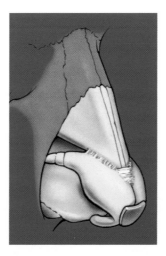

The infralobular graft primarily increases infratip lobular definition and tip projection. These grafts are variably shaped, depending on the nasal tip anatomy and requirements, but they must have smooth, tapered edges. A shield-shaped graft is cut from the septal cartilage graft so that the upper graft is approximately 8 mm in width. The width of the base of the graft is the same as the distance between the caudal margins of the medial crura. The length of the graft is 10 to 12 mm. The graft is placed so that it extends 2 to 3 mm beyond the tip-defining points. Key to reducing the incidence of secondary revision is removing the sharp edges of the graft and securing the tip graft in place with at least two 5-0 PDS sutures. The graft is sutured in placed with 5-0 PDS at the caudal margins of the dome and medial crura. Usually three sutures are required to stabilize the graft.

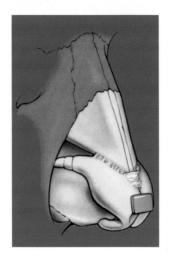

Onlay tip grafts increase tip projection and tip definition. Often the cephalic trim removed from the lower lateral cartilage can be used as a domal cap graft with great success. These are stacked as needed, but they must be firmly suture stabilized in place with 5-0 PDS. A 6 × 8 mm onlay tip graft is contoured from the septal cartilage and suture stabilized with two 5-0 PDS sutures to the tip-defining points of the dome. The sutures are placed in a horizontal mattress fashion with the knots tied on the underside of the dome areas.

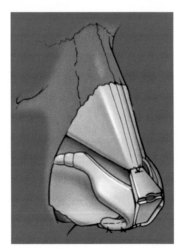

Additionally, combinations of the columellar, infratip lobular, and onlay tip cartilage grafts can be fashioned into a combination graft. This visible graft is reserved for the difficult primary rhinoplasty patient with inadequate tip projection, the thick-skinned patient, and the secondary rhinoplasty patient with inadequate tip projection.

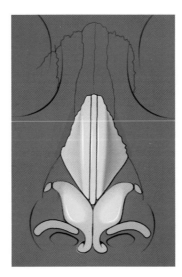

Alar contour grafts are used as a simple and effective method to correct primary alar notching/pinching after correction of the tip deformity. A subcutaneous tunnel is made with a sharp Stevens scissor below the infracartilaginous incision. The pocket should span the alar notched area and overlay it by 2 to 3 mm on either side. A 4 × 10 mm straight septal cartilage graft is contoured and placed into the pocket to correct the alar notch and secured medially with a 5-0 chromic suture.

Percutaneous Osteotomies

Percutaneous osteotomies are performed to narrow a wide bony vault, to close an open-roof defect, or to straighten deviated nasal bones (see Chapter 32). We prefer a transcutaneous discontinuous osteotomy via a lateral 2 mm incision. The incision is placed in the respective nasofacial groove and swept laterally to the bony nasofacial groove to avoid injury to the angular vessels. The discontinuous osteotomy is performed inferiorly, preserving the nasal aperture, to superiorly at the level of the medial canthus. A superior oblique osteotomy is then done. This is generally done in a low-low fashion, especially in a thin-skinned patient, to prevent a palpable or visible shadow/deformity.

Infrequently medial osteotomies are performed to narrow the bony nasal septum or if an open roof is not present after dorsal hump reduction. The dorsal skin is retracted with an Aufricht retractor. A medial osteotomy is performed on the right side, placing a 7 mm osteotome on the edge of the nasal bone where it meets the dorsal septum and angling it laterally 15 degrees. The osteotomy is performed by lightly tapping the osteotome with a mallet, stopping at the level of the medial canthus. Once the osteotomies have been performed bilaterally, the fracture is gently completed using slight digital pressure only.

Closure

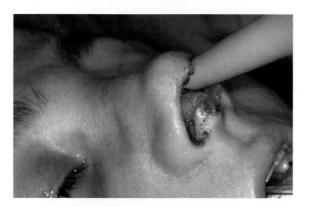

All debris is carefully removed with a final bulb syringe normal saline irrigation prior to closure. The osseocartilaginous contour should be inspected for a smooth, harmonious appearance. A final three-point dorsum contour test is done and any irregularities/depressions corrected with morselized onlay cartilage grafts. The soft tissue envelope is redraped and the supratip break assessed.

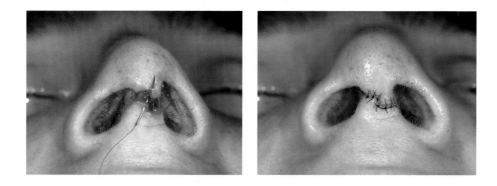

A 6-0 black nylon suture on a PC-3 needle is used to close the transcolumellar incision centrally with two sutures at the stair-step incision followed by a lateral vestibular margin suture. This is a meticulous effort to prevent notching or a noticeable scar, particularly at the vestibular margin when performing the final closure after open rhinoplasty. The infracartilaginous incision is closed with a 5-0 chromic suture on a PC-3 needle using interrupted sutures. Particular care is taken to reapproximate the mucosa at the middle crus region. Poor healing or inadequate closure in this area can result in distortion of the soft triangle and infratip area as well as a web deformity.

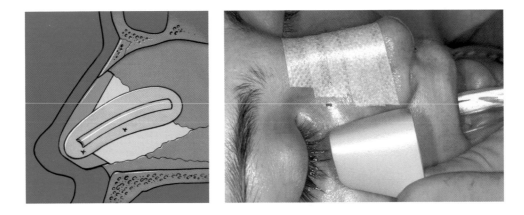

Internal nasal splints coated with an antistaphylococcal ointment are placed and fixed anteriorly with a transseptal 3-0 nylon suture. Dorsal taping of the soft tissue envelope is performed followed by placement of a dorsal nasal splint. A 2 × 2 cm drip pad is affixed with ½-inch flesh-colored paper tape under the alar base and fixed to the cheek. One-inch flesh-colored paper tape over the malar areas prevents skin maceration from frequent nasal dressing changes, especially for the first 2 to 3 days postoperatively. The throat pack is carefully removed, and suction is applied to the orogastric tube as it is slowly backed out to remove any pooled blood and secretions. This helps minimize/prevent postoperative nausea and sore throat.

Depressor Septi Muscle Translocation

If the patient has a tension tip that on animation causes a foreshortened upper lip and a decrease in tip projection, then the depressor septi muscle is released through a gingivolabial sulcus approach (see Chapter 47). An 8 to 10 mm horizontal incision centered over the upper labial frenulum is made using a pinpoint Colorado tip electrocautery with the setting on 8.

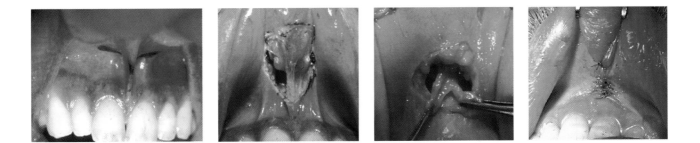

The depressor septi is easily visualized superiorly and released from its orbicularis and/or periosteal insertion. The muscle is identified along its course and is released and separated with electrocautery. Once each depressor septi muscle is released and transposed end to end with sutures, the mucosal incision is closed vertically to further elongate and add fullness to the central upper lip.

Alar Base Surgery

Abnormalities requiring alar base modification include nostril flaring, elongated nasal sidewalls, widened nasal base, large alae, and alar asymmetry. Alar abnormalities are carefully identified preoperatively to select the proper alar contouring procedure. Alar flaring is the most common indication for alar base modification. The measured alar plane and the nostril circumference dictate the surgical approach.

Alar Flaring Correction Only

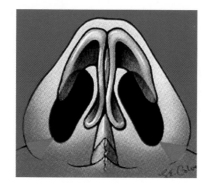

If the patient has alar flaring only and normal nostrils, the flaring is corrected by limiting the excised tissue to the alar flare, leaving at least 1 to 2 mm of the alar base. This prevents alar base notching. The incision is not carried into the vestibule. The wound is closed with 6-0 nylon on a PC-3 needle using the "halving principle" since the alar groove incision is longer than the one on the alar surface.

Alar Flaring and Nostril Shape Correction

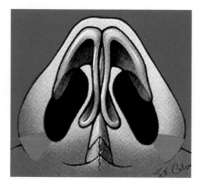

Conversely, resecting a complete wedge reduces the nostril circumference when done for nostril asymmetry or excessively large nostrils. Straight-line closure is avoided to prevent notching or a distorted nostril. The inferior resection extends into the nasal vestibule 2 mm above the alar groove. When making the medial incision at the sill a No. 11 scalpel is used and angled 30 degrees laterally. This will result in a small flap medially. The full-thickness lateral rim is resected superiorly as well. This is everted during closure with 6-0 nylon using the halving principle to avoid a depressed scar across the nostril sill.

Harvesting Autologous Cartilage Grafts

With increasing finesse in nasal analysis and in treating iatrogenically induced nasal deformities, the emphasis has been on augmentation rhinoplasty rather than the traditional reduction rhinoplasty. Hence there is a growing requirement for suitable donor sites that provide consistent and effective autologous supportive tissue (see Chapter 57). I only use autologous tissue in the nose and do not feel that alloplasts are indicated in rhinoplasty (Table 65-2).

Septal cartilage remains the cartilage of choice in that it is available in the same operative field and easily contoured for dorsal augmentation, columellar struts, or tip grafts as needed. It does not have the convolutions found in other cartilage such as ear cartilage. Sometimes, however, especially in secondary rhinoplasty patients, it is not present or sufficient for nasal reconstruction.

Ear cartilage grafts provide a large volume of cartilage, but because of their flaccidity and convolutions, they are best used when these characteristics are desired, especially in reconstructing the lower lateral cartilages. Rib cartilage is used when a large volume or length is required, such as in dorsal augmentation, but warping may be a problem as discussed below. (See Chapter 57 for details on graft harvesting techniques.)

Table 65-2. Preferred Use of Cartilage/Bone Grafts

Septal Cartilage	Ear Cartilage	Rib Cartilage
Tip graft	Alar cartilage	Dorsal onlay graft
Dorsal onlay graft	Dorsal onlay graft	Columellar strut
Columellar strut	Tip graft	Tip graft
Spreader graft		Spreader graft
		Alar cartilage graft

CASE ANALYSES

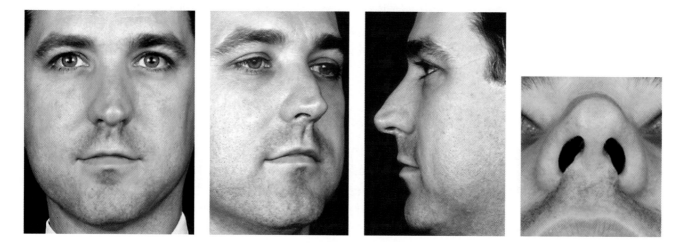

This 35-year-old man sought primary rhinoplasty because of the following complaints, which are listed in order of their importance to him: (1) nasal airway obstruction, (2) a pinched and asymmetric nasal tip, and (3) deviation of the nose to the left. The analysis revealed adequate facial proportions on the frontal view. The nose was deviated to the left. In addition, the nasal tip was asymmetric and had a concave, pinched appearance bilaterally. On the lateral and oblique views a slight dorsal hump and a low radix were noted. There was adequate tip projection. The tip concavity was confirmed on these views. On the basal view the nasal deviation was confirmed and a wide alar base revealed. The columellar/lobular ratio was acceptable. The intranasal examination revealed pink mucosa with a septal deflection to the left without perforation.

The operative goals included:
- Correction of nasal airway obstruction
- Correction of tip asymmetry and increase in projection
- Correction of nasal deviation
- Correction of the low radix

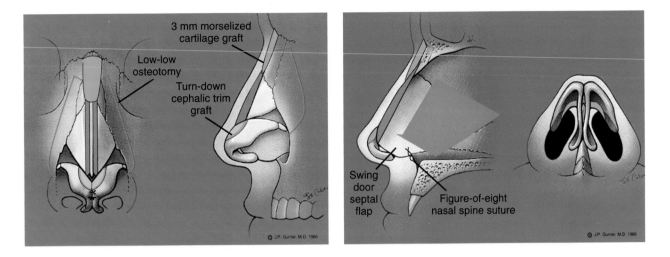

The surgical plan called for:
- External approach with transcolumellar incision and infracartilaginous extensions
- Exposure of nasal framework
- Exposure of nasal septum and harvest of septal cartilage
- Application of 3 mm morselized cartilage onlay radix graft to correct low radix and appearance of slight nasal hump
- Minimal dorsal reduction
- Low-low osteotomies to reposition bony nasal base
- Placement of turnover flaps of cephalic portion of lower lateral cartilages to correct pinched, asymmetric appearance of tip
- Placement of intercrural and interdomal sutures in graduated approach to increase tip projection
- Scoring of septum and creation of a swing-door septal flap with figure-of-eight suture to contralateral periosteum of anterior nasal spine with 5-0 PDS to correct septal deviation

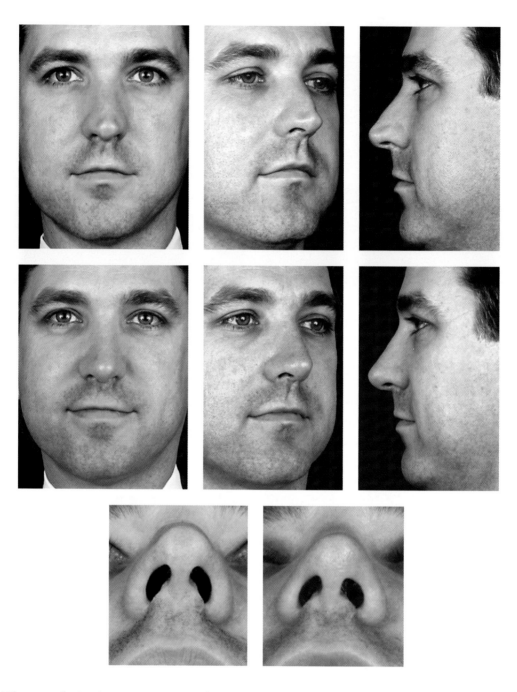

The result is shown 5 years after surgery. Analysis of the preoperative and postoperative frontal views reveals straight dorsal aesthetic lines and a balanced tip and dorsum. The nasal tip is more symmetric. The lateral preoperative and postoperative views confirm that balance has been established between the tip and the dorsum. Moreover, the low radix has been corrected, resulting in a smooth, straight dorsum. Tip projection is good with a nasolabial angle of approximately 90 degrees. The alar-columellar relationship is normal. The improved nasal balance is confirmed on the oblique views, especially in the area of the midvault. The basal views demonstrate a balanced tip with a 2:1 columellar/lobular ratio. The transcolumellar scar is nearly imperceptible.

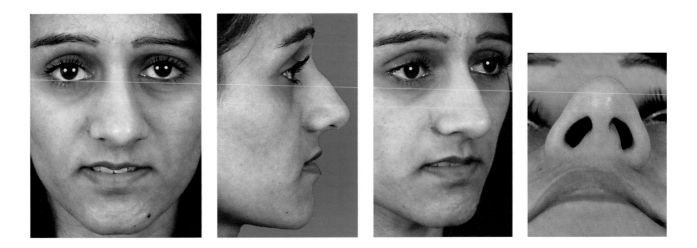

This 22-year-old woman requesting primary rhinoplasty had a history of a dorsal septal reverse C-shaped deviation, a bulbous tip, a dorsal hump, and a short upper lip. The frontal view showed she has Fitzpatrick III type skin (thick) with a reverse C-shaped deviated nose. Her facial proportions were good. The nasal tip deviated to the left and there was a wide nasal base as well. She had a bulbous tip with slight alar flaring (left greater than the right). The lateral view showed a normal radix with a 4 mm medial dorsal hump. Tip projection and nasal length were normal. She also had a short upper lip. The intranasal examination revealed nasal airway obstruction (more on the left than the right) with obstructive anteroinferior septal deviation and inferior turbinate hypertrophy on the right side. The oblique view confirmed the dorsal hump and nasal bulbous tip. The basal view revealed a left caudal septal deviation, a bulbous tip, and slight alar flaring.

The operative goals included:
- Correction of nasal airway obstruction
- Correction of dorsally deviated nose
- Correction of bulbous tip and refinement of nasal tip
- Narrowing of nasal base
- Correction of short upper lip

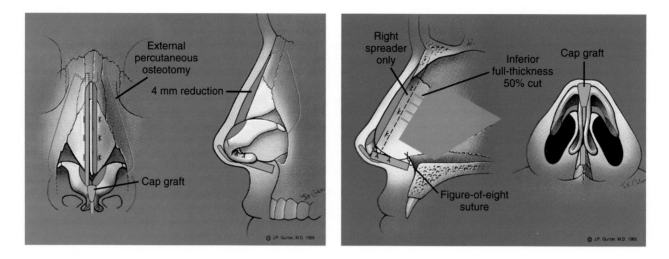

The surgical plan called for:
- Open approach via transcolumellar stair-step incision
- Exposure of dorsal framework
- Separation of upper lateral cartilage from septum proper
- Component dorsal hump reduction (4 mm cartilage and bony reduction)
- Septal reconstruction and harvest of remaining 10 mm caudal and dorsal strut
- Straightening of dorsum with 50% full-thickness inferior cuts from the deviated L-strut segment inferiorly
- Right spreader graft to keep L-strut straight and strengthen septal dorsal aesthetic lines
- Figure-of-eight suture in caudal septum to correct caudal septal deviation
- Cephalic trim (retaining 5 mm of lower lateral cartilage)
- Columellar strut secured with 5-0 PDS intercrural sutures
- Tip refinement with interdomal and transdomal sutures and placement of cap graft from cephalic trim
- External percutaneous osteotomies (low-low)
- Release and transposition of depressor septi muscle via upper lip transfrenulum incision

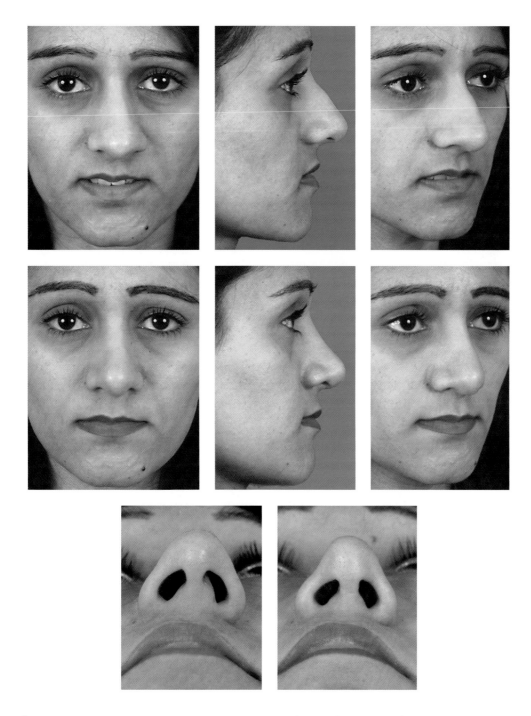

The patient is seen 2 years postoperatively with a straight nose, improved dorsal aesthetic lines, and a refined nasal tip as seen from the frontal view. The lateral view shows a smooth, straight dorsum with a slight supratip break and improved nasal length along with a normal radix and tip projection. She has a 95-degree nasolabial angle and an improved alar-columellar relationship. In addition, the subtle increase in upper lip length achieved by the depressor septi release has enhanced the tip-lip relationship. The oblique view demonstrates the improved nasal dorsal and tip balance. The basal view also shows the improved alar-columellar relationship, straight columella, and aesthetic triangular nasal tip.

OUTCOMES
Aesthetic

Although statistics have been complied to analyze the results of primary rhinoplasty, aesthetic surgery does not lend itself readily to statistical analysis given its largely subjective character. In my practice about 1 in 25 primary rhinoplasty patients benefit from operative revision and about 1 in 20 secondary rhinoplasty patients benefit from revision for aesthetic or functional complications. Five to ten percent is considered an acceptable number. In my experience the most unfavorable results are found in the lower third of the nose, specifically the tip area, followed by the middle vault, and then the upper third or dorsum. These unfavorable results include knuckling/asymmetry/deviation of the lower lateral cartilages, the parrotbeak and pinched supratip in the middle third, and excessive dorsal reduction and dorsal irregularities in the upper third.

Functional

Nasal airway obstruction is the primary consideration in rhinoplasty. In the immediate postoperative period nasal airway obstruction is typically due to persistent edema or crusting and is usually self-limited. Allergy or disturbance of the neuromuscular control of the nasal mucosal circulation may cause prolonged obstruction. I have found obstructive symptoms are commonly the result of undiagnosed or untreated inferior turbinate hypertrophy. Septal deviation is less of a functional problem, especially if not significantly deviated anteriorly and inferiorly.

External valve pathology may result in long-term nasal airway obstruction. Problems with the external valve may occur after excessive resection of the lower lateral cartilages and septum resulting in loss of tip support. They also result from poorly placed intranasal incisions that cause vestibular stenosis.

Index